Glomerulopathies: Advanced Concepts and Treatment

Glomerulopathies: Advanced Concepts and Treatment

Edited by **Ida Waddell**

New Jersey

Published by Foster Academics,
61 Van Reypen Street,
Jersey City, NJ 07306, USA
www.fosteracademics.com

Glomerulopathies: Advanced Concepts and Treatment
Edited by Ida Waddell

© 2015 Foster Academics

International Standard Book Number: 978-1-63242-198-2 (Hardback)

Printed in the United States of America.

Contents

Permissions

List of Contributors

Preface

Glomerulopathy is a kidney disease. This book is a comprehensive overview of current developments in clinical features and therapeutic options in glomerulopathies physiology. This book has several chapters which discuss various topics regarding this subject. It explains fundamental autoimmune diseases and vasculitides which are the main reasons of glomerular disease. Furthermore, this book presents several aspects of the glomerular participation in some main metabolic and systemic situations. The book explains several miscellaneous aspects of this disorder. This book intends to help students and experts in gaining more knowledge regarding this disease.

The researches compiled throughout the book are authentic and of high quality, combining several disciplines and from very diverse regions from around the world. Drawing on the contributions of many researchers from diverse countries, the book's objective is to provide the readers with the latest achievements in the area of research. This book will surely be a source of knowledge to all interested and researching the field.

In the end, I would like to express my deep sense of gratitude to all the authors for meeting the set deadlines in completing and submitting their research chapters. I would also like to thank the publisher for the support offered to us throughout the course of the book. Finally, I extend my sincere thanks to my family for being a constant source of inspiration and encouragement.

Editor

Part 1

Vasculitis and Autoimmune Glomerulopathies

Lupus Glomerulonephritis

Chi Chiu Mok

Department of Medicine, Tuen Mun Hospital and Center for Assessment and
Treatment of Rheumatic Diseases, Pok Oi Hospital, Hong Kong,
SAR China

1. Introduction

Systemic lupus erythematosus (SLE) is a multi-systemic autoimmune disease of unknown etiology. The onset of SLE is believed to be triggered by ill-defined environmental factors in genetically susceptible individuals (Mok, 2003a). Although the exact pathogenetic mechanisms have yet to be elucidated, recent works have revealed a myriad of immunological abnormalities in patients with SLE. These include aberrant apoptosis and defective clearance of apoptotic materials such as nuclear autoantigens and nucleosomes, and immune complexes by macrophages and the complement system (Katsiari, 2010), increased maturation of myeloid dendritic cells which drive the development of the proinflammatory Th17 cells (Fransen, 2010), and defective functions of the regulatory T cells (Tregs) leading to hyperactivity of the helper T cells and autoreactive B cells causing production of autoantibodies (Tucci, 2010).

Of the numerous clinical manifestations of SLE, renal disease is one of the commonest and most serious. Lupus renal disease appears to be more prevalent in certain ethnic groups such as the African and Hispanic Americans, as well as the Asians (Mok, 2005a). Renal involvement in SLE adversely affects its ultimate prognosis as reflected by the rates of patient survival and renal survival (survival without the need for renal replacement therapy), and is a major determinant for morbidity and impairment of quality of life (Mok, 1999).

The glomerulus is the commonest site of kidney involvement by lupus. However, the renal interstitium and tubules, as well as the vessels may also be affected (Cross, 2005). The presentation of renal disease in SLE is variable, ranging from no symptoms, trace proteinuria or urinary sediments to frank nephrotic syndrome, chronic renal insufficiency, and nephritic syndrome with rapid progression leading to acute renal failure. Early recognition of renal disease and close monitoring of renal parameters for progress after treatment is an essential part of the management. Conventional serological markers and clinical renal parameters for active lupus nephritis are not sensitive or specific enough, and novel biomarkers for early detection of renal disease and prediction of renal prognosis are under ongoing evaluation. It is believed that a combination of conventional parameters with one or more serological or urine biomarkers may yield better sensitivity and specificity for predicting renal activity or flare of nephritis in patients with SLE. This may help to abate the need for more invasive investigations such as renal biopsy in the assessment of renal activity and allow early institution of therapy (Mok, 2010a).

Therapy of lupus nephritis should target at symptomatic control, preservation of renal function, reduction of renal flares, prevention of treatment-related complications, and ultimately reduction in mortality (Mok, 2003b). The treatment schedule of lupus nephritis is now divided into an induction phase and a maintenance phase. Induction treatment aims at controlling inflammation and minimizing glomerular injury, whereas maintenance therapy is to reduce the risk of renal flares and renal function decline in the long-run. A combination of glucocorticoids with a non-glucocorticoid immunosuppressive agent has been shown to be more effective than glucocorticoid monotherapy in reducing the risk of progression into end stage renal failure in lupus nephritis (Austin, 1986). Of the many non-glucocorticoid immunomodulating agents, mycophenolate mofetil (MMF) has emerged to be the first-line treatment of lupus nephritis around the world because studies have shown that it is associated with fewer adverse effects than cyclophosphamide, particularly on the ovarian functions (Ginzler, 2005). Recent evidence also reveals that maintenance therapy with MMF is more effective than azathioprine in reducing the composite endpoint of renal flare and deterioration of renal function (Wolfsy, 2010).

In this chapter, the prevalence, presentation and significance of renal involvement in patients with SLE is discussed. An update on the current therapies of lupus nephritis is also presented based on the results of recent randomized controlled trials. Finally, promising biomarkers for the detection and monitoring of lupus nephritis is briefly reviewed.

2. Prevalence of renal disease in SLE

Lupus renal disease appears to be more prevalent in certain ethnic groups such as the African and Hispanic Americans, as well as the Asians (Mok, 2005a; Dooley, 1997). In a comparative study of the clinical manifestations of SLE in three ethnic groups, it was reported that renal disease, as defined by the American College of Rheumatology (ACR) criteria, namely persistent daily proteinuria of more than 500mg, presence of cellular casts or biopsy evidence of lupus nephritis, occurred in 45% of African American, 42% of Chinese and 30% of Caucasian patients, respectively (Mok, 2005a). Another multi-ethnic US cohort of SLE patients reported that renal disease occurred in 51% of Africans and 43% of Hispanics but only in 14% of Caucasians (Bastian, 2002). In a prospective study of 216 Chinese patients with new onset SLE, 31% patients had active renal disease at the time of initial presentation (Mok, 2004). Of 148 patients without overt renal disease at SLE onset, 33% developed active renal disease after a median of 14 months. The overall cumulative incidence of renal disease as defined according to the ACR renal criteria in this cohort of patients was 60% at 5 years post-SLE diagnosis (Mok, 2004). The actual incidence of renal disease might have been underestimated as the renal definition does not include subtle renal involvement such as proteinuria of less than 500mg/day or microscopic hematuria, or both. These studies illustrate that lupus renal involvement is more common in the Africans, Hispanics and Chinese than the Caucasians.

3. Clinical presentation of lupus renal disease

The presentation of renal disease in SLE is variable, ranging from no symptoms (detected by routine renal biopsy or "silent" lupus nephritis), trace proteinuria or active urinary sediments (microscopic hematuria, pyuria or cellular casts), to more serious proteinuria (nephrotic syndrome), and acute nephritic syndrome with rapid progression to acute renal failure. Occasionally, patients may present with chronic renal failure, isolated renal insufficiency and hypertension as the initial manifestation.

The wide range of presentations of lupus nephritis does not necessarily correlate with the histological findings from renal biopsy. "Silent" lupus nephritis has long been recognized in the literature. A retrospective study of 21 SLE patients with low level of proteinuria (<1gm/day) who underwent renal biopsy showed that proliferative lupus nephritis was present in 57% patients (Christopher-Stine, 2007). This emphasizes the frequent discordance of the histological severity with clinical presentation, and the need for renal biopsy, especially for new onset renal disease as evidenced by abnormal urinalysis and/or renal function impairment.

4. Renal biopsy

Renal biopsy is the gold standard of confirming the diagnosis of lupus glomerulonephritis. The finding of positive staining for immunoglobulin G, A and M, together with C1q, C3 and C4, constitutes the "full house" staining pattern for lupus nephritis. In addition to establishment of the diagnosis of lupus renal disease and confirming renal flares, renal biopsy also provides information on the histological classes of lupus nephritis, and the degree of inflammation and damage in the kidneys so as to guide therapeutic decision. Renal biopsy should be considered in SLE patients with new onset of proteinuria of more than 1g/day with and without active urinary sediments, especially in the presence of active lupus serology or impaired renal function. Some experts recommend renal biopsy at a lower threshold of proteinuria (eg. ≥500mg/day).

Patients with lupus nephritis that is refractory to treatment should be evaluated for other possible causes for the persistence of proteinuria or deterioration in renal function such as the nephrotoxic side effects of medications (eg. the calcineurin inhibitors and non-steroidal anti-inflammatory drugs), renal vein thrombosis, infections, overdiuresis and poorly controlled hypertension. Treatment compliance should be checked. A repeat renal biopsy should be considered in patients with persistently active serological markers because it provides information on the following: (1) histological transformation of the classes of lupus nephritis; (2) the degree of residual activity in the kidneys; and (3) the extent of chronic irreversible changes and its progression since the initiation of immunosuppressive treatment. These data may help to guide further treatment decisions.

5. Histological classification of lupus glomerulonephritis

The histological classification of lupus nephritis has undergone several modifications. The first WHO classification was formulated in 1974 and was last revised in 1995. According to this system, lupus glomerulonephritis was classified according to the extent and pattern of immune deposits and inflammation, which were detected by immunohistochemistry on light microscopy. There were 5 histological subtypes of lupus nephritis (class I to V) in the 1974 WHO classification (McCluskey, 1975). The differentiation of class III and class IV disease was based on the percentage of glomeruli affected by proliferative lesions (>50% was classified as Class IV). No qualitative differences between class III and class IV lesions were described. Tubulointerstitial and vascular lesions were not included in the classification.

The WHO classification was revised in 1982 (Churg, 1982). Class I disease was subdivided into 2 subclasses based on the presence and absence of immune deposits on immunofluorescence or electron microscopy. Class III was denoted focal segemental glomerulonephritis and Class IV was referred to diffuse proliferative glomerulonephritis. There were no description on the percentage of involvement of glomeruli for the differentiation between class III and class IV disease. Class III and IV disease was subdivided into active, chronic, or mixed types of glomerular injury. Class V was denoted membranous glomerulonephritis, which was subdivided into 4 subclasses: pure membranous nephropathy without or with mesangial hypercellularity (Va and Vb, respectively), membranous nephropathy with segmental endocapillary proliferation and/or necrosis (Vc) and membranous nephropathy with diffuse endocapillary proliferation and/or necrosis (Vd). Class VI was introduced to denote advanced sclerosing glomerulonephritis.

The WHO system was further revised in 1995 (Churg, 1995), with the emphasis of segmental glomerular capillary wall necrosis to be the defining feature of class III lesions, regardless of the percentage of glomeruli affected. For membranous lupus nephropathy, as the long-term prognosis is dependent on the proliferative than membranous component, the 1995 WHO classification removed Vc and Vd to be included into class III and class IV lupus nephritis, respectively. Class V retained only the subclasses Va and Vb, under the category "diffuse membranous glomerulonephritis".

The histological classification system was modified once again in 2003 by the International Society of Nephrology and the Renal Pathology Society (Weening, 2004) (Table 1). One of the reasons was the demonstration of the poor outcome of diffuse segmental necrotizing glomerulonephritis involving over 50% of glomeruli, (a "severe" form of class III disease), as compared to class IV lupus nephritis. Class III disease referred to focal lupus nephritis, which was defined as involvement of less than 50% of glomeruli by segmental endocapillary proliferative lesions, with or without capillary wall necrosis and crescents, and subendothelial deposits. Class IV disease was denoted diffuse lupus nephritis which involved more than 50% of the glomeruli. This class is subdivided into diffuse segmental lupus nephritis (class IVS) when >50% of the involved glomeruli showed segmental lesions, and diffuse global lupus nephritis (class IVG) when >50% of the glomeruli having global lesions. The proportion of glomeruli with active and chronic lesions, fibrinoid necrosis or crescents, tubulointerstitial and vascular pathology should be separated reported.

Class V, or membranous lupus nephritis, was defined as global or segmental continuous granular subepithelial immune deposits, often in the presence of concomitant mesangial immune deposits and hypercellularity. The distinction between pure membranous nephropathy and membranous nephropathy superimposed on mesangial changes was eliminated. When a diffusely distributed membranous lesion is associated with an active lesion of class III or IV, both diagnoses are reported ('V+III' or 'V+IV'). Finally, minimal change nephropathy (class I) was renamed minimal mesangial lupus nephritis, which was characterized by normal light microscopy of the glomeruli with accumulation of mesangial immune complexes identified by immunofluorescence and/or electron microscopy. A complete lack of renal abnormalities by light microscopy, immunofluorescence, and electron microscopy no longer qualified Class I lupus nephritis.

Class I	Minimal mesangial lupus nephritis
	Normal glomeruli by light microscopy, but mesangial immune deposits by immunofluorescence
Class II	Mesangial proliferative lupus nephritis
	Purely mesangial hypercellularity of any degree or mesangial matrix expansion by light microsocpy, with mesangial immune deposits. A few isolated subepithelial or subendothelial deposits may be visible by immunofluorescence or electron microscopy, but not by light microscopy
Class III	Focal lupus nephritis
	Active or inactive focal, segmental or global endo- or extracapillary glomerulonephritis involving <50% of all glomeruli, typically with focal subendothelial immune deposits, with or without mesangial alterations
III (A)	Active lesions: focal proliferative lupus nephritis
III (A/C)	Active and chronic lesions: focal proliferative and sclerosing lupus nephritis
III (C)	Chronic inactive lesions with glomerular scars: focal sclerosing lupus nephritis
Class IV	Diffuse lupus nephritis
	Active or inactive diffuse, segmental or global endo- or extracapillary glomerulonephritis involving ≥50% of all glomeruli, typically with diffuse subendothelial immune deposits, with or without mesangial alterations. This class is divided into diffuse segmental (IV-S) lupus nephritis when ≥50% of the involved glomeruli have segmental lesions, and diffuse global (IV-G) lupus nephritis when ≥50% of the involved glomeruli have global lesions. Segmental is defined as a glomerular lesion that involves less than half of the glomerular tuft. This class includes cases with diffuse wire loop deposits but with little or no glomerular proliferation.
IV-S (A)	Active lesions: diffuse segmental proliferative lupus nephritis
IV-G (A)	Active lesions: diffuse global proliferative lupus nephritis
IV-S (A/C)	Active and chronic lesions: diffuse segmental proliferative and sclerosing lupus nephritis
IV-G (A/C)	Active and chronic lesions: diffuse global proliferative and sclerosing lupus nephritis
IV-S (C)	Chronic inactive lesions with scars: diffuse segmental sclerosing lupus nephritis
IV-G (C)	Chronic inactive lesions with scars: diffuse global sclerosing lupus nephritis
Class V	Membranous lupus nephritis
	Global or segmental subepithelial immune deposits or their morphologic sequelae by light microscopy and by immunofluorescence or electron microscopy, with or without mesangial alterations.
	Class V lupus nephritis may occur in combination with class III or IV in which case both will be diagnosed
	Class V lupus nephritis may show advanced sclerosis
Class VI	Advanced sclerotic lupus nephritis
	≥90% of glomeruli globally sclerosed without residual activity

Table 1. ISN/RPS 2003 classification of lupus nephritis

6. Prognosis of lupus renal disease

Renal involvement of SLE carries significant morbidity and mortality. The renal survival (survival without dialysis) rates of lupus nephritis in the 1990's range from 83-92% in 5 years and 74-84% in 10 years (Mok, 1999; Donadio, 1995; Bono, 1999; Neumann, 1995). The risks of end stage renal failure were particularly high in patients with diffuse proliferative glomerulonephritis, with figures ranging from 11-33% in 5 years (Mok, 1999; Dooley, 1997, Donadio, 1995; Neumann, 1995; Bakir, 1994; Nossent, 2000; Korbet, 2000). The prognosis of lupus nephritis depends on a large number of demographic, racial, genetic, histopathological, immunological and time-dependent factors (Mok, 2005b). Renal disease that fails to remit with conventional immunosuppressive therapies is a major risk factor for subsequent deterioration of renal function and poor outcome (Mok, 1999; Korbet, 2000; Mok, 2006b). Other unfavorable prognostic factors for lupus neprhitis include younger age, male sex, histological cellular crescents, fibrinoid necrosis, subendothelial deposits, glomerular scarring, tubular atrophy and interstitial fibrosis, impaired renal function at presentation, persistent hypertension, hypocomplementemia, low hematocrit, as well as delay in treatment due to problems of access to health care and poor compliance (Mok, 2005b).

A recent hospital registry study of 5686 patients with SLE showed that there was a loss in life expectancy of 20 years in female and 27 years in male patients, respectively (Mok, 2011). Among 514 lupus deaths, direct complications of renal disease accounted for 9% of all cases (Mok, 2011). This reiterates that the prognosis of renal disease in SLE has yet to be improved by novel therapies in the future.

7. Current treatment of lupus glomerulonephritis

The immunosuppressive therapy of lupus nephritis is divided into an induction phase which targets at reducing inflammation and glomerular injury and a maintenance phase that aims to reduce the long-term risk of renal flares and renal function decline. Adjunctive therapies such as vigorous control of blood pressure to less than 120/80mmHg may retard the deterioration of renal function. The early use of renal protection agents such as the angiotensin converting enzyme inhibitors (ACEIs) and the angiotensin II receptor antagonists is mandatory. Hyperlipidemia should also be aggressively controlled to offer protection against accelerated vascular disease, especially in the membranous type of lupus nephritis. Calcium and vitamin D should be adequately supplemented to reduce the risk of aggravation of disease activity related to vitamin D deficiency, and to protect against loss in bone mineral density. Low-dose aspirin should be considered in patients with histological evidence of antiphospholipid syndrome nephropathy, although there is still no published evidence that this will protect against renal function decline. Anticoagulation may be considered in patients with persistent nephrotic range of proteinuria and the presence of the antiphospholipid antibodies.

8. Induction therapy for lupus nephritis

Milder form of lupus nephritis (ISN/RPS Class I, II) is usually manageable with corticosteroids (Mok, 2010b). Azathioprine (AZA) can be added as a corticosteroid sparing agent and for the treatment of concomitant extra-renal manifestations. Mild class V disease can be treated with ACEIs. Proliferative lupus nephritis (class III and IV or mixed III/V and IV/V) and more serious class V (nephrotic range of proteinuria or deteriorating renal function) disease requires more aggressive induction regimens consisting of corticosteroids and a non-corticosteroid immunosuppressive agent.

The standard therapy for severe proliferative lupus nephritis has been a combination of high-dose glucocorticoid and cyclophosphamide (CYC). From the series of randomized controlled trial conducted by the National Institute of Health (NIH), it was demonstrated that prednisone combined with intravenous (IV) pulse CYC offered better long-term protection against renal function decline than prednisone alone (Austin, 1986; Gourley, 1996; Illei, 2001). However, the use of CYC is associated with a number of untoward side effects, which include infection, ovarian and bladder toxicities, leukopenia, increased risk of cervical intraepithelial neoplasia and malignancy. Some of these toxicities are dose dependent, with a higher risk related to a higher cumulative dose (Mok, 1998). IV pulse CYC has gained popularity over continuous daily oral CYC because it is associated with less toxicity on the bladder and the gonads. Whether oral CYC is more efficacious than IV pulse CYC in lupus nephritis remains controversial because of the lack of large controlled trials (Austin, 1986; Mok, 2001). A recent analysis of a large cohort of patients with diffuse proliferative lupus nephritis showed a trend of better efficacy of oral CYC than IV pulse CYC in preserving renal function after a mean follow-up of 8.8 years (Mok, 2006b). In a multivariate model, the cumulative dose of CYC delivered instead of the route of CYC was an independent factor for a complete renal response. This suggests that the higher potency of the oral CYC regimen is probably related to the higher cumulative dose delivered instead of the route of administration per se. However, ovarian toxicity leading to premature menopause was more frequent in users of oral CYC.

Although the optimal route of CYC and duration of therapy in lupus nephritis remains to be defined, recent evidence supports the use of a shorter course and lower dose of CYC to minimize toxicities (Mok, 2001; Mok, 2002; Houssiau, 2010a). Houssiau et al. (2010a) compared the efficacy and toxicity of two less intensive intravenous pulse CYC regimens for the initial treatment of lupus nephritis. Eighty-four patients (predominantly Caucasians) were randomized to receive either 8 intravenous pulses of CYC ($0.5g/m^2$ to a maximum of 1.5gm) or 6 biweekly low dose pulses of CYC (500mg each). In both regimens, CYC was later substituted with AZA for long-term maintenance. Patients who participated in the study had milder renal disease compared to other lupus nephritis trials, as reflected by a lower proportion of patients having class IV disease, nephrotic syndrome and renal function impairment. After 10 years, rates of mortality, sustained doubling of serum creatinine and end stage renal disease did not differ between the two groups (36). The incidence of cardiovascular events and was also similar. Cancers, however, were numerically more common in patients who had received the low-dose regimen. Thus, for less serious lupus nephritis, a low-dose CYC regimen, followed by AZA is a viable strategy if there are no alternatives to CYC for initial treatment.

Nevertheless, CYC remains the treatment of choice for high-risk patients with proliferative lupus nephritis such as those with impaired or rapidly deteriorating renal function, histological cellular crescents or a combination of high activity and chronicity scores (Tang, 2009). The course of CYC should be limited to less than 6 months, with subsequent replacement by another immunosuppressive agent, to reduce the incidence of toxicities (Mok, 2002).

9. Recent controlled trials for induction therapy of severe lupus nephritis

Six randomized controlled trials comparing the efficacy and adverse effects of different treatment protocols for the induction therapy of severe lupus nephritis have recently been presented (Appel, 2009; Grootscholten, 2006, Bao, 2008; Chen, 2011; Mok, 2008; Furie, 2009). These are briefly summarized in Table 2.

In the largest lupus nephritis controlled trial to-date, called the Aspreva Lupus Management Study (ALMS), 370 patients with histologically ISN/RPS class III, IV or V lupus nephritis were randomized to receive either monthly IV pulse CYC (0.5-$1.0g/m^2$) or MMF (target 3g/day) on top of high-dose prednisone (60mg/day initially and then tapered) (Appel, 2009). Two-third of the participants had class IV disease. Asians and Hispanics comprised 33% and 35% of the participants, respectively. Three hundred and six (83%) patients completed the 24-week protocol. Clinical response, defined by a decrease in urine protein/creatinine ratio (P/Cr) to <3 in patients with baseline nephrotic range P/Cr ≥3, or by ≥50% in patients with subnephrotic baseline P/Cr (<3), and stabilization (±25%) or improvement in serum creatinine at 24 wk as adjudicated by a blinded clinical endpoints committee, was not significantly different between the CYC (53%) and MMF (56%) group. Subgroup analyses revealed that MMF was associated with a significantly higher response rate than CYC (60% vs 39%; p=0.03) in the non-Caucaisan non-Asians, which were mainly Hispanics. The rates of adverse events and serious adverse events were not significantly different between the two groups. Specifically, nausea, vomiting and alopecia were numerically more frequent in the CYC group, whereas diarrhea was more commonly reported in the MMF group. The induction phase of the ALMS study did not allow comparison of long-term side effects such as sustained amenorrhea and malignancies. There were 9 and 5 deaths in the MMF and CYC group, respectively. Of the 9 deaths in the MMF group, 7 were Asians (mainly Chinese), suggesting that Asian patients tolerated high-dose prednisone and MMF (3g/day) less well.

A controlled trial comparing the efficacy of CYC and azathioprine (AZA) in lupus nephritis was reported by Grootscholten et al. (2006). In this study, 87 patients with proliferative lupus nephritis (class III and IV) were randomized to receive either oral prednisone combined with intravenous pulse CYC ($750mg/m^2$ monthly for 6 months and then quarterly for another 7 doses) or intravenous pulse methylprednisolone (1 gram daily for 3 days for 9 pulses) together with AZA (2mg/kg/day). At the end of the third year, both groups of patients received AZA for long-term maintenance (2mg/kg/day). The dosage of AZA was reduced to 1mg/kg/day after 4 years of treatment. This cohort of patients consisted mainly of Caucasian patients (76%) who had serious renal disease as evidenced by a high proportion of patients having hypertension (57%), nephrotic syndrome (53%) and impaired creatinine clearance (56%) at presentation. In the first 2 years, no significant difference in the rates of complete and partial renal remission could be demonstrated between the two regimens. After a median follow-up of more than 5 years, significantly more patients in the AZA arm relapsed and there was a trend of higher incidence of doubling of serum creatinine in the AZA-treated patients. Interestingly, the incidence of herpes zoster infection was lower in the CYC than AZA arm during the first two years of treatment.

Although this was a randomized controlled trial, the number of patients assigned to the two treatment arms was unequal (50 patients in the CYC arm vs 37 patients in the AZA group). The corticosteroid regimens of the two treatment arms were also different, which confounded a proper interpretation of whether CYC was more effective than AZA by its own. However, taking the observation that relapse of nephritis and renal function decline was more common in AZA-treated patients despite the use of a more intensive corticosteroid regimen, it was not unreasonable to conclude for the superiority of CYC over AZA in the treatment of severe lupus nephritis.

Author, year	N	Study duration	Histological classes of lupus nephritis	Steroid regimen	Comparators	Primary end points	Adverse events
Houssiau, 2010a	84	10 yrs	WHO III, IV, Vc,Vd	Prednisolone (0.5mg/kg/d) for 4wks, then taper to 5-7.5mg/d for at least 30mths	IV CYC ($0.5g/m^2$ to a max of 1.5g) monthly for 8 doses vs 6 biweekly low dose pulses of 500mg, followed by AZA in both	Rates of mortality, sustained doubling of serum creatinine and end stage renal disease similar between the two groups	Cardiovascular events similar; but cancers were numerically more common in the low dose CYC group
Appel, 2009	370	24 wks	ISN/RPS III,IV,V	Prednisolone 60mg/day then taper	IV CYC (0.5-1.0g/m²) monthly for 6 doses vs MMF (3g/d)	Clinical response similar at 6 months; MMF higher reponse rate than CYC in non-Caucasians non-Asians	Nausea, vomiting and alopecia more common in CYC group; diarrhea more common with MMF; numerically more deaths in MMF group
Grootscholten, 2006	87	5.7 yrs	WHO III, IV, Vc, Vd	Prednisone 1mg/kg/day, tapered to 10mg/d after 6 mths vs IV MP for 9 doses + prednisone 20mg/d and taper	IV CYC (750mg/m²) monthly for 6 then 3-monthly for another 7 doses followed by AZA vs AZA (2mg/kg/d) following pulse MP	Complete and partial response rate similar at 2 years; at 5 years, significantly more relapses in AZA group with a higher incidence of doubling of serum creatinine	More herpes zoster in the AZA group than CYC; major infection rate similar; more ovarian toxicities in the CYC-treated patients
Bao, 2008	40	9 mths	Mixed IV+V	Pulse MP (0.5g/day x 3d) + prednisolone (0.6-0.8mg/kg/day) then taper	IV CYC (0.5-1g/m²/ monthly for 9 months) vs MMF (1g/d) + Tac (4mg/d)	Complete response rate significantly higher in MMF + Tac than CYC group at 6 and 9 mths	Gastrointestinal upset, leucopenia, alopecia, menstrual irregularities and upper respiratory tract infection more common in CYC group
Chen, 2011	81	6 mths	ISN/RPS III,IV,V	Prednisolone (1mg/kg/d) then taper	IV CYC (0.5-1g/m²/ monthly for 6 months) vs Tac (0.05mg/kg/d) titrating to a level of 5-10ng/ml	Clinical response at 6 months similar between the two groups	Infection rate similar; more leucopenia and gastrointestinal upset with CYC
Mok, 2008	130	6 mths	ISN/RPS III,IV,V	Prednisolone (0.6mg/kg/d) then taper	MMF (2-3g/d) vs Tac (0.1-0.06mg/kg/d)	Clinical response similar at 6 months	Herpes zoster more common with MMF; alopecia, tremor and reversible increase in serum creatinine more common with Tac
Furie, 2009	144	52 wks	ISN/RPS III,IV	High-dose prednisone	MMF (2-3g/d) in both; rituximab x 2 courses (1g x2 each course) vs placebo	Clinical efficacy similar at 52 wks	Infection rate and major infection rate similar between the two groups

Yrs = years; mths = months; CYC = cyclophosphamide; MMF = mycophenolate mofetil;
AZA = azathioprine; Tac = tacrolimus

Table 2. Recent randomized controlled trials of induction therapy for lupus nephritis

Bao et al. (2008) studied 40 patients with mixed proliferative and membranous lupus nephritis (ISN/RPS IV+V) by randomizing them to receive either IV pulse CYC (0.5-1g.m^2 monthly) (N=20) or low-dose combination of MMF (500mg BD) and tacrolimus (Tac) (2mg BD) (N=20), on top of high-dose prednisolone (0.6-0.8mg/kg/day) after 3 daily pulses of methylprednisolone (0.5g). The mean creatinine clearance at recruitment was 97.6ml/min and 85% patients had normal serum creatinine level. At 6 months, the rate of complete response, defined as daily proteinuria <0.4g/day with normal urinary sediments and stabilization of serum creatinine (<15% increase), was significantly higher in the MMF / Tac group (50%) than the CYC group (5%). The corresponding rates at 9 months of treatment were 65% and 15%, respectively. Leukopenia, gastrointestinal upset, upper respiratory tract infection, alopecia and irregular menses were more common in the CYC than MMF/Tac group of patients.

A randomized controlled trial comparing the short-term efficacy of IV pulse CYC with tacrolimus (Tac) in lupus nephritis were recently presented (Chen, 2011). In this study, 81 patients with class III, IV or V lupus nephritis were randomized to receive IV pulse CYC (0.5-1g.m^2 monthly) (N=39) or Tac (0.05mg/kg/day titrating to a level of >5ng/mL) (N=42) in combination with high-dose prednisolone (1mg/kg/day). The study population consisted of moderate to high-risk patients as shown by a high proportion of class IV disease (77%) and impaired renal function (11%) at presentation. At 6 months, the rate of complete remission, which was defined as proteinuria <0.3g/day, stabilization of serum creatinine and normalization of urinary sediments, was not significantly different between the CYC and Tac group of patients (38% vs 52%, p=0.2). Regarding adverse events, gastrointestinal upset and leucopenia were significantly more frequent in the CYC group but the rate of infection was similar between the CYC- and Tac-treated patients. Transient increase in serum creatinine was reported in 8% of patients receiving Tac.

Our group has conducted a controlled trial comparing the efficacy of MMF (2g/day, titrating to 3g/day if response suboptimal at 3 months) with Tac (0.1mg/kg/day in first 2 months with tapering to 0.06mg/kg/day) in combination of high-dose prednisolone (0.6mg/kg/day for 6 weeks and taper) for lupus nephritis (Mok, 2008). Up to March 2011, 130 patients with ISN/RPS class III, IV or V lupus nephritis were recruited. Our preliminary analysis showed that the clinical complete and partial response rates were not significantly different between the two treatment arms at month 6. The rate of infection, in particular herpes zoster reactivation, was higher in MMF than Tac-treated patients, whereas alopecia, tremor and reversible increase in serum creatinine was more frequent in the Tac group of patients. Dose-related neurological and metabolic adverse effects of Tac, and the possibility of early renal relapse upon completion of the induction phase and substitution of Tac have to be carefully monitored.

The LUNAR study is a phase III randomized, double-blind, placebo-controlled multicenter study to evaluate the efficacy and safety of rituximab in patients with active proliferative lupus nephritis (Furie, 2009). Patients with ISN/RPS Class III or IV lupus nephritis and urine protein to creatinine (UP/Cr) ratio >1 were randomized to receive rituximab (1000mg) or placebo infusion on days 1, 15, 168 (week 24) and 182 (week 26), on top of corticosteroid and MMF (>2g/day). Seventy-two patients were recruited in each treatment arm. Two-third of the patients had class IV nephritis and the mean UP/Cr at entry was 4.0±2.8. At week 52, no statistically significant differences in the primary and secondary endpoints were observed between the rituximab and placebo groups of patients, although there were numerically more responders in the rituximab group (57% vs 46% in the placebo group). Africans and Hispanics treated with rituximab tended to have better response compared to placebo than the Whites. Rituximab had a greater effect than placebo on anti-dsDNA and complement levels at week 52. Serious adverse events and infection rates were similar between the two groups but two deaths occurred in the rituximab-treated patients.

Taken the evidence from these recent studies together, it appears that MMF should be used as the first line treatment in combination with corticosteroids for severe lupus nephritis because of its stronger evidence (largest sample size) compared to other agents and lower incidence of toxicities compared to conventional CYC. Although Tac has similar efficacy with either CYC or MMF, it has been tried in a smaller population of patients and disadvantages such as transient and long-term nephrotoxicity, as well as higher relapse rate upon substitution with another immunosuppressive agent are of concern. However, Tac is a definite option when patients are contraindicated for or intolerant to MMF. Moreover, Tac is indicated as salvage therapy for refractory lupus nephritis. Tac is preferred to cyclosporin A for the lower incidence of cosmetic side effects. The initial results of the B cell depleting agents such as rituximab are disappointing. Although evidence does not support an additional benefit of rituximab on top of MMF treatment for lupus nephritis, rituximab is an option to be considered in recalcitrant lupus nephritis, as evidenced by a number of uncontrolled case series (Jonsdottir, 2010; Melander, 2009; Vigna-Perez, 2006).

10. Maintenance therapy for lupus nephritis

There are no randomized controlled trials with the main objective of delineating whether maintenance therapy of lupus nephritis is effective or not. However, some indirect evidence suggests that maintenance therapy is probably necessary in severe lupus nephritis. In a long-term follow-up of 145 patients who participated in the NIH lupus nephritis studies, renal flares occurred in 45% of the patients when immunosuppression was completely stopped (Illei, 2002). A recent retrospective review of 32 patients with predominantly diffuse proliferative lupus nephritis described a relapse of lupus activity in 53% of patients after immunosuppression was discontinued (Moroni, 2006). In our experience with 212 patients with diffuse proliferative lupus nephritis (Mok, 2006b), despite maintenance treatment was given to 73% of patients, more than one-third of patients still had renal flares which might be serious. The use of maintenance therapy for more than 3 years was independently associated with an increased likelihood of having the composite outcome of doubling of serum creatinine, end stage renal failure or death (hazard ratio 4.62 [1.35-15.8]; p=0.02).

In a 2006 retrospective review of 32 patients with proliferative lupus nephritis in whom immunosuppressive therapy was stopped for a median of 203 months, clinical remission persisted in 47% of patients (Moroni, 2006). Patients who experienced sustained remission had received a longer total median duration of immunosuppressive treatment since renal biopsy than those who did not experience remission (median 57 months vs 30 months; p<0.01). This finding, coupled with the observation that maintenance treatment for less than 3 years after successful cyclophosphamide induction was a predictor of poor renal outcome in proliferative lupus nephritis (Mok, 2006b), suggests that maintenance immunosuppressive therapy should be continued for at least 3 years after a complete clinical response is achieved.

Four recent randomized controlled trials compare the efficacy of different immunosuppressive agents in maintaining remission in lupus nephritis (summarized in Table 3). Contreras et al. (2004) randomized 59 patients with lupus nephritis (mainly African and Hispanic Americans; 78% had class IV disease) to receive one of the three treatment arms after induction with 4-7 pulses of intravenous CYC: (1) MMF (0.5-3g/day); (2) quarterly pulse CYC; (3) AZA (1-

3mg/kg/day). Long-term observation showed that either MMF or AZA was superior to CYC in the prevention of the composite outcome of renal failure and death. MMF was more efficacious than pulse CYC in the prevention of renal flares. Moreover, maintenance treatment with CYC was associated with more side effects such as nausea, vomiting and infection. Although the sample size is small, this study shows that maintenance treatment of lupus nephritis with either AZA or MMF is safe and effective. However, whether MMF is more cost-effective than AZA is not clear because significant difference in all outcomes is not apparent between MMF- and AZA-treated patients. Moroni et al. (2006) studied 69 patients (mainly Caucasians) with lupus nephritis and compared the efficacy of cyclosporin A (CSA) with AZA for maintenance therapy. After initial induction treatment with pulse methylprednisolone, prednisone and oral CYC (91.5±23.8 mg/day for a median of 3 months), patients were randomized to receive either cyclosporin A (Neoral; 4.0 to 2.5-3.0mg/kg/day) (N=36) or AZA (2mg/kg/day) (N=33) for maintenance. At 4 years of follow-up, flare occurred in 24% of AZA-treated and 19% of CSA-treated patients, respectively (no significant difference). Minor infections and leucopenia were more commonly reported with AZA treatment whilst arthralgia and gastrointestinal symptoms were more common in CSA-treated patients.

Author, year	N	Follow-up duration	Histological classes of lupus nephritis	Induction regimen	Comparators	Primary end points	Adverse events
Contreras, 2004	59	Beyond 5 yrs	WHO III, IV, Vb	IV CYC (0.5-1g/m²) for 4-7 pulses	IV CYC (0.5-1g/m²) every 3 months vs MMF (0.5-3g/d) vs AZA (1-3mg/kg/d)	Renal flare and renal function deterioration was significantly more common with CYC than MMF; MMF no better than AZA in the above outcomes	Nausea, vomiting, major infection rate and sustained amenorrhea more common with CYC than the other 2 groups
Moroni, 2006	69	4 yrs	Class IV nephritis	Pulse MP + high dose prednisone + oral CYC for 3 mths	CSA (4mg/kg/d) and taper to 2.5-3mg/kg/d vs AZA 2mg/kg/d	7 flares in CSA (19%) vs 8 flares in AZA (24%) group; reduction in proteinuria, blood pressure and creatinine clearance similar in both groups	Gum hypertrophy, hypertrichosis, hypertension, arthralgia, gastrointestinal symptoms more common with CSA; Infections and leucopenia more common with AZA
Houssiau, 2011	105	53 mths	WHO class III, IV, Vc, Vd	Pulse MP + high dose prednisone + IV CYC (500mg) x 6 doses	AZA (2mg/kg/d) vs MMF (2g/d)	Frequency of renal and extra-renal flares, doubling of serum creatinine similar in both groups	Infection rate similar; but drug-related cytopenias more common with AZA; withdrawal due to pregnancy wish more common with MMF
Wofsy, 2010	227	2.1 yrs	ISN/RPS III,IV,V	High dose prednisone + either IV CYC (6 pulses) or MMF (3g/d) x 6 mths	AZA (2mg/kg/d) vs MMF (2g/d)	Treatment failure, defined as the composite outcome of renal flares, doubling of serum creatinine or end stage renal failure, death or need for rescue therapy significantly less common in MMF than AZA group	No information yet

Yrs = years; mths = months; CYC = cyclophosphamide; MMF = mycophenolate mofetil; AZA = azathioprine; CSA = cyclosporin A

Table 3. Recent randomized controlled trials of maintenance therapy for lupus nephritis

In the MAINTAIN study conducted by Houssiau et al. (2010b), 105 patients with class III, IV, Vc and Vd lupus nephritis were randomized to receive either MMF (2g/day) (N=53) or AZA (2mg/kg/day) (N=52) after an initial induction regimen that consisted of IV pulse methylprednisolone, high-dose prednisone and IV pulse CYC (500mg 2-weekly for 6 doses). Participants were mainly Caucasians and 10% of patients had impaired renal function at study entry. After a mean follow-up of 53 (15-65) months, 24 (23%) patients withdrew from the study mainly because of pregnancy wish (in the MMF group) and adverse effects. Frequency of renal and extra-renal flares, doubling of serum creatinine and incidence of infections occurred at similar frequency in the two arms. However, drug-related cytopenias were more common with AZA.

Results of the maintenance phase of the ALMS study was released in the 9th International Lupus Congress at Vancouver in 2010 (Wofsy 2010). Two hundred and twenty-seven patients who had completed the induction phase of the ALMS (IV pulse CYC or MMF 3g/day) were randomized to receive either MMF (2g/day) (N=116) or AZA (2mg/kg/day) (N=111) for maintenance treatment. The mean daily doses received by the patients were 1.87 ± 0.43g and 120 ± 48mg, respectively, for MMF and AZA. After a mean follow-up of 2.1 years, the rate of treatment failure, defined as renal flare, doubling of serum creatinine or end stage renal disease, need for rescue therapy or death, was significantly less common in MMF than AZA-treated patients. The results were similar in patients induced by CYC or MMF at recruitment.

Taken these studies together, it appears that MMF is the preferred agent for long-term maintenance therapy for lupus nephritis. However, the cost-effectiveness of this approach has to be evaluated in future analysis. AZA and CSA are alternative options for patients who are intolerant to MMF or plan for pregnancy. The long-term use of the calcineurin inhibitors such as Tac and CSA is not encouraged because of the increased risk of nephrotoxicity, hyperlipidemia and atherosclerosis.

11. Membranous lupus nephropathy

Membranous lupus nephropathy (MLN), defined as global or segmental continuous granular subepithelial immune deposits, often in the presence of mesangial immune deposits and mesangial hypercellularity, comprises only one-fifth of all cases of histologically confirmed lupus nephritis (Mok, 2009). Reported rates of patient survival and end-stage renal disease in MLN vary considerably, because of substantial heterogeneity among the published studies. The risk of progression of MLN to renal failure is generally reduced in the absence of proliferative lesions, but patients are nevertheless at risk of thromboembolic complications.

The optimal therapy for MLN remains elusive because of the paucity of clinical trials. Mixed membranous and proliferative lupus nephritis should be treated in the same way as pure proliferative lupus nephritis. If MLN is not accompanied by proliferative lesions but is associated with clinically relevant proteinuria, renal insufficiency or failure to respond to supportive therapies, immunosuppressive treatment is indicated. In addition, cardiovascular protection and blockade of the renin-angiotensin system should be instituted early in all patients.

Austin et al. (2009) randomized 42 patients (71% Blacks or Hispanics) with MLN to receive one of the following regimens: (1) alternate day prednisone (1mg/kg/day for 8 weeks and taper to 0.25mg/kg/day throughout); (2) similar prednisone regimen plus IV pulse CYC (0.5-1.0g/m² every two months); or (3) similar prednisone regimen plus CSA (5mg/kg/day). At 12 months, the cumulative probability of complete (<0.3g/day proteinuria) or partial (<2.0g/day proteinuria or improvement by 50% from baseline) remission was highest with CSA (83%), followed by IV pulse CYC (60%) and prednisone alone (27%). The response rates of either CSA or CYC were significantly better than prednisone alone. However, relapse of nephrotic syndrome was significantly more common after discontinuation of treatment with CSA than IV pulse CYC. Adverse effects during the 12-month period included insulin-requiring diabetes (one with prednisone and two with CsA), pneumonia (one with prednisone and two with CsA), and localized herpes zoster (two with IVCY).

A recent pooled analysis of 65 patients with pure membranous lupus nephritis recruited for two randomized controlled trials and completed 24 weeks of treatment (Ginzler, 2005; Appel, 2009) showed that there were no differences in the measured end points, response rate, mortality and withdrawal rate between MMF and IV pulse CYC (Radhakrishnan, 2010). There was also no difference in the change in proteinuria or partial response rate between MMF and CYC in those patients presenting with nephritic syndrome.

Therefore, similar to the proliferative types of lupus nephritis, more serious MLN should be treated with a combination of glucocorticoids and non-glucocorticoid immunosuppressive agent. A number of uncontrolled series have reported efficacy of various regimens for MLN such as AZA, tacrolimus and MMF in combination with glucocorticoids (Mok, 2009). Taken these together, possible options for MLN include MMF, IV pulse CYC, CSA, AZA and tacrolimus. Many specialists will start with MMF or AZA for their lower incidence of adverse effects, reserving other agents for salvage therapy when the clinical response is not optimal. Controlled trials comparing existing immunosuppressive agents and experimental modalities such as rituximab, infliximab and sirolimus should be undertaken in the future (Jonsdottir, 2011).

12. Refractory lupus nephritis

There is no international consensus on the definitions of remission and treatment refractoriness in lupus nephritis. In the absence of reliable and readily available biomarkers for ongoing activity / inflammation in the kidneys and histological / immunological data from routine post-therapy renal biopsy, true remission of lupus nephritis is difficult to define. Despite the discrepancies in the clinical criteria used, up to 20% of patients with lupus nephritis are reported to be resistant to initial immunosuppressive therapy (Mok, 2006a). They are more likely to be patients with multiple unfavorable prognostic factors such as the African ethnicity, delayed institution of CYC, poor treatment compliance, impaired serum creatinine, severe nephrotic syndrome, arterial hypertension at presentation, and the presence of active crescents and a higher degree of chronicity in renal histology (Mok, 2005b).

Using the similar renal response criteria as suggested by the NIH investigators (Boumpas, 1998), we reported that 14% of a cohort of 212 patients with diffuse proliferative lupus nephritis did not respond to either continuous oral or intermittent pulse CYC therapy at the end of the induction courses (Mok, 2006b). The failure to respond to immunosuppressive treatment in the first year is associated with increased risk of renal function decline and the development of end stage renal disease (Mok, 1999).

Controlled trials in refractory lupus nephritis are unavailable. Open-labeled studies have reported success of newer immunosuppressive drugs, immunomodulatory therapies and the biological agents such as MMF, calcineurin inhibitors (CSA and tacrolimus), leflunomide, intravenous immunoglobulin, immunoadsorption and rituximab in the treatment of CYC-refractory lupus nephritis. More aggressive CYC regimens such as daily oral CYC and the immunoablative CYC protocol have been used in lupus nephritis, but at the expense of more toxicities (Petri, 2010). Novel biological agents that are undergoing clinical trials in renal and non-renal lupus include epratuzumab, ocrelizumab, belimumab, abatacept and atacicept (summarized in Table 4) (Mok, 2010c).

B cell depletion
Fludarabine, rituximab, epratuzumab, ocrelizumab, belimumab, atacicept
B cell tolerization
Abetimus sodium
Blockade of the co-stimulatory pathways
Abatacept (CTLA4-Ig)
Neutralization of cytokines
IL-10, TNF, IL-6, type I interferons
Anti-complement
anti-C5b (eculizumab)

Table 4. Biological therapies for renal and non-renal lupus

13. Biomarkers for lupus nephritis

Current laboratory markers for lupus nephritis such as proteinuria, urine protein-to-creatinine ratio, creatinine clearance, anti-dsDNA and complement levels are unsatisfactory. They lack sensitivity and specificity for differentiating renal activity and damage in lupus nephritis. Significant kidney damage can occur before renal function is impaired and first detection by laboratory parameters. Persistent proteinuria may not necessarily indicate ongoing inflammation in the kidneys; and may be contributed by pre-existing chronic lesions or recent damage in the kidneys during the course of the disease. Flares of nephritis can occur without any observable and recent increase in the degree of proteinuria. Renal biopsy is the gold standard for providing information on the histological classes of lupus nephritis and the relative degree of activity and chronicity in the glomeruli. However, it is invasive and serial biopsies are impractical in the monitoring of lupus nephritis. Thus, novel biomarkers that are able to discriminate lupus renal activity and its severity, predict renal flares, monitor treatment response and disease progress, and stratify prognosis are necessary.

A biomarker refers to a biologic, biochemical or molecular event that can be assayed qualitatively and quantitatively by laboratory techniques. An ideal biomarker for lupus nephritis should possess the following properties: (1) Good correlation with renal activity as reflected by the degree of proteinuria and urine sediments; (2) Sensitive to change so that it can be used for serial monitoring of disease activity in the kidneys and defining treatment response and clinical remission; (3) Ability to predict renal activity / flares before an obvious change in conventional clinical parameters occurs so that early treatment / preventive strategies can be considered; (4) Specific to nephritis among patients with SLE; and (5) Specific to SLE for aiding early diagnosis of lupus nephritis. In addition, a useful biomarker should be easy to assay, simple to interpret and readily available in most laboratories with a reasonable cost.

Hitherto, quite a number of serum and urine biomarkers have been studied in lupus nephritis (summarized in Table 5). Many of these markers have only been tested in cross-sectional studies with small sample size, and none has been rigorously validated in large-scale longitudinal cohorts of patients with different ethnic background. It is unlikely at this juncture that a candidate biomarker stand-alone can replace conventional clinical parameters to monitor disease progress and detect early renal flares. Urine biomarkers appear to be more encouraging than serum biomarkers possibly because they are the direct products or consequences of kidney inflammation or injury. Future directions in SLE biomarker research should focus on a combination of novel markers with conventional clinical parameters to enhance the sensitivity and specificity for the prediction of renal flares and prognosis in lupus nephritis (Mok, 2010a).

Urinary monocyte chemoattractant protein-1 (uMCP-1)
Plasma and urine neutrophil gelatinase–associated lipocalin (NGAL)
Urinary tumor necrosis factor (TNF)-like inducer of apoptosis (uTWEAK)
Urine proteomics
Hepcidin
Anti-C1q antibodies
Anti-nucleosome antibodies
Anti-α-actinin antibodies
MAGE-B2 antibodies
Anti-CRP antibody
Serum and urine IL-12
Peripheral blood leukocyte chemokine transcriptional levels
Serum apoCIII
Serum ICAM-1
Anti-endothelial cell antibody
Urine osteoprotegerin (OPG)
FOXP3 mRNA expression in urinary sediments
Urine endothelin-1
Urine CXCR3+CD4+T cells
Urine VCAM-1, P-selectin, TNFR-1 and CXCL16
Urine TGFβ-1
TGFβ and MCP-1 mRNA expression in urine sediments
Chemokine and growth factor mRNA level in urinary sediments
Serum nitrate and nitrite level
Anti-ribosomal P antibody
Urine glycoprotein panel

Table 5. Novel biomarkers for lupus nephritis

14. Conclusions

Renal involvement is a major determinant of the prognosis of SLE. Lupus renal disease is more frequent in certain ethnic groups such as the Africans, Hispanics and Asians. Of the various histological types of lupus nephritis, diffuse proliferative lupus nephritis carries the worst prognosis. Treatment of lupus nephritis should target at disease remission, prevention of relapse and complications, and long-term preservation of renal function. The main stay of treatment of lupus nephritis is immunosuppression using a combination of high-dose glucocorticoid and a non-glucocorticoid immunosuppressive agent. Mycophenolate mofetil combined with prednisone has emerged to be the standard regimen. Intravenous pulse or daily oral cyclophosphamide is reserved for more serious or refractory cases of lupus nephritis. The evidence for calcineurin inhibitors in lupus nephritis is less strong and these agents are reserved for patients intolerant or recalcitrant to standard therapies. B cell modulation is emerging as novel therapeutic modalities for lupus nephritis. While further evidence from controlled trials is eagerly awaited, the current use of B cell modulating agents is confined to recalcitrant lupus renal disease. Conventional markers for activity of lupus nephritis are neither sensitive nor specific. Novel biomarkers are being studied for earlier detection of renal flares and better prognostic stratification so that intervention can be instituted early to minimize damage to renal function.

15. References

Appel GB, Contreras G, Dooley MA, Ginzler EM, Isenberg D, Jayne D, et al. ; Aspreva Lupus Management Study Group (2009). Mycophenolate mofetil versus cyclophosphamide for induction treatment of lupus nephritis. J Am Soc Nephrol. 20(5):1103-12.

Austin HA III, Klippel JH, Balow JE, le Riche NG, Steinberg AD, Plotz PH, et al. (1986). Therapy of lupus nephritis: controlled trial of prednisone and cytotoxic drugs. New Engl J Med. 314:614-619.

Austin HA 3rd, Illei GG, Braun MJ, Balow JE (2009). Randomized, controlled trial of prednisone, cyclophosphamide, and cyclosporine in lupus membranous nephropathy. J Am Soc Nephrol. 20(4):901-11.

Bakir AA, Levy PS, Dunea G (1994). The prognosis of lupus nephritis in African-Americans: a retrospective analysis. Am J Kidney Dis. 24:159-171.

Bao H, Liu ZH, Xie HL, Hu WX, Zhang HT, Li LS (2008). Successful treatment of class V+IV lupus nephritis with multitarget therapy. J Am Soc Nephrol. 19(10):2001-10.

Bastian HM, Roseman JM, McGwin G Jr, et al.; LUMINA Study Group. LUpus in MInority populations: NAture vs nurture (2002). Systemic lupus erythematosus in three ethnic groups. XII. Risk factors for lupus nephritis after diagnosis. Lupus. 11:152-60.

Bono L, Cameron JS, Hicks JA. The very long-term prognosis and complications of lupus nephritis and its treatment (1999(. QJM. 92:211-218.

Boumpas DT, Balow JE (1998). Outcome criteria for lupus nephritis trials: a critical overview. Lupus. 7:622-629.

Chen W, Tang X, Liu Q, Chen W, Fu P, Liu F, et al (2011). Short-term outcomes of induction therapy with tacrolimus versus cyclophosphamide for active lupus nephritis: A multicenter randomized clinical trial. Am J Kidney Dis. 57(2):235-44.

Christopher-Stine L, Siedner M, Lin J, Haas M, Parekh H, Petri M, et al (2007). Renal biopsy in lupus patients with low levels of proteinuria. J Rheumatol. 34:332-5

Churg J, Sobin LH: Renal Disease (1982). Classification and Atlas of Glomerular Disease, Tokyo, Igaku-Shoin.

Churg J, Bernstein J, Glassock RJ (1995). Renal Disease: Classification and Atlas of Glomerular Diseases, 2nd Ed., New York, Igaky-Shoin.

Contreras G, Pardo V, Leclercq B, et al (2004). Sequential therapies for proliferative lupus nephritis. N Engl J Med. 350:971-80.

Cross J, Jayne D (2005). Diagnosis and treatment of kidney disease. Best Pract Res Clin Rheumatol. 19(5):785-98.

Donadio JV Jr, Hart GM, Bergstralh EJ, Holley KE (1995). Prognostic determinants in lupus nephritis: a long-term clinicopathologic study. Lupus. 4:109-115.

Dooley MA, Hogan S, Jennette C, Falk R (1997). Cyclophosphamide therapy for lupus nephritis: poor renal survival in black Americans. Glomerular Disease Collaborative Network. Kidney Int. 51:1188-95

Fransen JH, van der Vlag J, Ruben J, Adema GJ, Berden JH, Hilbrands LB (2010). The role of dendritic cells in the pathogenesis of systemic lupus erythematosus. Arthritis Res Ther. 12:207.

Furie R, Looney RJ, Rovin B, et al (2009). Efficacy and Safety of Rituximab in Subjects with Active Proliferative Lupus Nephritis (LN): Results From the Randomized, Double-Blind Phase III LUNAR Study. ACR abstract [number 1149]

Ginzler EM, Dooley MA, Aranow C, et al (2005). Mycophenolate mofetil or intravenous cyclophosphamide for lupus nephritis. N Engl J Med. 353:2219-28.

Gourley MF, Austin HA 3rd, Scott D, et al (1996). Methylprednisolone and cyclophosphamide, alone or in combination, in patients with lupus nephritis. A randomized, controlled trial. Ann Intern Med. 125:549-557.

Grootscholten C, Ligtenberg G, Hagen EC, van den Wall Bake AW, de Glas-Vos JW, Bijl M, et al; Dutch Working Party on Systemic Lupus Erythematosus (2006). Azathioprine/methylprednisolone versus cyclophosphamide in proliferative lupus nephritis. A randomized controlled trial. Kidney Int. 70(4):732-42.

Houssiau FA, Vasconcelos C, D'Cruz D, Sebastiani GD, de Ramon Garrido E, Danieli MG, et al (2010a). The 10-year follow-up data of the Euro-Lupus Nephritis Trial comparing low-dose and high-dose intravenous cyclophosphamide. Ann Rheum Dis. 69(1): 61-4.

Houssiau FA, D'Cruz D, Sangle S, Remy P, Vasconcelos C, Petrovic R, et al; MAINTAIN nephritis trial group (2010b). Azathioprine versus mycophenolate mofetil for long-term immunosuppression in lupus nephritis: results from the MAINTAIN Nephritis Trial. Ann Rheum Dis. 69(12):2083-9.

Illei GG, Austin HA, Crane M, et al (2001). Combination therapy with pulse cyclophosphamide plus pulse methylprednisolone improves long-term renal outcome without adding toxicity in patients with lupus nephritis. Ann Intern Med. 135:248-257.

Illei GG, Takada K, Parkin D, et al (2002). Renal flares are common in patients with severe proliferative lupus nephritis treated with pulse immunosuppressive therapy: long-term followup of a cohort of 145 patients participating in randomized controlled studies. Arthritis Rheum. 46:995-1002.

Jónsdóttir T, Gunnarsson I, Mourão AF, Lu TY, van Vollenhoven RF, Isenberg D (2010). Clinical improvements in proliferative vs membranous lupus nephritis following B-cell depletion: pooled data from two cohorts. Rheumatology (Oxford). 49(8):1502-4.

Jónsdóttir T, Sundelin B, Welin Henriksson E, van Vollenhoven RF, Gunnarsson I (2011). Rituximab-treated membranous lupus nephritis: clinical outcome and effects on electron dense deposits. Ann Rheum Dis. 70(6):1172-3.

Katsiari CG, Liossis SN, Sfikakis PP (2010). The pathophysiologic role of monocytes and macrophages in systemic lupus erythematosus: a reappraisal. Semin Arthritis Rheum. 39:491-503.

Korbet SM, Lewis EJ, Schwartz MM, Reichlin M, Evans J, Rohde RD (2000). Factors predictive of outcome in severe lupus nephritis. Lupus Nephritis Collaborative Study Group. Am J Kidney Dis. 35:904-914.

McCluskey RT (1975). Lupus nephritis. In Kidney Pathology Decennial 1966-1975, edited by Sommers SC, East Norwalk, CT, Appleton-Century-Crofts, 1975, pp 435-450.

Melander C, Sallée M, Trolliet P, Candon S, Belenfant X, Daugas E, et al (2009). Rituximab in severe lupus nephritis: early B-cell depletion affects long-term renal outcome. Clin J Am Soc Nephrol. 4(3):579-87.

Mok CC, Lau CS, Wong RWS (1998). Risk factors for ovarian failure in patients with systemic lupus erythematosus receiving cyclophosphamide therapy. Arthritis Rheum. 41:831-7.

Mok CC, Wong WS, Lau CS (1999). Lupus nephritis in Southern Chinese patients: clinicopathologic findings and long-term outcome. Am J Kidney Dis. 34(2):315-23.

Mok CC, Ho CT, Siu YP, et al (2001). Treatment of diffuse proliferative lupus glomerulonephritis: a comparison of two cyclophosphamide-containing regimens. Am J Kidney Dis. 38:256-264.

Mok CC, Ho CTK, Chan KW, et al (2002). Outcome and prognostic indicators of diffuse proliferative lupus glomerulonephritis treated with sequential oral cyclophosphamide and azathioprine. Arthritis Rheum. 46:1003-1013.

Mok CC Lau CS (2003a). Pathogenesis of systemic lupus erythematosus. J Clin Pathol. 56(7):481-90.

Mok CC, Wong RW, Lai KN (2003b). Treatment of severe proliferative lupus nephritis: the current state. Ann Rheum Dis. 62(9):799-804.

Mok CC, Tang SK (2004). Incidence and predictors of renal disease in Chinese patients with systemic lupus erythematosus. Am J Med. 117:791-5

Mok CC, Tang SS, To CH, Petri M (2005a). Incidence and risk factors of thromboembolism in systemic lupus erythematosus: a comparison of three ethnic groups. Arthritis Rheum. 52(9):2774-82.

Mok CC (2005b). Prognostic factors in lupus nephritis. Lupus. 14:39-44.

Mok CC (2006a). Therapeutic options for resistant lupus nephritis. Semin Arthritis Rheum. 36(2):71-81.

Mok CC, Ying KY, Ng WL, Lee KW, To CH, Lau CS, et al (2006b). Long-term outcome of diffuse proliferative lupus glomerulonephritis treated with cyclophosphamide. Am J Med. 119(4):355.e25-33.

Mok CC, Ying KY, Tong KH, Siu YP, To CH, Yim CW, Ng WL (2008). Mycophenolate mofetil versus tacrolimus for active lupus nephritis: an extended observation of a randomized controlled trial. Arthritis Rheum. 58(9 Suppl):S566

Mok CC (2009). Membranous nephropathy in systemic lupus erythematosus: a therapeutic enigma. Nat Rev Nephrol. 5(4):212-20.

Mok CC (2010a). Biomarkers for lupus nephritis: a critical appraisal. J Biomed Biotechnol. 2010:638413.

Mok CC, Cheung TT, Lo WH (2010b). Minimal mesangial lupus nephritis: a systematic review. Scand J Rheumatol. 39(3):181-9.

Mok CC (2010c). Update on emerging drug therapies for systemic lupus erythematosus. Expert Opin Emerg Drugs. 15(1):53-70

Mok CC, Kwok CL, Ho LY, Chan PT, Yip SF (2011). Life expectancy, standardized mortality ratios and causes of death of six rheumatic diseases in Hong Kong, China. Arthritis Rheum. 63(5):1182-9

Moroni G, Doria A, Mosca M, Alberighi OD, Ferraccioli G, Todesco S, et al (2006). A randomized pilot trial comparing cyclosporine and azathioprine for maintenance therapy in diffuse lupus nephritis over four years. Clin J Am Soc Nephrol. 1(5):925-32.

Moroni G, Gallelli B, Quaglini S, et al (2006). Withdrawal of therapy in patients with proliferative lupus nephritis: long-term follow-up. Nephrol Dial Transplant. 21:1541-8.

Neumann K, Wallace DJ, Azen C, Nessim S, Fichman M, Metzger AL, et al (1995). Lupus in the 1980s: III. Influence of clinical variables, biopsy, and treatment on the outcome in 150 patients with lupus nephritis seen at a single center. Semin Arthritis Rheum. 25:47-55.

Nossent HC, Koldingsnes W (2000). Long-term efficacy of azathioprine treatment for proliferative lupus nephritis. Rheumatology (Oxford). 39:969-974.

Petri M, Brodsky RA, Jones RJ, Gladstone D, Fillius M, Magder LS (2010). High-dose cyclophosphamide versus monthly intravenous cyclophosphamide for systemic lupus erythematosus: a prospective randomized trial. Arthritis Rheum. 62(5):1487-93.

Radhakrishnan J, Moutzouris DA, Ginzler EM, Solomons N, Siempos II, Appel GB (2010). Mycophenolate mofetil and intravenous cyclophosphamide are similar as induction therapy for class V lupus nephritis. Kidney Int. 77(2):152-60.

Tang Z, Wang Z, Zhang HT, Hu WX, Zeng CH, Chen HP, et al (2009). Clinical features and renal outcome in lupus patients with diffuse crescentic glomerulonephritis. Rheumatol Int. 30(1):45-9.

Tucci M, Stucci S, Strippoli S, Silvestris F (2010). Cytokine overproduction, T-cell activation, and defective T-regulatory functions promote nephritis in systemic lupus erythematosus. J Biomed Biotechnol. 2010:457146.

Vigna-Perez M, Hernández-Castro B, Paredes-Saharopulos O, Portales-Pérez D, Baranda L, Abud-Mendoza C, et al (2006). Clinical and immunological effects of Rituximab in patients with lupus nephritis refractory to conventional therapy: a pilot study. Arthritis Res Ther. 8(3):R83.

Weening JJ, D'Agati VD, Schwartz MM, Seshan SV, Alpers CE, Appel GB, et al. (2004) The classification of glomerulonephritis in systemic lupus erythematosus revisited. J Am Soc Nephrol. 15:241-50.

Wofsy D, Appel GB, Dooley MA, Ginzler EM, Isenberg DA, Jaynes D, et al; ALMS Study Group (2010). Aspreva Lupus Management maintenance results. Lupus. 19S1:p27.

2

Anti-Glomerular Basement Membrane Disease

Kouichi Hirayama and Kunihiro Yamagata
Tokyo Medical University Ibaraki Medical Center,
University of Tsukuba
Japan

1. Introduction

Anti–glomerular basement membrane (anti-GBM) disease is a rare autoimmune disorder characterized by rapidly progressive glomerulonephritis (RPGN) with diffuse crescentic formation on renal biopsy, and it is a well-characterized cause of glomerulonephritis.

In 1919, an autopsy of an 18-year-old male patient, who had developed hemoptysis and acute renal failure after experiencing flu-like symptoms, revealed massive alveolar hemorrhage, glomerulonephritis with fibrinous exudates in Bowman's capsule and necrotizing vasculitis in the spleen and gut (Goodpasture, 1919). Stanton and Tange reported 9 cases with alveolar hemorrhage and RPGN as Goodpasture's syndrome (Stanton & Tange, 1958). Anti-GBM disease was defined as the presence of serum autoantibodies to the noncollagenous domain of the alpha 3 chain of type IV collagen or a linear binding of IgG to glomerular capillary walls as detected by direct immunofluorescence in patients with RPGN. Anti-GBM disease was divided into two types: anti-GBM disease without alveolar hemorrhage was regarded as renal-limited anti-GBM disease, and that with alveolar hemorrhage was defined as Goodpasture's syndrome.

This review focuses on anti-GBM disease by comparing international differences in prevalence, clinical features, treatments and outcomes in order to improve the prognosis of anti-GBM disease.

2. Prevalence

Anti-GBM disease is relatively rare, with an estimated annual incidence of about 0.5-1.0/million population (Table 1). It has been estimated to cause 0.2-2.4% of biopsy-proven glomerulonephritis cases in Europe, but less than 0.2% in Asia. It causes about 10% of RPGN (or necrotizing and/or crescentic glomerulonephritis) in Europe, more than 10% of RPGN in the United States, and less than 10% in Asia. In Japan, to improve the prognosis of patients with RPGN, a nation-wide survey of patients with RPGN in 365 hospitals between 1989 and 2000 was conducted, and clinical characteristics including initial symptoms, laboratory findings and histological findings were investigated along with treatment methods and outcomes (Hirayama et al., 2008). Among patients with RPGN, 6.6% had anti-GBM disease. In comparison with foreign countries, this Japanese rate of anti-GBM disease in RPGN was lower.

Authors	Year	Nation	Incidence (/million/yr)	Frequency (%) GN	2nd GN	RPGN
Rychlík et al.	2004	Czech	0.17	0.31 *	1.2 *	
Heaf et al.	1999	Denmark	0.6			12.8 +
Andrassy et al.	1991	Germany	0.55			7.9
Daly et al.	1996	Ireland		2.4 *		
Schena et al.	1997	Italy	0.1	0.20 *	1.5 *	
Grcevska et al.	1995	Macedonia				3.6 +
Naumovic et al.	2009	Serbia	0.02	0.18 *	0.74 *	
Rivera et al.	2002	Spain				14.6 +
Saxena et al.	1991	Sweden				13.4 +
Williams et al.	1988	United Kingdom	1.12(0.2 – 4.0)			
Angangco et al.	1994	United Kingdom		0.81 *		11.2 +
Parfrey et al.	1985	Canada				11.5 +
Wilson and Dixon	1973	United States		7.0 *		
Jennette	1993	United States				14.6 +
Briganti et al.	2001	Australia	0.99	0.8 *		
NZGS	1989	New Zealand		5.9 *		
Date et al.	1987	India		0.04 *		
Sumethkul et al.	1999	Thai		0.10 *		3.3 +
Tang et al.	2003	China		0.15 *		8.7 +
Li, FK. et al.	2004	China(HongKong)	0.6			
Li, LS. et al.	2004	China		0.21 *	0.86 *	
Hirayama et al.	2008	Japan				6.6

The incidence of patients with anti-GBM disease is expressed as the number per 1 million population per year. The frequencies of patients with anti–GBM disease in glomerulonephritis, secondary glomerulonephritis or rapidly progressive glomerulonephritis are expressed as percentages. *Biopsy-proven glomerulonephritis. Blanks are unavailable data. Abbreviations: yr, years; GN, glomerulonephritis; 2nd GN, secondary glomerulonephritis; RPGN, rapidly progressive glomerulonephritis (including +necrotizing and/or crescentic glomerulonephritis); NZGS, The New Zealand Glomerulonephritis Study.

Table 1. Prevalence of anti–GBM disease in various countries.

All age groups are affected, but the peak incidence of anti-GBM disease is in the third decade in young men, with a second peak in the sixth and seventh decades affecting men and women equally (Figure 1). Alveolar hemorrhage is more common in younger men, while isolated renal disease is more frequent in the elderly, with a near-equal gender distribution. In that survey (Hirayama et al., 2008), the mean age at onset of renal-limited anti-GBM disease was 52.6±17.0 years. There was only one peak incidence of anti-GBM disease, and this peak occurred in the fifth and sixth decades. The gender distribution was nearly equal in renal-limited anti-GBM disease (male: female = 1: 0.94).

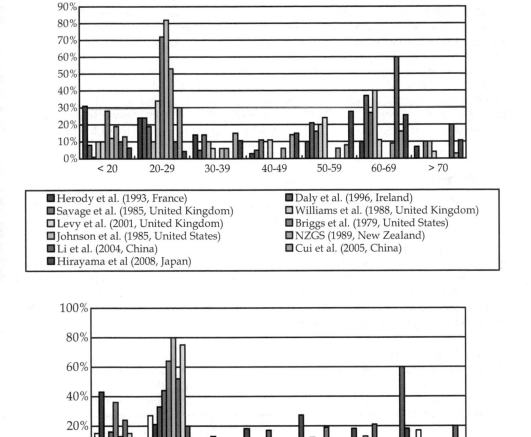

Fig. 1. Investigations of age distribution in anti-GBM disease (upper) and Goodpasture's syndrome (lower).

The histograms show the number of patients with anti-GBM disease classified by patient age at the onset of the disease. Abbreviations: GN, glomerulonephritis; Biopsy, biopsy-proven glomerulonephritis; RPGN, rapidly progressive glomerulonephritis; NZGS, The New Zealand Glomerulonephritis Study; N.A., not available.

Alveolar hemorrhage is observed in 35-62% of patients with anti-GBM disease in Europe, the United States, and China, and it is more common in younger patients and in men, whereas renal-limited anti-GBM disease is more common in older patients and in women. In Japan, alveolar hemorrhage of patients with anti-GBM disease was less frequent (23.4%) and the age at onset of Goodpasture's syndrome was lower (49.4±14.4 years), but it was more common in females (male: female = 1: 1.75).

This disease appears to be more common in Caucasians and very rare in those of African origin (Pusey, 2003; Ooi et al., 2008). There is apparently a higher incidence of onset of Goodpasture's disease in the spring and summer, as well as localized clustering of the disease, perhaps suggesting an infectious relationship (Pusey, 2003). Anecdotal associations with urinary tract infections and lithotripsy, which may subclinically affect the glomerular basement membrane, have also been reported (Pusey, 2003; Ooi et al., 2008).

3. Pathogenesis

In 1934, Masugi reported nephrotoxic glomerulonephritis induced by anti-kidney serum in an experimental model (Masugi, 1934), after which a linear binding of IgG to glomerular capillary walls was detected by direct immunofluorescence (Ortega & Mellors, 1956). In 1964, a linear immunostaining of IgG was observed in 2 patients with Goodpasture's syndrome (Scheer & Grossman, 1964), and in another study the kidney serum of patients with Goodpasture's syndrome and of patients with crescentic glomerulonephritis without alveolar hemorrhage contained antibodies that reacted with the GBM of humans and animals (Lerner et al., 1967). Those authors also demonstrated that those anti-GBM antibodies caused glomerulonephritis when injected into animals.

3.1 Structure of GBM

GBM, which exists between endothelial cells and podocytes, consists of type IV collagen, heparansulphate proteoglycan, laminine and fibronectin. Type IV collagen, which consists of 3 of 6 alpha-chains ($\alpha 1$ to $\alpha 6$) encoded by three pairs of genes on chromosomes 2, 13 and X, and its molecules were trimeric ($\alpha 1 \alpha 1 \alpha 2$, $\alpha 3 \alpha 4 \alpha 5$ and $\alpha 5 \alpha 5 \alpha 6$). This basement membrane, found in kidney, lung, cochlea and eye, comprises the surface on which epithelial cells rest. In kidneys, $\alpha 3 \alpha 4 \alpha 5$ molecules were found in the GBM, particularly the epithelial side; $\alpha 1 \alpha 1 \alpha 2$ molecules were in the mesangium, the endothelial side of the GBM, tubular basement membranes and Bowman's capsule; and $\alpha 5 \alpha 5 \alpha 6$ molecules were in tubular basement membranes and Bowman's capsule. Each alpha-chain was made by one long collagenous domain and two terminal noncollagenous globular domains: the C-terminal noncollagenous (NC1) domain and the N-terminal domain (the 7S domain). Mature GBM is a lattice-like structure comprised in part by heterotrimers of $\alpha 3$, 4 and 5 chains, which form a triple helix with short NC1 and 7S domains (Sado et al., 1998). The NC1 domain of the $\alpha 3$ chain of a tissue-specific type IV collagen [$\alpha 3$(IV)NC1] monomer is structured into the collagen IV network through the association of $\alpha 3$, $\alpha 4$ and $\alpha 5$ chains to form a triple helical protomer and through the oligomerization of these protomers via end-to-end associations and intertwining of triple helixes (Hudson et al., 2003).

3.2 Anti-GBM antibodies

The target of the anti-GBM antibodies was identified as $\alpha 3$(IV)NC1 (Saus et al., 1988). The two conformational epitopes of anti-GBM antibodies have been defined as E_A and E_B

(Kalluri et al., 1996; Borza et al., 2000). The E_A epitope is 17-31 amino acids on the N-terminal side, and the E_B epitope is 127-141 amino acids on the C-terminal side (Netzer et al., 1999). Alterations of the amino acid sequence translated by the COL4A3 gene, which encodes α3(IV)NC1, are not major factors, because no mutation of the COL4A3 gene was found (Persson et al., 2004). It was suggested that E_A and E_B, as cryptic B-cell epitopes, were enclosed in the quaternary structure of the hexamers created by sulfilimine crosslinks between the trimers of adjacent NC1 chains (Vanacore et al., 2008, 2009). Recently, in patients with Goodpasture's disease, elevated autoantibody titers to α3(IV)NC1 and α5(IV)NC1 monomers at diagnosis were associated with the eventual loss of renal function (Pedchenko et al., 2010). In that study, these anti-GBM antibodies bound to specific epitopes that encompassed region E_A in the α5(IV)NC1 monomer and regions E_A and E_B in the α3(IV)NC1 monomer, but did not bind to the native crosslinked α345(IV)NC1 hexamer. Thus, it is a dissociation of the NC1 hexamers that expose the pathogenic epitopes on the α3 and α5 chains, precipitating the production of anti-GBM antibodies (Pedchenko et al., 2010). It was suggested that the autoantibody itself may subsequently alter antigen conformation and expose further epitopes, causing an epitope-spreading phenomenon (Salant, 2010).

3.3 Crescent formations

The anti-GBM antibody bound to GBM ligates Fc receptors, leading to the activation of monocytes, neutrophils, eosinophils, basophils and macrophages. These release chemokines that attract a further influx of neutrophils into glomeruli, causing severe tissue injury, including the disruption of the GBM. Renal injury in anti-GBM disease is amplified by the activation of complements and protease after the binding (Sheerin et al., 1997; Baricos et al., 1991). The release of reactive oxygen species by neutrophils is also probably an important pathogenic mechanism of tissue injury.

The histogenesis and origin of cellular crescents, which are cap-like multilayered accumulations of proliferating cells, have remained controversial. Although early ultrastructural studies suggested that crescents are formed by proliferating epithelial cells (Morita et al., 1973; Min et al., 1974), subsequent histochemical studies with antibodies against leukocytes identified the presence of monocytes-macrophages in cellular crescents (Atkins et al., 1976; Thomson et al., 1979). It was demonstrated that epithelial cells predominated in crescents of patients during the early phases of disease; later phases were characterized by rupture of the basement membrane of Bowman's capsule and subsequent infiltration of cellular crescents, predominantly by macrophages (Boucher et al., 1987). The composition of cellular crescents may change during the progression of disease after the inciting glomerular injury (Ophascharoensuk et al., 1998).

The main stimulus to the migration of macrophages and neutrophils is probably the exudation of fibrin in Bowman's space caused by the disruption of the GBM and Bowman's capsule (Tipping et al., 1988). Several possible causes of acute renal injury in anti-GBM disease were identified, including the functional roles of a number of macrophage proinflammatory mediators, such as IL-1 (Lan et al., 1993), TNF-alpha (Lan et al., 1997; Le Hir et al., 1998) and matrix metalloproteinase (Kaneko et al., 2003). In epithelial crescent formation in the glomerulus, thrombin generated by coagulation (He et al., 1991) and growth-factor cytokines (IL-1 and IL-2) released by monocytes and platelets (Adler et al., 1990) stimulate the migration of epithelial cells. Moreover, interleukin-12 (Kitching et al., 1999) and interferon-γ (Timoshanko et al., 2002) are also involved.

3.4 Environmental and genetic factors

Environmental factors are thought to play a role in triggering the disease. In the first case of Goodpasture's syndrome, intercurrent infection amplifies the intensity of inflammatory responses and can aggravate disease and so make it clinically apparent. There are a number of case reports of clusters of patients with anti-GBM disease (Perez et al., 1974), which may implicate an infective agent; however, no clear viral association has been identified. Group A type 12 streptococcal cell membrane shares some cross-reactivity with the human glomerular basement membrane, generating another hypothesis: that infection may initiate anti-GBM antibody production (Blue & Lange, 1975).

Goodpasture's syndrome has been noted to occur more frequently in smokers (Salama et al., 2001). Lazor et al. (2007) reported that 89% of their patients with Goodpasture's syndrome were active smokers. In another study, alveolar hemorrhage was present in 100% of patients who smoked and in only 20% of nonsmokers with Goodpasture's disease (Donaghy & Rees, 1983). No significant difference in circulating anti-GBM antibody titers was found between smokers and nonsmokers, suggesting that cigarette smoking may increase the permeability of lung capillaries and thus expose alveolar basement membranes to circulating anti-GBM antibodies (Donaghy & Rees, 1983; Klasa et al., 1988). Other inhaled substances may also be associated with anti-GBM disease, including cocaine (García-Rostan y Pérez et al., 1997; Lazor et al., 2007), hard metals such as inert tungsten carbide and cobalt (Lechleitner et al., 1993), smoke inhalation (Klasa et al., 1988) and possibly volatile hydrocarbon solvents (Beirne & Brennan, 1972; Bombassei & Kaplan, 1992). In particular, hydrocarbon exposure may influence the development of alveolar hemorrhage (Churchill et al., 1983; Bonzel et al., 1987). Another environmental factor, alemtuzumab, which is a humanized anti-CD52 monoclonal antibody, recently was identified as a cause of anti-GBM disease (Clatworthy et al., 2008).

Genetic factors appear to play a role in susceptibility to anti-GBM disease. As a genetic factor of anti-GBM disease, the human leukocyte antigen (HLA) complexes are known to influence susceptibility to anti-GBM disease. A strong association with HLA-DR2 specificity has been confirmed (Rees et al., 1978). In HLA genotyping, DRB1*1501 (the serologically defined HLA-DR2 gene) and DRB1*1502 (HLA-DR15 gene) allele at the DRB1 locus is associated with anti-GBM disease in Caucasians (Fisher et al., 1997), Chinese (Yang et al., 2009) and Japanese (Kitagawa et al., 2008). The strongest association was with HLA DRB1*1501 but, when the effect of this gene was excluded, subsequent analysis revealed an increased frequency of DRB1*04 and DRB1*03 and a decreased frequency of DRB1*07 and DRB1*01 (Phelps & Rees, 1999). Other genetic influences of anti-GBM disease have been identified, including the immunoglobulin heavy chain Gm locus that encodes the constant region of the IgG heavy chain (Rees et al., 1984), polymorphisms of FCGR genes that encode the Fc receptor for IgG (FcγR) (Zhou et al., 2010a, 2010b) and kallikrein genes (Liu et al., 2009).

4. Clinical symptoms

General malaise (fatigue), weight loss, fever, arthralgia or myalgia may be the initial features of anti-GBM disease in a pattern similar to but much less prominent than that in systemic vasculitis. Symptoms relating to anemia may also occur even in the absence of significant hemoptysis.

Authors	Year	Nation	symptoms					
			fatigue	fever	dys-pnea	hemo-ptysis	macro hemat uria	oligo-anuria
Shah et al. *	2002	Various	15% (8/54)	28% (15/54)	26% (14/54)	65% (35/54)	7% (4/54)	17% (9/54)
Lazor et al.	2007	France & Switzerland	64% (18/28)	43% (12/28)	79% (22/28)	75% (21/28)	36% (10/28)	18% (5/28)
Merkel et al.	1994	Germany	40% (14/35)	28% (10/35)	14% (5/35)	51% (18/35)	20% (7/35)	N.A.
Daly et al.	1996	Ireland	N.A.	N.A.	N.A.	25% (10/40)	35% (14/40)	50% (20/40)
Williams et al.	1988	United Kingdom	N.A.	N.A.	10% (1/10)	10% (1/10)	10% (1/10)	60% (6/10)
Proskey et al. *	1970	United States	51% (29/56)	22% (12/56)	57% (32/56)	82% (46/56)	12% (7/56)	N.A.
Wilson et al.	1973	United States	34% (17/50)	14% (7/50)	32% (16/50)	46% (23/50)	42% (21/50)	10% (5/50)
Briggs et al.	1979	United States	22% (4/18)	11% (2/18)	44% (8/18)	50% (9/18)	56% (10/18)	N.A.
Walker et al.	1985	Australia	N.A.	N.A.	N.A.	62% (13/21)	N.A.	62% (13/21)
Teague et al. *	1978	New Zealand	68% (19/28)	26% (7/27)	78% (21/27)	86% (25/29)	43% (12/28)	N.A.
Li et al.	2004	China (Hong Kong)	N.A.	N.A.	N.A.	40% (4/10)	N.A.	40% (4/10)
Cui et al.	2005	China	N.A.	N.A.	N.A.	59% (57/97)	27% (26/97)	52% (50/97)
Hirayama et al.	2008	Japan	53% (25/47)	57% (27/47)	6% (3/47)	15% (7/47)	19% (9/47)	28% (13/47)

The frequencies of patients with each symptom are expressed as percentages. *All investigated patients had Goodpasture's syndrome. Abbreviations: N.A., not available.

Table 2. Investigations of clinical symptoms in anti-GBM disease at the initial presentation.

The principal clinical features relate to the development of renal failure due to RPGN or alveolar hemorrhage (Table 2). Hemoptysis is the predominant symptom of alveolar hemorrhage. Alveolar hemorrhage may cause severe impairment of oxygenation, so intensive care and artificial ventilation are sometimes needed. The mild lung symptoms are only dry cough and shortness of breath. Although one-third to two-thirds of patients with anti-GBM disease demonstrate alveolar hemorrhage in general, in our survey, 23.4% (11/47) of patients with anti-GBM disease suffered from alveolar hemorrhage (Hirayama et al., 2008). A minority of patients exhibited macrohematuria. Anirua or oliguria was seen in 17-62% of patients at presentation, and these findings suggested a poorer prognosis (Levy et al., 2001; Hudson et al., 2003).

5. Laboratory examinations

In general, all patients with anti-GBM disease had microscopic hematuria on urinalysis. Proteinuria is modest, but can be heavier when the disease has a more subacute course. In our survey (Hirayama et al., 2008), the mean 24-hour excretion of urinary protein in renal-limited anti-GBM disease was 2.1±3.0 g and that of Goodpasture's syndrome was 3.7±3.2 g.

Authors	Year	Nation	Urinary protein (g/day)	Serum creatinine (mg/dL)	ESRD (%)
Shah et al.	2002	Various	N.A.	6.62 (N.A.)	35% (27/78)
Herody et al.	1993	France	N.A.	N.A.	55% (16/29)
Lazor et al.	2007	France & Switzerland	1.2 (0 – 35.0)	1.27 (0.61 – 21.47)	41% (11/28)
Andrassy et al.	1991	Germany	6.4 (0 – 15.3)	12.8 (6.1 – 16.5)	67% (2/3)
Merkel et al.	1994	Germany	N.A. (0.2 – 3.5)	11.41 ± 5.64 (0.19 – 22.96)	71% (20/28)
Daly et al.	1996	Ireland	N.A.	5.1 ± 6.8 (N.A.)	50% (20/40)
Segelmark et al.	2003	Sweden	N.A.	8.94 (5.44 – 12.34)	46% (36/79)
Savage et al.	1986	United Kingdom	N.A.	N.A.	64% (69/108)
Williams et al.	1988	United Kingdom	N.A.	11.80 ± 4.67 (1.60 – 18.37)	70% (7/10)
Levy et al.	2001	United Kingdom	N.A.	3.59 (0.6 – 10.9)	55% (39/71)
Briggs et al.	1979	United States	2.6 ± 0.5 (1.9 – 3.5)	5.94 ± 7.11 (0.8 – 30.0)	33% (6/18)
Johnson et al.	1985	United States	4.3 ± 5.2 (0 – 22.0)	4.87 ± 6.93 (0.9 – 25.0)	12% (2/17)
Jennette	2003	United States	1.67 ± 3.35 (0.20- 16.20)	9.7 ± 7.2 (0.8 - 50)	N.A.
Walker et al.	1985	Australia	1.4 (0.4 – 5.4)	6.56 (1.24 – 32.35)	45% (10/22)
Simpson et al.	1982	New Zealand	N.A.	5.37 ± 5.22 (0.68 – 19.80)	10% (2/20)
Teague et al.	1978	New Zealand	N.A.	N.A.	14% (4/29)
Li et al.	2004	China (Hong Kong)	N.A.	6.96 ± 6.41 (1.19 – 22.09)	50% (5/10)
Cui et al.	2005	China	N.A.	N.A.	71% (69/97)
Hirayama et al	2008	Japan	2.4 ± 3.0 (0.1 – 12.2)	7.29 ± 4.19 (1.00 – 16.80)	60% (28/47)

Amounts of urinary protein and serum creatinine levels are expressed as means ± standard deviation or medians with ranges. Frequency of end-stage renal failure at presentation is expressed as a percentage. To convert serum creatinine in mg/dL to μmol/L, multiply by 88.4. Abbreviations: ESRD, end-stage renal disease; N.A., not available.

Table 3. Investigations of renal findings in anti-GBM disease at the initial presentation.

Unfortunately, most patients with anti-GBM disease had renal failure at the time of diagnosis, and the number of patients needing dialysis was not a few (Table 3). In our survey (Hirayama et al., 2008), the mean serum creatinine (s-Cr) level in renal-limited anti-GBM disease was 7.07±4.21 mg/dl, while that in Goodpasture's syndrome was 7.99±4.31 mg/dl. Hemodialysis therapy had already been initiated in 59.6% (28/47) of the anti-GBM disease patients before the start of immunosuppressive treatments.

Anemia was observed in most patients with anti-GBM disease, and the mean hemoglobin concentration in renal-limited anti-GBM disease was 8.8±1.7 g/dl, while that in Goodpasture's syndrome was 7.5±1.1 g/dl. The mean erythrocyte sedimentation rate (ESR) in renal-limited anti-GBM disease was 105±44 mm/h, and that in Goodpasture's syndrome was 82±45 mm/h. The mean serum C-reactive protein (CRP) level in renal-limited anti-GBM disease was 8.5±7.2 mg/dl, and that in Goodpasture's syndrome was 8.2±8.1 mg/dl. In comparison with other forms of RPGN, such as micropolyangiitis (MPA) and Wegener's granulomatosis (WG), there was no difference in inflammation markers such as leukocyte count, ESR and serum CRP. However, in patients with anti-GBM disease, the mean level of s-Cr at the time of diagnosis was higher than that in patients with MPA (4.54±3.13 mg/dl) or WG (3.84±3.24 mg/dl). Therefore, early diagnosis of anti-GBM disease is very important.

Although obvert hemoptysis may not be immediately present in patients with Goodpasture's syndrome and alveolar hemorrhage may not be immediately obvious in radiological examinations, an elevated alveolo-arterial oxygen difference ($AaPO_2$) can be a sensitive indicator of alveolar hemorrhage. An elevated red blood cell count in bronchoalveolar lavages, as detected by bronchoscopy, is useful information for the diagnosis of alveolar hemorrhage, but lung biopsy does not contribute to this diagnosis (Lazor et al., 2007).

The diagnosis of anti-GBM disease is dependent on the detection of anti-GBM antibodies in either the circulation or the kidney tissue. These serum antibodies are usually detected using an enzyme-linked immunosorbent assay or radioimmunoassay method. The antibodies have not been reported to occur in the absence of disease, and false negatives are rare when appropriate checks are performed. In our survey (Hirayama et al., 2008), 91.5% (43/47) of patients with anti-GBM disease were diagnosed via the detection of serum anti-GBM antibodies.

In serological examinations, other autoantibodies were not usually detected. However, in our survey (Hirayama et al., 2008), anti-nuclear antibodies were detected in 11.8% of renal-limited anti-GBM disease and in 27.3% of patients with Goodpasture's syndrome. Anti-DNA antibody was not detected in renal-limited anti-GBM disease, but it was detected in 22.2% of patients with Goodpasture's syndrome. Moreover, anti-neutrophil cytoplasmic antibodies (ANCA) were detected in 12.8% (5/39) of patients with anti-GBM disease; a perinuclear pattern was detected in all five anti-GBM disease patients with ANCA, and a cytoplasmic pattern was detected in one. Anti-GBM antibody and ANCA coexisted in 15 - 50% of cases of anti-GBM disease described in the previous literature (Jayne et al., 1990; Bosch et al., 1991; Yang et al., 2005; Rutgers et al., 2005; Levy et al., 2004). Other studies revealed that patients with double-positive antibodies were predominantly MPO-ANCA, older and male (Jayne et al., 1990; Bosch et al., 1991; Yang et al., 2005; Rutgers et al., 2005). In our survey (Hirayama et al., 2008), the age at onset of patients with double-positive antibodies was higher (mean age, 52.6 years), but female-dominant (male : female = 1 : 4). The prognosis of patients with double-positive antibodies varied; the renal and patient survival rates of patients with double-positive antibodies were reported to be either better (Jayne et al., 1990; Bosch et al., 1991), not significantly different (Yang et al., 2005), or worse (Rutgers et al., 2005; Levy et al., 2004) than those of patients with anti-GBM antibody alone. In our survey (Hirayama et al., 2008), the prognosis of patients with double-positive antibodies was poor; two died and the remaining three required maintenance hemodialysis. Alveolar hemorrhage was observed in two of five patients with double-positive antibodies, and three of them had interstitial pneumonitis.

6. Imaging examinations

Kidneys were usually normal-sized or enlarged due to inflammation. In our survey (Hirayama et al., 2008), ultrasonography showed that 61.0% of patients with anti-GBM disease had kidneys of normal size, while atrophic kidneys were observed in 12.2% of patients and enlarged kidneys were observed in 26.8%. There were no specific morphological abnormalities on any type of renal imaging examinations.

In cases with Goodpasture's syndrome, shadows usually involve the central lung fields with peripheral and upper-lobe sparing on chest radiography or computed tomography (Figure 2). Although the shadows are generally symmetrical, they can be markedly asymmetrical.

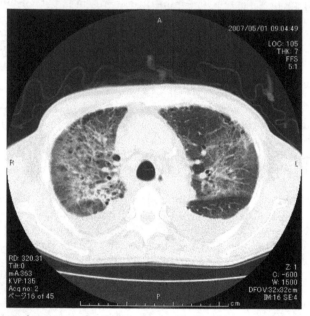

Fig. 2. Chest computed tomography in a patient with Goodpasture's syndrome.

Symmetrical shadows involved the central lung fields with peripheral sparing. Bilateral pleural effusions due to hypervolemia in acute kidney injury were also observed.

7. Pathological findings

A renal biopsy is essential in suspected anti-GBM disease both to confirm the diagnosis and to assess the renal prognosis. Glomerular fibrinoid necrosis and crescent formation with linear staining of the glomerular capillary walls for IgG are the histological hallmarks of anti-GBM disease.

7.1 Light microscopic findings

The histological pattern of disease starts with mesangial expansion and hypercellularity. It progresses to focal and segmental glomerulonephritis with infiltration by inflammatory cells, accompanied by segmental necrosis with prominent breaks in the GBM. Later, glomeruli develop an extensive crescent formation composed of parietal epithelial cells and macrophages in association with the destruction of the GBM (Figure 3). The crescents are usually at the same stage of evolution.

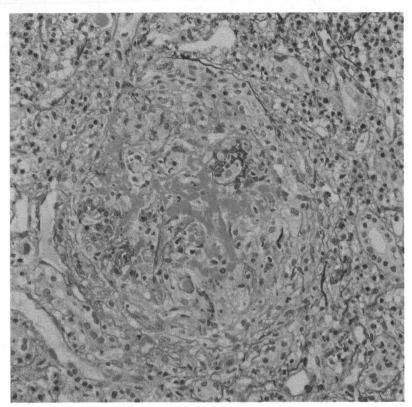

Fig. 3. Periodic acid-Schiff methenamine silver (PAM)−stained glomerulus in a patient with anti-GBM disease.

The disruption of the capillary walls, segmental necrosis and cellular crescent formation are observed. Rupture of the basement membrane of Bowman's capsule and periglomerular infiltration of inflammatory cells are also observed. Interstitial edema with infiltration of inflammatory cells is revealed.

Various degrees of crescent formation are observed in more than 90% of patients with anti-GBM disease. In Europe, the United States and Asian-Pacific, including Japan, the mean percentage of glomeruli showing crescent formation ranged from 40% to 100%, and about 70% to 100% of patients with anti-GBM disease had more than 50% crescentic glomeruli (Figure 4). Anti-GBM disease is pathologically the most severe form of glomerulonephritis (Holdsworth et al., 1985; Jennette, 2003, Hirayama et al., 2008).

Although tubules are usually normal, epithelial flattening is revealed in the severe acute phase. In the chronic phase, tubules in the area of severe injury undergo atrophy and some disappear. Acute tubulitis sometimes occurs if there is a linear staining of tubular basement membranes for IgG. Interstitial edema with infiltration of inflammatory cells is predominant in the acute phase, whereas interstitial fibrosis is revealed in the chronic phase. Interstitial infiltrates are composed of neutrophils, eosinophils, lymphocytes, monocytes and macrophages. If Bowman's capsules are disrupted, inflammatory cells infiltrate around glomeruli and have a granulomatous appearance. Acute inflammation of renal vessels, except for glomerular capillaries, is not typical for anti-GBM disease, unless the case has concurrent ANCA (Bosch et al., 1991).

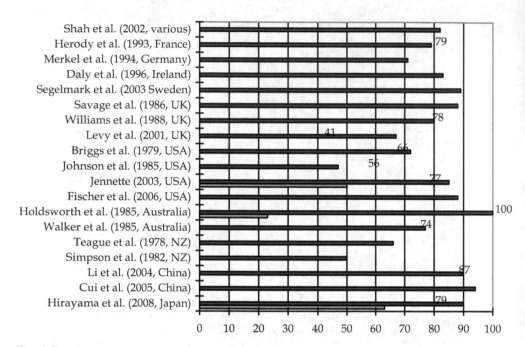

Fig. 4. Previous investigations of crescent formation in anti-GBM disease and ANCA-associated vasculitis.

Each bar shows the frequency of patients with 50% or more crescents in anti-GBM disease (purple) and ANCA-associated vasculitis (blue). The numbers show the mean percentage of glomeruli showing crescent formation in anti-GBM disease. Abbreviations: UK, United Kingdom; USA, United States; NZ, New Zealand.

7.2 Immunofluorescence findings

The immunohistologic feature of anti-GBM disease is linear staining of the glomerular capillary walls for IgG (Figure 5). IgG1 is the predominant IgG subclass in staining of the glomerular capillary walls (Bowman et al., 1987; Segelmark et al., 1990). Linear staining for IgM and IgA is less common, but rare cases with anti-GBM disease have linear staining only for IgA and circulating IgA-class anti-GBM antibodies in the absence of IgG-class anti-GBM antibodies in the serum or staining in glomeruli (Border et al., 1979; Gris et al., 1991; Borza et al., 2005). Granular or discontinuous linear staining for C3 is observed in most cases with anti-GBM disease, but glomerular staining for C3 is negative for some cases (Wilson and Dixon, 1973). Irregular staining for fibrin is observed in portions of glomerular necrosis and cellular crescents.

Linear staining of tubular basement membranes for IgG sometimes occurs (Lehman et al., 1975; Andres et al., 1978).

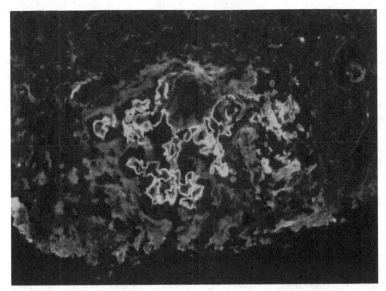

Fig. 5. Direct immunofluorescence for IgG in a patient with anti-GBM disease.

Linear staining for IgG along glomerular capillary walls is observed, but staining for IgG at the part of the cellular crescent is not.

7.3 Electroscopic findings
The rupture of GBM with variable degrees of endothelial swelling and lucent expansion of the subendothelial zone is common urtrasturactural findings in the acute phase of anti-GBM disease. Rupture of Bowman's capsule, focal effacement of epithelial foot processes and accumulation of epithelial cells and macrophages in Bowman's spaces are also observed. Occasionally, neutrophils are identified in capillaries, especially at sites where GBM is disrupted. Those findings are also observed in pauci-immune crescentic glomerulonephritis, but electron-dense deposits are absent, unlike the case with immune complex-type crescentic glomerulonephritis.

8. Treatments

As the pathogenesis of anti-GBM disease became clear, treatment regimens were designed to remove the circulating pathogenic anti-GBM antibodies by therapeutic plasma exchange, attenuate the pathogenic antibody-mediated glomerular inflammatory responses by administration of corticosteroids and suppress further production of these pathogenic antibodies by the use of immunosuppressive agents.

8.1 Therapeutic plasmapheresis
To remove the circulating pathogenic anti-GBM antibodies, therapeutic plasma exchange is recommended as the initial treatment. The effectiveness of therapeutic plasmapheresis for improving renal function has been reported. In the most commonly used regimens, plasma exchange of 4 L of plasma for 5% human albumin was performed daily for 14 days or until

the circulating anti-GBM antibodies were no longer detected (Lockwood et al., 1976). In the presence of alveolar hemorrhage, 300-400 ml of fresh-frozen plasma was given at the end of each treatment.

To reduce the replacement of plasma, anti-GBM antibody removal has been modified. Immunoadsorption to remove circulating IgG immunoglobulins without the need for protein substitution during daily treatments may also be beneficial in Goodpasture's disease. Anecdotal case reports suggest that it may be an alternative to plasmapheresis in patients with severe renal failure (Laczika et al., 2000). There was a case report of Goodpasture's syndrome that we treated with double filtration plasmapheresis combined with immunosuppression therapy (Nagasu et al., 2009). In that therapy, the removal efficiency for the anti-GBM antibody was 24 to 60% for each procedure.

8.2 Corticosteroids

To attenuate the pathogenic antibody-mediated glomerular inflammatory responses, corticosteroid is also a key element of this treatment. According to the most commonly used regimens, oral dosing of prednisolone at 1 mg/kg/day ideal body weight (maximum 80 mg daily) continues for at least 2 weeks, after which the dose is reduced every second week to 30 mg by 8 weeks. After that, the dosages of prednisolone are tapered to 2.5-5.0 mg/week and maintained at 7.5-10 mg/kg/day. Oral corticosteroids have generally been continued for at least 6 months. Intravenous administration of methylprednisolone 10 mg/kg (500-1000 mg) once daily for 1-3 days has been advocated for patients with severe alveolar hemorrhage or very rapid deterioration of renal function (Johnson et al., 1985).

8.3 Immunosuppressive agents

To further suppress the production of pathogenic anti-GBM antibodies, a combination of immunosuppressive agents is usually given. Among these immunosuppressive agents, cyclophosphamide is usually administered. According to the most commonly used regimens, the oral dose is 2-3 mg/kg/day (this is rounded down to the nearest 50 mg; reduced to 2 mg/kg/day in patients over 55 years) for 3 months. This administration is stopped if white blood cell counts fall below $4,000/\mu L$. In such cases the agent is restarted at a lower dose once the white blood cell counts return above $4,000/\mu L$. Intravenous cyclophosphamide (IVCY) is not usually administered, but it may be useful for a refractory case of the standard therapy (Baumgartner et al., 1995).

Although azathioprine is sometimes used as maintenance therapy, it alone does not provide adequate immunosuppression to modify the disease.

8.4 Therapeutic options for refractory diseases

There is very little study on the treatment of refractory anti-GBM disease. Cyclosporine is controversial; at 6 mg/kg/day it was effective for an anti-GBM disease patient treated with corticosteroid, cyclophosphamide and plasma exchange (Querin et al., 1992), whereas it was not useful (Pepys et al., 1982). Small numbers of case reports of successful outcomes with mycophenolic acid or mycophenolate mofetil in patients unresponsive to or intolerant of standard therapy have been published (Garcia-Canton et al., 2000; Kiykim et al., 2010; Malho et al., 2010). Rituximab, a chimeric monoclonal anti-CD20 antibody, was effective for a case of relapsed anti-GBM disease that was resistant to standard treatment (Arzoo et al., 2002). In that case, rituximab (375 mg/m^2) was administered once a week for 6 consecutive weeks; the symptoms completely resolved and anti-GBM antibody titers were decreased from 51 U/mL to the undetectable range. However, these treatments cannot yet be recommended as a first-line therapy because no randomized controlled trials have been carried out.

9. Prognosis

Most patients without treatment died shortly after diagnosis of anti-GBM disease; the survival rate at 12 months was 4%, and the renal survival rate was 2% (Benoit et al., 1963). Although mortality has improved by the introduction of intense immunosuppression, renal survival remains very poor because of the delayed diagnosis of anti-GBM disease or delayed initiation of induction therapies.

9.1 Outcomes

The prognosis for patients with anti-GBM disease is poor; the survival rate at 6-12 months was 67-94%, but the renal survival rate was 15-58% in Europe, the United States, China and Japan (Table 4).

Authors	Year	Nation	Treatment	N	AH (%)	1-year survival (%)	
						Patient	Renal
Herody et al.	1993	France	OCS+CYC+AZA	29	50	93	41
Lazor et al.	2007	France & Switzerland	OCS+CYC+PE	24	100	100	58
Merkel et al.	1994	Germany	OCS+CYC+PE	35	57	89	29
Daly et al.	1996	Ireland	IS+PE	40	67	98	20
Segelmark et al.	2003	Sweden	OCS+CYC+PE	79	24	66	25
Peters et al.	1982	United Kingdom	IS+PE	41	56	76	39
Savage et al.	1986	United Kingdom	IS+PE	108	52	78	20
Levy et al.	2001	United Kingdom	OCS+CYC+PE	71	62	77	53
Proskey et al.	1970	United States	IS	56	100	77	23
Wilson et al.	1973	United States	IS	53	60	53	13
Beirne et al.	1977	United States	IS	29	54	42	17
Briggs et al.	1979	United States	IS(+PE)	18	61	84	22
Johnson et al	1985	United States	OCS+CYC	9	78	89	22
			OCS+CYC+PE	8	100	100	75
Walker et al.	1985	Australia	IS+PE	22	62	59	45
Teague et al.	1978	New Zealand	IS+PE	29	100	64	31
Simpson et al.	1982	New Zealand	no treatment	8	100	63	25
			OCS+AZA	4	100	100	50
			OCS+CYC+PE	8	100	100	63
Li et al.	2004	China (Hong Kong)	IS+PE	10	40	70	15
Cui et al.	2005	China	IS+PE	97	58	92	22
Hirayama et al	2008	Japan	OCS+CYC	21	14	86	24
			OCS+CYC+PE	22	36	68	14

Abbreviations: N, number of patients; AH, alveolar hemorrhage; IS, immunosuppressants (including methylprednisolone pulse therapy, oral corticosteroids, cyclophosphamide or azathioprine); PE, plasma exchange; OCS, oral corticosteroids; CYC, cyclophosphamide; AZA, azathioprine.

Table 4. Investigations of treatments for anti–GBM antibody disease.

Renal function improves in 15-75% of patients with anti-GBM disease through the combination of plasma exchange with corticosteroids and immunosuppressive agents, whereas the renal survival rates of anti-GBM disease patients treated with immunosuppressive agents alone ranged from 2-22%. Improvement of renal function is usually evident within days of the start of plasma exchange. However, it should be emphasized that this regimen has never been properly assessed by a prospective randomized controlled trial because of the rarity and acuteness of the condition. The only reported randomized controlled trial was very small and used lower doses of both plasma exchange and cyclophosphamide than those that are generally used in practice.

Although the effectiveness of treatment using therapeutic plasma exchange combined with immunosuppressive agents to improve renal function has been reported, only half of patients with anti-GBM disease had been treated with plasma exchange in our survey (Hirayama et al., 2008). Therefore, there was no significant difference in the renal survival rates between anti-GBM antibody disease patients treated with and without plasma exchange (P = 0.683 by the Log-rank Mantel-Cox test). Moreover, there was no significant difference in mortality between anti-GBM antibody disease patients treated with and without plasma exchange (P = 0.109).

9.2 Predictors of survival

The best predictors of renal survival are s-Cr at the initiation of treatment and the mean percentage of crescent formations. Renal function improves coincidentally with the introduction of plasma exchange in about 80-95% of patients with s-Cr levels less than or equal to 5.7-6.8 mg/dL (500-600 µmol/L), but in far fewer of those with higher s-Cr levels or those who require dialysis. Unfortunately, most patients with anti-GBM disease had renal failure at the time of diagnosis, and the mean percentage of crescent formation was high in anti-GBM disease patients. Therefore, in most patients with anti-GBM disease, the diagnosis may have been made too late to improve renal function by combination therapy.

9.3 Relapse/recurrence

Relapses of anti-GBM disease are rarely observed, in contrast to most other autoimmune kidney diseases. The anti-GBM antibodies seem to disappear spontaneously after 12-18 months (Levy et al., 1996). However, several reports demonstrated recurring cases with anti-GBM disease (Adler et al., 1981; Hind et al., 1984; Klasa et al., 1988; Levy et al., 1996). In our survey (Hirayama et al., 2008), relapse or recurrence was also rare in patients with anti-GBM disease (13.9%) in comparison with patients with ANCA-associated vasculitis, such as WG (29.4%) and MPA (29.3%). Therefore, remission induction therapy is more important in anti-GBM disease. The mean time to recurrence is estimated to be 4.3 years (range, 1-10 years), and that late recurrence may occur with a frequency of 2-14%. During relapses, circulating anti-GBM antibodies often reappear. The combination of plasmapheresis and immunosuppressive agents as re-remission induction therapy is also successful in relapsing cases (Levy et al., 1996).

10. Conclusion

Anti-GBM disease is a rare but well-characterized glomerulonephritis. It occurs across all racial groups but is most common in Caucasians. Although the effectiveness of treatment using therapeutic plasma exchange combined with immunosuppressive agents to improve renal function has been reported, the prognosis for patients with this disease is poor. To improve the prognosis, it may be necessary to detect this disease in earlier stages and to treat it without delay.

11. Acknowledgment

The authors acknowledge the participants in this Japanese nationwide survey and the members of the RPGN Clinical Guidelines Committee of Japan. The authors thank Dr. Miho Nagai, Dr. Yujiro Ogawa, Dr. Shogo Fujita, Dr. Homare Shimohata and Prof. Masaki Kobayashi (Tokyo Medical University Ibaraki Medical Center) and Dr. Joichi Usui (University of Tsukuba) for their assistance. The Japanese nationwide RPGN survey was supported by a grant-in-aid from the Research Fund for the Special Study Group on Progressive Glomerular Disease, the Ministry of Health, Labor and Welfare, Japan.

12. References

Adler, S.; Bruns, F.J., Fraley, D.S. & Segel, D.P. (1981). Rapid progressive glomerulonephritis: relapse after prolonged remission. *Archives of Internal Medicine*, Vol.141, No.7, (June 1981), pp. 852-854, ISSN 0003-9926

Adler, S.; Chen, X. & Eng, B. (1990). Control of rat glomerular epithelial cell growth in vitro. *Kidney International*, Vol.37, No.4, (April 1990), pp. 1048-1054, ISSN 0085-2538

Andrassy, K.; Küster, S., Waldherr, R. & Ritz, E. (1991). Rapidly progressive glomerulonephritis: analysis of prevalence and clinical course. *Nephron*, Vol.59, No.2, (October 1991), ISSN 0028-2766

Andres, G.; Brentjens, J., Kohli, R., Anthone, R., Anthone, S., Baliah, T., Montes, M., Mookerjee, B.K., Prezyna, A., Sepulveda, M., Venuto, R. & Elwood, C. (1978). Histology of human tubulo-interstitial nephritis associated with antibodies to renal basement membranes. *Kidney International*, Vol.13, No. 6, (June 1978), pp. 480-491, ISSN 0085-2538

Angangco, R.; Thiru, S., Esnault, V.L., Short, A.K., Lockwood, C.M. & Oliveira, D.B. (1994). Does truly 'idiopathic' crescentic glomerulonephritis exist? *Nephrology Dialysis Transplantation*, Vo.9, No.6, (June 1994), pp.630-636, ISSN 0931-0509

Arzoo, K.; Sadeghi, S. & Liebman, H.A. (2002). Treatment of refractory antibody mediated autoimmune disorders with an anti-CD20 monoclonal antibody (rituximab). *Annals of the Rheumatic Diseases*, Vol.61, No.10, (October 2002), pp. 922-924, ISSN 0003-4967

Atkins, R.C.; Holdsworth, S.R., Glasgow, E.F. & Matthews, F.E. (1976). The macrophage in human rapidly progressive glomerulonephritis. *The Lancet*, Vol.1, No.7964, (April 1976), pp. 830-832, ISSN 0140-6736

Baricos, W.H.; Cortez, S.L., Le, Q.C., Wu, L.T., Shaw, E., Hanada, K. & Shah, S.V. (1991). Evidence suggesting a role for cathepsin L in an experimental model of glomerulonephritis. *Archives of Biochemistry and Biophysics*, Vol.288, No.2, (August 1991), pp. 468-472, ISSN 0003-9861

Baumgartner, I.; Gmür, J., Fontana, A., Widmer, U. & Walter, E. (1995). Recovery from life threatening pulmonary hemorrhage in Goodpasture's syndrome after plasmapheresis and subsequent pulse dose cyclophosphamide. *Clinical Nephrology*, Vol.43, No.1, (January 1995), pp. 68-70, ISSN 0301-0430

Beirne, G.J.; Wagnild, J.P., Zimmerman, S.W., Macken, P.D. & Burkholder, P.M. (1977). Idiopathic crescentic glomerulonephritis. *Medicine (Baltimore)*, Vol.56, No.5, (September 1977), pp.349–381, ISSN 0025-7974

Beirne, G.J. & Brennan J.T. (1972). Glomerulonephritis associated with hydrocarbon solvents: mediated by antiglomerular basement membrane antibody. *Archives of Environmental Health*, Vol.25, No.5, (November 1972), pp. 365–369, ISSN 0003-9896

Benoit, F.L.; Rulon, D.B., Theil, G.B., Doolan, P.D. & Watten, R.H. (1963). Goodpasture's syndrome: A clinicopathologic entity. *The American Journal of Medicine*, Vol.58, (September 1963), pp. 424–444, ISSN 0002-9343

Blue, W.T. & Lange, C.F (1975). Increased immunologic reactivity between human glomerular basement membrane and group A type 12 streptococcal cell membrane after carbohydrase treatment. *Journal of Immunology*, Vol.114, No.1, (January 1975), pp. 306–309, ISSN 0022-1767

Bombassei, G.J. & Kaplan, A.A. (1992). The association between hydrocarbon exposure and anti-glomerular basement membrane antibody-mediated disease (Goodpasture's syndrome). *American Journal of Industrial Medicine*, Vol.21, No.2, (February 1992), pp. 141–153, ISSN 0271-3586

Bonzel, K.E.; Müller-Wiefel, D.E., Ruder, H., Wingen, A.M., Waldherr, R. & Weber, M. (1987). Anti-glomerular basement membrane antibody-mediated glomerulonephritis due to glue sniffing. *European Journal of Pediatrics*, Vol.146, No.3, (May 1987), pp. 296-300, ISSN 0340-6199

Border, W.A.; Baehler, R.W., Bhathena, D. & Glassock, R.J. (1979). IgA antibasement membrane nephritis with pulmonary hemorrhage. *Annals of Internal Medicine*, Vol.91, No.1, (July 1979), pp. 21-25, ISSN 0003-4819

Borza, D.B.; Netzer, K.O., Leinonen, A., Todd, P., Cervera, J., Saus, J. & Hudson, B.G. (2000). The Goodpasture autoantigen. Identification of multiple cryptic epitopes on the NC1 domain of the alpha3(IV) collagen chain. *The Journal of Biological Chemistry*, Vol.275, No.8, (February 2000), pp. 6030–6037, ISSN 0021-9258

Borza, D.B.; Chedid, M.F., Colon, S., Lager, D.J., Leung, N. & Fervenza, F.C. (2005). Recurrent Goodpasture's disease secondary to a monoclonal IgA1-kappa antibody autoreactive with the alpha1/alpha2 chains of type IV collagen. *American Journal of Kidney Diseases*, Vol.45, No.2, (February 2005), pp. 397-406, ISSN 0272-6386

Bosch, X.; Mirapeix, E., Font, J., Borrellas, X., Rodríguez, R., López-Soto, A., Ingelmo, M. & Revert, L. (1991). Prognostic implication of anti-neutrophil cytoplasmic autoantibodies with myeloperoxidase specificity in anti-glomerular basement membrane disease. *Clinical Nephrology*, Vol.36, No.3, (September 1991), pp. 107-113, ISSN 0301-0430

Boucher, A.; Droz, D., Adafer, E. & Noel, L.H. (1987). Relationship between the integrity of Bowman's capsule and the composition of cellular crescents in human crescentic glomerulonephritis. *Laboratory Investigation*, Vol.56, No.5, (May 1987), pp. 526–533, ISSN 0023-6837

Bowman, C.; Ambrus, K. & Lockwood, C.M. (1987). Restriction of human IgG subclass expression in the population of auto-antibodies to glomerular basement membrane. *Clinical and Experimental Immunology*, Vol.69, No.2, (August 1987), pp. 341-349, ISSN 0009-9104

Briganti, E.M.; Dowling, J., Finlay, M., Hill, P.A., Jones, C.L., Kincaid-Smith, P.S., Sinclair, R., McNeil, J.J. & Atkins, R.C. (2001). The incidence of biopsy-proven glomerulonephritis in Australia. *Nephrology Dialysis Transplantation*, Vol.16, No.7, (July 2001), pp. 1364–1367, ISSN 0931-0509

Briggs, W.A.; Johnson, J.P., Teichman, S., Yeager, H.C. & Wilson, C.B. (1979). Antiglomerular basement membrane antibody-mediated glomerulonephritis and Goodpasture's syndrome. *Medicine (Baltimore)*, Vol.58, No.5, (September 1979), pp. 348–361, ISSN 0025-7974

Churchill, D.N.; Fine, A. & Gault, M.H. (1983). Association between hydrocarbon exposure and glomerulonephritis. An appraisal of the evidence. *Nephron*, Vol.33, No.3, (June 1983), pp. 169-172, ISSN 0028-2766

Clatworthy, M.R.; Wallin, E.F. & Jayne, D.R. (2008). Anti-glomerular basement membrane disease after alemtuzumab. *The New England Journal of Medicine*, Vol.359, No.7, (August 2008), pp. 768-769, ISSN 0028-4793

Cui, Z.; Zhao, M.H., Xin, G. & Wang, H.Y. (2005). Characteristics and prognosis of Chinese patients with anti-glomerular basement membrane disease. *Nephron Clinical Practice*, Vol.99, No.2, (February 2005), pp. c49-c55, ISSN 1660-2110

Daly, C.; Conlon, P.J., Medwar, W. & Walshe, J.J. (1996). Characteristics and outcome of anti-glomerular basement membrane disease: a single-center experience. *Renal Failure*, Vol.18, No.1, (January 1996), pp. 105-112, ISSN 0886-022X

Date, A.; Raghavan, R., John, T.J., Richard, J., Kirubakaran, M.G. & Shastry, J.C.N. (1987). Renal disease in adult Indians: a clinicopathological study of 2827 patients. *The Quarterly Journal of Medicine*, Vol.64, No.245, (September 1987), pp. 729-737, ISSN 0033-5622

Donaghy, M. & Rees, A.J. (1983). Cigarette smoking and lung haemorrhage in glomerulonephritis caused by autoantibodies to glomerular basement membrane. *The Lancet*, Vol. 2, No.8364, (December 1983), pp. 1390–1393, ISSN 0140-6736

Fisher, M.; Pusey, C.D., Vaughan, R.W. & Rees, A.J. (1997). Susceptibility to anti-glomerular basement membrane disease is strongly associated with HLA-DRB1 genes. *Kidney International*, Vol.51, No.1, (January 1997), pp. 222–229, ISSN 0085-2538

Fischer, E.G. & Lager, D.J. (2006). Anti-glomerular basement membrane glomerulonephritis: a morphologic study of 80 cases. *American Journal of Clinical Patholology*, Vol.123, No.3, (March 2006), pp. 445-450, ISSN 0002-9173

García-Cantón, C.; Toledo, A., Palomar, R., Fernandez, F., Lopez, J., Moreno, A., Esparza, N., Suria, S., Rossique, P., Diaz, J.M. & Checa, D. (2000). Goodpasture's syndrome treated with mycophenolate mofetil. *Nephrology Dialysis Transplantation*, Vol.15, No.6, (June 2000), pp. 920-922, ISSN 0931-0509

García-Rostan y Pérez, G.M.; García Bragado, F. & Puras Gil, A.M. (1997). Pulmonary hemorrhage and antiglomerular basement membrane antibody-mediated glomerulonephritis after exposure to smoked cocaine (crack): a case report and review of the literature. *Pathology International*, Vo.47, No.10, (October 1997), pp. 692-697, ISSN 1320-5463

Goodpasture E.W. (1919). The significance of certain pulmonary lesions in relation to the etiology of influenza. *The American Journal of the Medical Sciences*, Vol.158, No.6, (1919), pp. 863-870, (republished in *The American Journal of the Medical Sciences*, Vol.338, No.2, (August 2009), pp. 148-151), ISSN 0002-9629

Grcevska, L. & Polenakovic, M. (1995). Crescentic glomerulonephritis as renal cause of acute renal failure. *Renal Failure*, Vol.17, No.5, (September 1995), pp. 595-604, ISSN 0886-022X

Gris, P.; Pirson, Y., Hamels, J., Vaerman, J.P., Quoidbach, A. & Demol, H. (1991). Antiglomerular basement membrane nephritis induced by IgA1 antibodies. *Nephron*, Vol.58, No.4, (August 1991), pp. 418-424, ISSN 0028-2766

He, C.J.; Rondeau, E., Medcalf, R.L., Lacave, R., Schleuning, W.D. & Sraer, J.D. (1991). Thrombin increases proliferation and decreases fibrinolytic activity of kidney glomerular epithelial cells. *Journal of Cellular Physiology*, Vol.146, No.1, (January 1991), pp. 131-140, ISSN 0021-9541

Heaf, J.; Løkkegaard, H. & Larsen, S. (1999). The epidemiology and prognosis of glomerulonephritis in Denmark 1985-1997. *Nephrology Dialysis Transplantation*, Vol.14, No.8, (August 1999), pp. 1889-1897, ISSN 0931-0509

Herody, M.; Bobrie, G., Gouarin, C., Grünfeld, J.P. & Noel, L.H. (1993). Anti-GBM disease: Predictive value of clinical, histological and serological data. *Clinical Nephrology*, Vol.40, No.5, (November 1993), pp. 249–255, ISSN 0301-0430

Hind, C.R.K.; Bowman, C., Winearles, C.G. & Lockwood, C.M. (1984). Recurrence of circulating anti-glomerular basement membrane antibody three years after immunosuppressive treatment and plasma exchange. *Clinical Nephrology*, Vol.21, No.4, (April 1984), pp. 244-246, ISSN 0301-0430

Holdsworth, S.; Boyce, N., Thomson, N.M. & Atkins, R.C. (1985). The clinical spectrum of acute glomerulonephritis and lung haemorrhage (Goodpasture's syndrome). *The Quarterly Journal of Medicine*, Vol.55, No.216, (April 1985), pp. 75-86, ISSN 0033-5622

Hudson, B.G.; Tryggvason, K., Sundaramoorthy, M. & Neilson, E.G (2003). Alport's syndrome, Goodpasture's syndrome, and type IV collagen. *The New England Journal of Medicine*, Vol.348, No.25, (June 2003), pp. 2543–2556, ISSN 0028-4793

Jayne, D.R.; Marshall, P.D., Jones, S.J. & Lockwood, C.M. (1990). Autoantibodies to GBM and neutrophil cytoplasm in rapidly progressive glomerulonephritis. *Kidney International*, Vol.37, No.3, (March 1990), pp. 965-970, ISSN 0085-2538

Jennette, J.C. (2003). Rapidly progressive crescentic glomerulonephritis. *Kidney International*, Vol.63, No.3, (March 2003), pp. 1164-1177, ISSN 0085-2538

Johnson, J.P.; Moore, J. Jr., Austin, H.A. 3rd., Balow, J.E., Antonovych, T.T. & Wilson, C.B. (1985). Therapy of anti-glomerular basement membrane antibody disease: analysis of prognostic significance of clinical, pathologic and treatment factors. *Medicine (Baltimore)*, Vol.64, No.4, (July 1985), pp. 219-227, ISSN 0025-7974

Kalluri, R.; Sun, M.J., Hudson, B.G. & Neilson, E.G. (1996). The Goodpasture autoantigen. Structural delineation of two immunologically privileged epitopes on alpha3(IV) chain of type IV collagen. *The Journal of Biological Chemistry*, Vol.271, No.15, (April 1996), pp. 9062–9068, ISSN 0021-9258

Kaneko, Y.; Sakatsume, M., Xie, Y., Kuroda, T., Igashima, M., Narita, I. & Gejyo, F. (2003). Macrophage metalloelastase as a major factor for glomerular injury in anti-glomerular basement membrane nephritis. *Journal of Immunology*, Vol.170, No.6, (March 2003), pp. 3377–3385, ISSN 0022-1767

Kitagawa, W.; Imai, H., Komatsuda, A., Maki, N., Wakui, H., Hiki, Y. & Sugiyama, S. (2008). The HLA-DRB1*1501 allele is prevalent among Japanese patients with anti-glomerular basement membrane antibody-mediated disease. *Nephrology Dialysis Transplantation*, Vol. 23, No.10, (October 2008), pp. 3126–3129, ISSN 0931-0509

Kitching, A.R., Tipping, P.G. & Holdsworth, S.R. (1999). IL-12 directs severe renal injury, crescent formation and Th1 responses in murine glomerulonephritis. *European Journal of Immunology*, Vol.29, No.1, (January 1999), pp. 1–10, ISSN 0014-2980

Kiykim, A.A.; Horoz, M. & Gok, E. (2010). Successful treatment of resistant antiglomerular basement membrane antibody positivity with mycophenolic acid. *Internal Medicine*, Vol.49, No.6, (June 2010), pp. 577-580, ISSN 0918-2918

Klasa, R.J.; Abboud, R.T., Ballon, H.S. & Grossman, L. (1988). Goodpasture's syndrome: recurrence after a five-year remission. Case report and review of the literature. *The American Journal of Medicine*, Vol.84, No.4, (April 1988), pp. 751–755, ISSN 0002-9343

Laczika, K.; Knapp, S., Derfler, K., Soleiman, A., Horl, W.H. & Druml, W. (2000). Immunoadsorption in Goodpasture's syndrome. *American Journal of Kidney Diseases*, Vol.36, No.2, (August 2000), pp. 392–395, ISSN 0272-6386

Lan, H.Y.; Nikolic-Paterson, D.J., Zarama, M., Vannice, J.L. & Atkins, R.C. (1993). Suppression of experimental crescentic glomerulonephritis by the interleukin-1 receptor antagonist. *Kidney International*, Vol.43, No.2, (February 1993), pp. 479–485, ISSN 0085-2538

Lan, H.Y.; Yang, N., Metz, C., Mu, W., Song, Q., Nikolic-Paterson, D.J., Bacher, M., Bucala, R. & Atkins, R.C. (1997). TNF-alpha up-regulates renal MIF expression in rat crescentic glomerulonephritis. *Molecular Medicine*, Vol.3, No.2, (February 1997), pp. 136–144, ISSN 1076-1551

Lazor, R.; Bigay-Gamé, L., Cottin, V., Cadranel, J., Decaux, O., Fellrath, J.M. & Cordier, J.F.; Groupe d'Etudes et de Recherche sur les Maladies Orphelines Pulmonaires (GERMOP); Swiss Group for Interstitial and Orphan Lung Diseases (SIOLD). (2007). Alveolar hemorrhage in anti-basement membrane antibody disease: a series of 28 cases. *Medicine (Baltimore)*, Vol.86, No.3, (March 2007), pp. 181-193, ISSN 0025-7974

Le Hir, M.; Haas, C., Marino, M. & Ryffel, B. (1998). Prevention of crescentic glomerulonephritis induced by anti-glomerular membrane antibody in tumor necrosis factor-deficient mice. *Laboratory Investigation*, Vol.78, No.12, (December 1998), pp. 1625–1631, ISSN 0023-6837

Lechleitner, P.; Defregger, M., Lhotta, K., Tötsch, M. & Fend, F. (1993). Goodpasture's syndrome. Unusual presentation after exposure to hard metal dust. *Chest*, Vol.103, No.3, (March 1993), pp. 956–957, ISSN 0012-3692

Lehman, D.H.; Wilson, C.B. & Dixon, F.J. (1975). Extraglomerular immunoglobulin deposits in human nephritis. *American Journal of Medicine*, Vol.58, No.6, (June 1975), pp. 765-796., ISSN 0002-9343

Lerner, R.A.; Glassock, R.J. & Dixon, F.J. (1967). The role of anti-glomerular basement membrane antibody in the pathogenesis of human glomerulonephritis. *The Journal of Experimental Medicine*, Vol.126, No.6, (December 1967), pp. 989-1004. 0022-1007

Levy, J.B.; Lachmann, R.H. & Pusey, C.D. (1996). Recurrent Goodpasture's disease. *American Journal of Kidney Diseases*, Vol.27, No.4, (April 1996), pp. 573-578, ISSN 0272-6386

Levy, J.B.; Turner, A.N., Rees, A.J. & Pusey, C.D. (2001). Long-term outcome of anti-glomerular basement membrane antibody disease treated with plasma exchange and immunosuppression. *Annals of Internal Medicine*, Vol.134, No.11, (June 2001), pp. 1033-1042, ISSN 0003-4819

Levy, J.B.; Hammad, T., Coulthart, A., Dougan, T. & Pusey, C.D. (2004). Clinical features and outcome of patients with both ANCA and anti-GBM antibodies. *Kidney International*, Vol.66, No.4, (October 2004), pp. 1535-1540, ISSN 0085-2538

Li, F.K.; Tse, K.C., Lam, M.F., Yip, T.P., Lui, S.L., Chan, G.S., Chan, K.W., Chan, E.Y., Choy, B.Y., Lo, W.K., Chan, T.M. & Lai, K.N. (2004). Incidence and outcome of antiglomerular basement membrane disease in Chinese. *Nephrology (Carlton)*, Vol.9, No.2, (April 2004), pp. 100-104, ISSN 1320-5358

Li, L.S. & Liu, Z.H. (2004). Epidemiologic data of renal diseases from a single unit in China: analysis based on 13,519 renal biopsies. *Kidney International*, Vol.66, No.3, (September 2004), pp. 920–923, ISSN 0085-2538

Liu, K.; Li, Q.Z., Delgado-Vega, A.M., Abelson, A.K., Sánchez, E., Kelly, J.A., Li, L., Liu, Y., Zhou, J., Yan, M., Ye, Q., Liu, S., Xie, C., Zhou, X.J., Chung, S.A., Pons-Estel, B., Witte, T., de Ramón, E., Bae, S.C., Barizzone, N., Sebastiani, G.D., Merrill, J.T., Gregersen, P.K., Gilkeson, G.G., Kimberly, R.P., Vyse, T.J., Kim, I., D'Alfonso, S., Martin, J., Harley, J.B., Criswell, L.A.; Profile Study Group; Italian Collaborative Group; German Collaborative Group; Spanish Collaborative Group; Argentinian Collaborative Group; SLEGEN Consortium, Wakeland, E.K., Alarcón-Riquelme, M.E. & Mohan, C. (2009). Kallikrein genes are associated with lupus and glomerular basement membrane-specific antibody-induced nephritis in mice and humans. *The Journal of Clinical Investigation*, Vol.119, No.4, (April 2009), pp. 911-923, ISSN 0021-9738

Lockwood, C.M.; Rees, A.J., Pearson, T.A., Evans, D.J., Peters, D.K. & Wilson, C.B. (1976). Immunosuppression and plasma-exchange in the treatment of Goodpasture's syndrome. *The Lancet*, Vol.1, No.7962, (April 1976), pp. 711-715, ISSN 0140-6736

Malho, A.; Santos, V., Cabrita, A., Silva, A.P., Pinto, I., Bernardo, I. & Neves, P.L. (2010). Severe relapsing Goodpasture's disease successfully treated with mycophenolate mofetil. *International Journal of Nephrology*, Vol.16, (August 2010), pp. 383548. ISSN 2090-2158

Masugi, M. (1939). Über die experimentelle glomerulonephritis durch das spezifische antinieren serum. Ein beiträg zur pathogenese der diffusen glomerulonephritis. *Beitrage zur pathologischen anatomie und allgemeinen pathologie*, Vol.92, pp. 429-466

Merkel, F.; Pullig, O., Marx, M., Netzer, K.O. & Weber, M. (1994). Course and prognosis of anti-basement membrane antibody (anti-BM-Ab)-mediated disease: Report of 35 cases. *Nephrology Dialysis Transplantation*, Vol.9, No.4, (April 1994), pp. 372–376, ISSN 0931-0509

Min, K.W.; Györkey, F., Györkey, P., Yium, J.J. & Eknoyan, G. (1974). The morphogenesis of glomerular crescents in rapidly progressive glomerulonephritis. *Kidney International*, Vol.5, No.1, (January 1974), pp. 47–56, ISSN 0085-2538

Morita, T.; Suzuki, Y. & Churg, J. (1973). Structure and development of the glomerular crescent. *The American Journal of Pathology*, Vol.72, No.3, (September 1973), pp. 349–368, ISSN 0002-9440

Nagasu, H., Abe, M., Kuwabara, A., Kawai, T., Nishi, Y., Okuda, N. & Sakaguchi, K. (2009). A case report of efficiency of double filtration plasmapheresis in treatment of

Goodpasture's syndrome. *Therapeutic Apheresis and Dialysis*, Vol.13, No.4, (August 2009), pp. 373–377, ISSN 1744-9979

Naumovic, R.; Pavlovic, S., Stojkovic, D., Basta-Jovanovic, G. & Nesic, V. (2009). Renal biopsy registry from a single centre in Serbia: 20 years of experience. *Nephrology Dialysis Transplantation*, Vol.24, No.3, (March 2009), pp. 877–885, ISSN 0931-0509

Netzer, K.O.; Leinonen, A., Boutaud, A., Borza, D.B., Todd, P., Gunwar, S., Langeveld, J.P. & Hudson, B.G. (1999). The Goodpasture autoantigen. Mapping the major conformational epitope(s) of alpha3(IV) collagen to residues 17-31 and 127-141 of the NC1 domain. *The Journal of Biological Chemistry*, Vol.274, No.16, (April 1999), pp. 11267-11274, ISSN 0021-9258

The New Zealand Glomerulonephritis Study Group. (1989). The New Zealand Glomerulonephritis Study: introductory report. *Clinical Nephrology*, Vol.31, No.5, (May 1989), pp. 239-246, ISSN 0301-0430

Ooi, J.D.; Holdsworth, S.R. & Kitching, A.R. (2008). Advances in the pathogenesis of Goodpasture's disease: from epitopes to autoantibodies to effector T cells. *Journal of Autoimmunity*, Vol.31, No.3, (November 2008), pp. 295–300, ISSN 0896-8411

Ophascharoensuk, V.; Pippin, J.W., Gordon, K.L., Shankland, S.J., Couser, W.G. & Johnson, R.J. (1998). Role of intrinsic renal cells versus infiltrating cells in glomerular crescent formation. *Kidney International*, Vol.54, No.2, (August 1998), pp. 416–425, ISSN 0085-2538

Ortega, L.G. & Mellors, R.C. (1956). Analytical pathology. IV. The role of localized antibodies in the pathogenesis of nephrotoxic nephritis in the rat. *The Journal of Experimental Medicine*, Vol.104, No.1, (July 1956), pp. 151-157, ISSN 0022-1007

Parfrey, P.S.; Hutchinson, T.A., Jothy, S., Cramer, B.C., Martin, J., Hanley, J.A. & Seely, J.F. (1985). The spectrum of disease associated with necrotizing glomerulonephritis and its prognosis. *American Journal of Kidney Diseases*, Vol.6, No.6, (December 1985), pp. 387-396, ISSN 0272-6386

Pedchenko, V.; Bondar, O., Fogo, A.B., Vanacore, R., Voziyan, P., Kitching, A.R., Wieslander, J., Kashtan, C., Borza, D.B., Neilson, E.G., Wilson, C.B. & Hudson, B.G. (2010). Molecular architecture of the Goodpasture autoantigen in anti-GBM nephritis. *The New England Journal of Medicine*, Vol.363, No.4, (July 2010), pp. 343-354, ISSN 0028-4793

Pepys, E.O.; Rees, A.J. & Pepys, M.B. (1982). Enumeration of lymphocyte populations in whole peripheral blood of patients with antibody-mediated nephritis during treatment with cyclosporin A. *Immunology Letters*, Vol.4, No.4, (April 1982), pp. 211-214, ISSN 0165-2478

Perez, G.O.; Bjornsson, S., Ross, A.H., Aamato, J. & Rothfield, N. (1974). A mini-epidemic of Goodpasture's syndrome clinical and immunological studies. *Nephron*, Vol.13, No.2, (August 1974), pp. 161–173, ISSN 0028-2766

Persson, U.; Hertz, J.M., Carlsson, M., Hellmark, T., Juncker, I., Wieslander, J. & Segelmark, M. (2004). Patients with Goodpasture's disease have two normal COL4A3 alleles encoding the NC1 domain of the type IV collagen alpha 3 chain. *Nephrology Dialysis Transplantation*, Vol.19, No.8, (August 2004), pp. 2030-2035, ISSN 0931-0509

Peters, D.K.; Rees, A.J., Lockwood, C.M. & Pusey, C.D. (1982). Treatment and prognosis in antibasement membrane antibody-mediated nephritis. *Transplantation Proceedings*, Vol.14, No.3, (September 1982), pp. 513-521, ISSN 0041-1345

Phelps, R.G. & Rees, A.J. (1999). The HLA complex in Goodpasture's disease: a model for analyzing susceptibility to autoimmunity. *Kidney International*, Vol.56, No.5, (November 1999), pp. 1638–1653, ISSN 0085-2538

Proskey, A.J.; Weatherbee, L., Easterling, R.E., Greene, J.A. Jr. & Weller, J.M. (1970). Goodpasture's syndrome. A report of five cases and review of the literature. *The American Journal of Medicine*, Vol.48, No.2, (February 1970), pp. 162-173, ISSN 0002-9343

Pusey, C.D. (2003). Anti-glomerular basement membrane disease. *Kidney International*, Vol.64, No.4, (October 2003), pp. 1535–1550, ISSN 0085-2538

Quérin, S.; Schürch, W. & Beaulieu, R. (1992). Ciclosporin in Goodpasture's syndrome. *Nephron*, Vol.60, No.3, (March 1992), pp. 355-359, ISSN 0028-2766

Rees, A.J.; Peters, D.K., Compston, D.A. & Batchelor, J.R. (1978). Strong association between HLA-DRW2 and antibody-mediated Goodpasture's syndrome. *The Lancet*, Vol.1, No.8071, (May, 1978), pp. 966–968, ISSN 0140-6736

Rees, A.J.; Demaine, A.G. &, Welsh, K.I. (1984). Association of immunoglobulin Gm allotypes with antiglomerular basement membrane antibodies and their titer. *Human Immunology*, Vol.10, No.4, (August 1984), pp. 213-220, ISSN 0198-8859

Rivera, F.; López-Gómez, J.M., Pérez-García, R. & Spanish Registry of Glomerulonephritis. (2002). Frequency of renal pathology in Spain 1994–1999. *Nephrology Dialysis Transplantation*, Vol.17, No.9, (September 2002), pp. 1594-1562, ISSN 0931-0509

Rutgers, A.; Slot, M., van Paassen, P., van Breda Vriesman, P., Heeringa, P. & Tervaert, J.W. (2005). Coexistence of anti-glomerular basement membrane antibodies and myeloperoxidase-ANCAs in crescentic glomerulonephritis. *American Journal of Kidney Diseases*, Vol.46, No.2, (August 2005), pp. 253-262, ISSN 0272-6386

Rychlík, I.; Jancová, E., Tesar, V., Kolsky, A., Lácha, J., Stejskal, J., Stejskalová, A., Dusek, J. & Herout V. (2004). The Czech registry of renal biopsies. Occurrence of renal diseases in the years 1994-2000. *Nephrology Dialysis Transplantation*, Vol.19, No.12, (December 2004), pp. 3040-3049, ISSN 0931-0509

Sado, Y.; Kagawa, M., Naito, I., Ueki, Y., Seki, T., Momota, R., Oohashi, T. & Ninomiya, Y. (1998). Organization and expression of basement membrane collagen IV genes and their roles in human disorders. *Journal of Biochemistry*, Vol.123, No.5, (May 1998), pp. 767-776, ISSN 0021-924X

Salama, A.D.; Levy, J.B., Lightstone, L. & Pusey, C.D. (2001). Goodpasture's disease. *The Lancet*, Vol.358, No.9285, (September 2001), pp. 917–920, ISSN 0140-6736

Salant, D.J. (2010). Goodpasture's disease – new secrets revealed. *The New England Journal of Medicine*, Vol.363, No.4, (July 2010), pp. 388-391, ISSN 0028-4793

Saus, J.; Wieslander, J., Langeveld, J.P., Quinones, S. & Hudson, B.G. (1988). Identification of the Goodpasture antigen as the α3(IV) chain of collagen IV. *The Journal of Biological Chemistry*, Vol.263, No.26, (September 1988), pp. 13374-13380, ISSN 0021-9258

Savage, C.O.S.; Pusey, C.D., Bowman, C., Rees, A.J. & Lockwood, C.M. (1986) Antiglomerular basement membrane antibody mediated disease in the British Isles 1980–4. *British Medical Journal*, Vol.292, No.6516, (February 1986), pp. 301–304, ISSN 0267-0623

Saxena, R.; Bygren, P., Rasmussen, N. & Wieslander, J. (1991). Circulating autoantibodies in patients with extracapillary glomerulonephritis. *Nephrology Dialysis Transplantation*, Vol.6, No.6, (June 1991), pp. 389-397, ISSN 0931-0509

Scheer, R.L. & Grossman, M.A. (1964). Immune aspects of the glomerulonephritis associated with pulmonary hemorrhage. *Annals of Internal Medicine*, Vol. 60, No.6, (June 1964), pp. 1009-1021, ISSN 0003-4819

Schena, F.P. & Survey of the Italian Registry of Renal Biopsies. (1997). Frequency of the renal diseases for 7 consecutive years. The Italian Group of Renal Immunopathology. *Nephrology Dialysis Transplantation*, Vol.12, No.3, (March 1997), pp. 418-426, ISSN 0931-0509

Segelmark, M.; Butkowski, R. & Wieslander, J. (1990) Antigen restriction and IgG subclasses among anti-GBM autoantibodies. *Nephrology Dialysis Transplantation*, Vol.5, No.12, (December 1990), pp. 991–996, ISSN 0931-0509

Segelmark, M.; Hellmark, T. & Wieslander, J. (2003) The prognostic significance in Goodpasture's disease of specificity, titre and affinity of anti-glomerular-basement-membrane antibodies. *Nephron Clinical Practice*, Vol.94, No., (2003), pp. c59-c68, ISSN 1660-2110

Shah, M.K. & Hugghins, S.Y. (2002). Characteristics and outcomes of patients with Goodpasture's syndrome. *South Medical Journal*, Vol.95, No.12, (December 2002), pp. 1411–1418, ISSN 0038-4348

Sheerin, N.S.; Springall, T., Carroll, M.C., Hartley, B. & Sacks, S.H. (1997). Protection against anti-glomerular basement membrane (GBM)-mediated nephritis in C3- and C4-deficient mice. *Clinical and Experimental Immunology*, Vol.110, No.3, (December 1997), pp. 403–409, ISSN 0009-9104

Simpson, I.J.; Doak, P.B., Williams, L.C., Blacklock, H.A., Hill, R.S., Teague, C.A., Herdson, P.B. & Wilson, C.B. (1982). Plasma exchange in Goodpasture's syndrome. *American Journal of Nephrology*, Vol.2, No.6, (December 1982), pp.301-311, ISSN 0250-8095

Stanton, M.C. & Tange, J.D. (1958). Goodpasture's syndrome (pulmonary haemorrhage associated with glomerulonephritis). *Australasian Annals of Medicine*, Vol.7, No.2, (May 1958), pp. 132-144, ISSN 0571-9283

Sumethkul, V.; Changsirikulchai, S., Radinahamed, P. & Chalermasnyakorn, P. (1999). Antineutrophil cytoplasmic antibody (ANCA) and rapidly progressive crescentic glomerulonephritis in Thai population. *Asian Pacific Journal of Allergy and Immunology*, Vol.17, No.4, (December 1999), pp. 281-287, ISSN 0125-877X

Tang, Z.; Wu, Y., Wang, Q., Zeng, C., Yao, X., Hu, W., Chen, H., Liu, Z. & Li, L. (2003). Clinical spectrum of diffuse crescentic glomerulonephritis in Chinese patients. *Chinese Medical Journal*, Vol.116, No.11, (2003), pp. 1737-1740, ISSN 0366-6999

Teague, C.A.; Doak, P.B., Simpson, I.J., Rainer, S.P. & Herdson, P.B. (1978). Goodpasture's syndrome: an analysis of 29 cases. *Kidney International*, Vol.13, No.6, (June 1978), pp. 492-504, ISSN 0085-2538

Thomson, N.M.; Holdsworth, S.R., Glasgow, E.F. & Atkins, R.C. (1979). The macrophage in the development of experimental crescentic glomerulonephritis. Studies using tissue culture and electron microscopy. *The American Journal of Pathology*, Vol.94, No.2, (February 1979), pp. 223-240, ISSN 0002-9440

Timoshanko, J.R.; Holdsworth, S.R., Kitching, A.R. & Tipping, P.G. (2002). IFN-gamma production by intrinsic renal cells and bone marrow-derived cells is required for full expression of crescentic glomerulonephritis in mice. *Journal of Immunology*, Vol.168, No.8, (April 2002), pp. 4135–4141, ISSN 0022-1767

Tipping, P.G.; Lowe, M.G. & Holdsworth, S.R. (1988). Glomerular macrophages express augmented procoagulant activity in experimental fibrin-related glomerulonephritis in rabbits. *The Journal of Clinical Investigation*, Vol.82, No.4, (October 1988), pp. 1253–1259, ISSN 0021-9738

Vanacore, R.M.; Ham, A.J., Cartailler, J.P., Sundaramoorthy, M., Todd, P., Pedchenko, V., Sado, Y., Borza, D.B. & Hudson, B.G. (2008). A role for collagen IV cross-links in conferring immune privilege to the Goodpasture autoantigen: structural basis for the crypticity of B cell epitopes. *The Journal of Biological Chemistry*, Vol.283, No.33, (August 2008), pp. 22737–22748, ISSN 0021-9258

Vanacore, R.M.; Ham, A.J., Voehler, M., Sanders, C.R., Conrads, T.P., Veenstra, T.D., Sharpless, K.B., Dawson, P.E. & Hudson, B.G. (2009). A sulfilimine bond identified in collagen IV. *Science*, Vol.325, No.5945, (September 2009), pp. 1230–1234, ISSN 0036-8075

Walker, R.G.; Scheinkestel, C., Becker, G.J., Owen, J.E., Dowling, J.P. & Kincaid-Smith, P. (1985). Clinical and morphological aspects of the management of crescentic anti-glomerular basement membrane antibody (anti-GBM) nephritis/Goodpasture's syndrome. *The Quarterly Journal of Medicine*, Vol.54, No.213, (January 1985), pp. 75–89, ISSN 0033-5622

Williams, P.S.; Davenport, A., McDicken, I., Ashby, D., Goldsmith, H.J. & Bone, J.M. (1988). Increased incidence of anti-glomerular basement membrane antibody (anti-GBM) nephritis in the Mersey Region, September 1984-October 1985. *The Quarterly Journal of Medicine*, Vol.68, No.257, (September 1988), pp. 727–733, ISSN 0033-5622

Wilson, C.B. & Dixon, F.J. (1973). Anti-glomerular basement membrane antibody-induced glomerulonephritis. *Kidney International*, Vol.3, No.2, (February 1973), pp. 74–89, ISSN 0085-2538

Yang, G.; Tang, Z., Chen, Y., Zeng, C., Chen, H., Liu, Z. & Li, L. (2005). Antineutrophil cytoplasmic antibodies (ANCA) in Chinese patients with anti-GBM crescentic glomerulonephritis. *Clinical Nephrology*, Vol.63, No.6, (June 2005), pp. 423-428, ISSN 0301-0430

Yang, R.; Cui, Z., Zhao, J. & Zhao, M.H. (2009). The role of HLA-DRB1 alleles on susceptibility of Chinese patients with anti-GBM disease. *Clinical Immunology*, Vol.133, No.2, (November 2009), pp. 245–250, ISSN 1521-6616

Zhou, X.J.; Lv, J.C., Yu, L., Cui, Z., Zhao, J., Yang, R., Han, J., Hou, P., Zhao, M.H. & Zhang, H. (2010a). FCGR2b gene polymorphism rather than FCGR2A, FCGR3A and FCGR3B is associated with anti-GBM disease in Chinese. *Nephrology Dialysis Transplantation*, Vol.25, No.1, (January 2010), pp. 97–101, ISSN 0931-0509

Zhou, X.J.; Lv, J.C., Bu, D.F., Yu, L., Yang, Y.R., Zhao, J., Cui, Z., Yang, R., Zhao, M.H. & Zhang, H. (2010b). Copy number variation of FCGR3A rather than FCGR3B and FCGR2B is associated with susceptibility to anti-GBM disease. *International Immunology*, Vol.22, No.1, (January 2010), pp. 45–51, ISSN 1460-2377

Hirayama, K.; Yamagata, K., Kobayashi, M., Koyama, A. (2008). Anti-glomerular basement membrane antibody disease in Japan: part of the nationwide rapidly progressive glomerulonephritis survey in Japan. *Clinical and Experimental Nephrology*, Vol.12, No.5, (October 2008), pp. 339-347, ISSN 1342-1751

3

Henoch-Schönlein Purpura Nephritis in Childhood

Marco Zaffanello
University of Verona
Italy

1. Introduction

Henoch-Schönlein purpura is one of the most common causes of systemic vasculitis. Henoch–Schönlein purpura typically affects children between the age of 3 and 10 years. The aetiology is unknown. Diagnosis includes palpable purpura (essential) in the presence of diffuse abdominal pain, acute arthritis/arthralgia, renal involvement characterized by haematuria and/or proteinuria (Ozen et al., 2006) and skin biopsy showing predominant IgΛ deposition in the walls of cutaneous vessels.

In the majority of cases it is a self-limiting disease. Therefore, up to 40% of children with Henoch–Schönlein purpura require hospitalization for management of acute disease manifestations which may include nephritis, hypertension, severe pain, gastrointestinal bleeding or arthritis. Purpura occurs in all cases, joint pains and arthritis in 80% of cases, and abdominal pain in 62% of cases.

The purpura typically appears on the legs and buttocks (Fig.1), but may also be seen on the arms, face and trunk. The abdominal pain is colicky, and may be accompanied by nausea, vomiting, constipation or diarrhea. There may be blood or mucus in the stools. Sometime finding includes a gastrointestinal haemorrhage, occurring in 33% of cases, due to intussusceptions (Saulsbury, 1999). The joints involved tend to be the ankles, knees, and elbows but arthritis in the hands and feet is possible; the arthritis is non-erosive and hence causes no permanent deformity. Problems in other organs, such as the central nervous system (brain and spinal cord) and lungs may occur, but much less commonly than the skin, bowel and kidneys (Saulsbury, 2001)

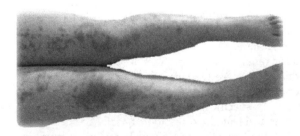

Fig. 1. Henoch-Schönlein purpura in a 8 years old female child

Paediatric patients may develop glomerulonephritis within 4 to 6 weeks of the initial purpura presentation (Saulsbury, 2007). Renal involvement in Henoch-Schönlein purpura is transitory in most cases. Therefore, the long-term prognosis in Henoch-Schönlein purpura depends on the severity of renal involvement and can be poor when complicated by severe nephritis and chronic renal failure.

2. Pathogenesis

Henoch-Schönlein purpura nephritis is a systemic immune-complex mediated disease according to the clinical or histological pattern of recurrences of Henoch-Schönlein purpura nephritis in some patients after transplantation (Soler et al., 2005). The histological hallmark of Henoch-Schönlein purpura is severe inflammation of small vessels, particularly post-capillary venules, with neutrophils, resulting in fibrinoid necrosis of vessel walls and extravasation of erythrocytes (Saulsbury, 1999). The clinical features are a consequence of general vasculitis due to IgA1 deposition in vessels and the renal measangium (Saulsbury, 1999). Therefore, the pathogenetic mechanisms are still not fully understood.

2.1 IgA immune complexes
Similarly to IgA nephropathy, deposits of IgA-binding M proteins of group A streptococci were found on Henoch-Schönlein purpura kidneys. All Henoch-Schönlein purpura patients have IgA1-circulating immune complexes of small molecular mass. Therefore, only those with nephritis have large-molecular-mass IgA1-IgG-containing circulating immune complexes (Levinsky & Barratt, 1979). Large-molecular mass IgA-IgG complexes in the circulation are the major factor responsible for the formation of the nephritogenic immune complexes in patients with Henoch-Schönlein purpura nephritis.

Some children with Henoch-Schönlein purpura nephritis subsequently have an episode or recurrent episodes of macroscopic hematuria, associated with upper respiratory tract infection without the other clinical features of Henoch-Schönlein purpura nephritis (Waldo, 1988). Thus, these children's clinical phenotype changes to that of IgA nephropathy. As the renal histologic and immunofluorescence microscopy findings in Henoch-Schönlein purpura nephritis are indistinguishable from those seen in patients with IgA nephropathy (Evans et al., 1973), it has long been ever speculated that Henoch-Schönlein purpura nephritis and IgA nephropathy have common pathogenetic mechanisms representing different ends of a continuous spectrum of disease (Waldo, 1988).

Henoch-Schönlein purpura nephritis is similar to IgA nephropathy since IgA1, but not IgA2, is found in the circulating immune complexes and in mesangial immune deposits (Novak et al., 2007). IgA1-containing immune complexes are excreted in elevated amounts in the urine in patients with IgA nephropathy and Henoch-Schönlein purpura nephritis and may provide a specific marker for disease activity and/or severity in these patients (Suzuki et al., 2008). IgA-binding M proteins may encounter circulatory IgA forming a complex with IgA-Fc that could deposit in renal tissues (Schmitt et al., 2010).

Reduced galactosylation of IgA1 O-glycans has been reported in patients with Henoch-Schönlein purpura nephritis (Allen et al., 1998). Glycosylation defects are due to complex changes in expression of specific glycosyltransferases with reduced expression of β1,3-galactosyltransferase and elevated expression of GalNAc-specific α2,6-sialyltransferase in patients with both IgA nephropathy and Henoch-Schönlein purpura nephritis, but not in patients with Henoch-Schönlein purpura without nephritis or healthy controls (Suzuki,

Moldoveanu et al., 2008). Due to their size, Galactose-deficient IgA1 containing immune complexes are less efficiently taken up by the asialoglycoprotein receptor in the liver and catabolised and their amounts increase in the circulation (Moura et al., 2004). Galactose-deficient IgA1 leads to the formation of the circulating immune complexes. These complexes may then deposit in the renal mesangium and incite, likely due to the binding to mesangial cells, to cellular activation (Lau et al., 2010). Consequently, mesangial cells start to proliferate and overproduce extracellular matrix components, cytokines and chemokines (Davin & Weening, 2003) leading to glomerular injury contributing to the pathogenesis of Henoch-Schönlein purpura nephritis.

Glomerular depositions of other components, including kappa and lambda light chains, are also variably demonstrated in Henoch-Schönlein purpura nephritis. In patients with IgA nephropathy, lambda light chains were found predominantly over kappa light chains (Lai et al., 1996).

2.2 Complement

Complement activation appears to play an important role in the pathogenesis of IgA nephropathy and Henoch-Schönlein purpura nephritis, as glomerular complement activation may initiate the inflammatory cascade and enhance glomerular injury (Wyatt et al., 1987). Therefore, hypocomplementemia has been reported in some patients with Henoch-Schönlein purpura nephritis, and it is usually transient and not related to the severity of the diseases (Motoyama & Litaka, 2005).

3. Incidence

The estimated annual incidence of Henoch-Schönlein purpura in children is 10–20 per 100,000 children (Rostoker, 2001). The annual incidence of Henoch-Schönlein purpura in Asian children [4.9 per 100,000] and African children [6.2 per 100,000] was significantly lower than Caucasian children [17.8 per 100,000].

In childhood Henoch-Schönlein purpura, the male:female ratio ranges from 1.2–1.6 (Yang et al., 2005).

Renal involvement occurs less frequently in children than adulthood (Yang et al., 2005; Pillebout et al., 2002). The incidence of nephritis in patients with Henoch-Schönlein purpura has been reported to be 15-62% with an estimated annual incidence of 20.4 per 100,000 children (Gardner-Medwin et al., 2002; Shenoy, Bradbury, et al. 2007; Bogdanovic, 2009).

The overall incidence of Henoch-Schönlein purpura nephritis and the severity of Henoch-Schönlein purpura nephritis in patients between 1987 and 1997 were similar to those in children between 1998 and 2008 and the number of patients with severe Henoch-Schönlein purpura nephritis has not decreased (Kawasaki et al., 2010). The overall incidence of Henoch-Schönlein purpura nephritis is rather stable over time.

It could be estimated that 1–2% of all Henoch-Schönlein purpura nephritis patients will ultimately develop chronic kidney disease (Stewart et al., 1988; Narchi, 2005). A variable percentage of children (0–19%) with Henoch-Schönlein purpura nephritis may progress to renal failure or end stage renal disease (Ronkainen et al., 2002; Coppo et al., 1997; Goldstein et al., 1992; Kawasaki et al., 2003; Pillebout et al., 2002). In children with Henoch-Schönlein purpura nephritis followed up at tertiary centres the risk for progression to chronic kidney disease or end-stage renal disease is predicted to be 5–18% at 5 years, 10–20% at 10 years and 20–32% at 20 years from the diagnosis (Goldstein et al., 1992; Coppo et al., 1997; Kaku et al., 1998; Bogdanovic, 2009).

4. Clinical patterns

The average duration of Henoch-Schönlein purpura symptoms is 4 weeks. The majority of patients experience resolution of symptoms within 2 to 3 months. Approximately 30% of patients have one or more recurrences after the resolution of initial symptoms (Saulsbury, 1999; Trapani et al., 2005). Therefore, purpura lasting longer than 1 month or relapsing disease are associated with the development of nephritis(Rigante et al., 2005; Shin, Park, et al., 2006). Patients showing abdominal pain as the initial symptom had a higher probability of developing nephrotic syndrome. Persistent rash was a poor prognostic factor for Henoch-Schönlein purpura nephritis (Hung et al., 2009).

Renal signs are manifested in the majority of Henoch-Schönlein purpura patients from 3 days to 17 months after onset of the disease (Kaku et al., 1998), occurring more frequently within the first 3 months (Sano et al., 2002). In few cases the renal disease may develop even years after the initial presentation (Mollica et al., 1992). While abnormalities on urinalysis may continue for a long time, only 1% of all Henoch-Schönlein purpura patients develop chronic kidney disease (Saulsbury, 2001).

Nephritis is the one feature of Henoch-Schönlein purpura that may have chronic consequences. The long-term prognosis is largely dependent on the severity of nephritis (Narchi, 2005; Mir et al., 2007). Renal manifestations of the disease ranged from mild, benign involvement, intermittent haematuria and proteinuria, to rapidly progressive or crescentic nephritis. Of the 40% of patients who develop kidney involvement, almost all have evidence (visible or on urinalysis) of blood in the urine. More than half also have proteinuria, which in one eighth is severe enough to cause nephrotic syndrome (Saulsbury, 2001). From a retrospective study, nephritis occurred in 46% of the Henoch-Schönlein purpura patients, consisting of isolated haematuria in 14%, isolated proteinuria in 9%, both haematuria and proteinuria in 56%, nephrotic-range proteinuria in 20% and nephrotic-nephritic syndrome in 1% (Jauhola et al., 2010).

Renal involvement is in most cases mild and self-limited in children. Henoch-Schönlein purpura nephritis in children had a lower risk of progression to renal insufficiency than adults. Gross hematuria and lower extremity edema were less frequent in the children than adults (Hung et al., 2009). Morbidity is low in patients with Henoch-Schönlein purpura who have hematuria and mild proteinuria at onset, while it is higher among those with more severe renal disease, as in a nephritic, nephrotic or a nephritic/nephrotic signs (Coppo et al., 2006; Ronkainen et al., 2002; Narchi, 2005; Goldstein et al., 1992). The main clinical signs of rapidly progressive Henoch-Schönlein purpura nephritis at presentation were edema, hypertension, gross hematuria, and oliguria (Oner, 1995). End-stage renal disease was associated with nephritic and/or nephrotic syndrome at presentation in nearly all children with Henoch-Schönlein purpura nephritis (Soylemezoglu et al., 2009). The highly variable clinical course of Henoch-Schönlein purpura nephritis has been related to the marked variability in histopathologic presentation at renal biopsy, with glomeruli ranging from histologically normal to diffuse proliferative and crescentic lesions (Assadi, 2009).

4.1 Classification

Five categories of Henoch-Schönlein purpura nephritis were identified according to renal manifestations at disease onset (Falkner et al., 2004): (A) micro/macroscopic hematuria or persistent mild proteinuria (< 1 g/L or urine albumin/creatinine ratio < 200 mg/mmol); (B) persistent mild proteinuria (< 1 g/L or urine albumin/creatinine ratio < 200 mg/mmol) and micro- or macroscopic hematuria; (C) nephritic syndrome (moderate proteinuria and urine albumin/creatinine ratio ≥ 200–400 mg/mmol), decreased glomerular filtration rate, hematuria and/or hypertension, or nephrotic syndrome (urinary albumin excretion > 40 mg/hour/m² body surface area or urine albumin/creatinine ratio ≥ 400 mg/mmol, serum albumin < 25 g/L; (D) acute progressive glomerular nephritis; (E) chronic glomerular nephritis. Classes A and B were considered as mild renal disease, and classes C to E as severe disease (Meadow et al., 1972).

Another clinical evaluation categorized the patients according to four stages. Stage (A) is considered normal: the patient was normal on physical examination, with normal urine and renal function; stage (B) had minor urinary abnormalities: the patient was normal on physical examination, with microscopic hematuria or proteinuria of less than 20 mg/m²/h; stage (C) had persistent nephropathy: the patient had proteinuria of 20 mg/m²/h or greater or hypertension and a 24-h creatinine clearance of 60 ml/ min/1.73 m² or greater; stage (D) had renal insufficiency: the patient had a 24-h creatinine clearance of less than 60 ml/min/1.73 m², including dialysis/transplant or death (Kawasaki et al., 2010).

4.2 Serum IgA

Although serum IgA levels are higher in children with Henoch-Schönlein purpura / Henoch-Schönlein purpura nephritis than in controls, this serum abnormality does not constitute a sensitive diagnostic marker of Henoch-Schönlein purpura with or without nephritis. In particular, over 40% children with Henoch-Schönlein purpura had elevated serum IgA levels at presentation. Therefore, the difference in serum IgA levels between patients with and without nephritis was not statistically significant.

4.3 Renal biopsy

Renal involvement can be severe but may resolve completely. Therefore, some children will develop long-term sequelae. The renal biopsy is helpful in determining the need for treatment with immunosuppression in the acute phase (McCarthy & Tizard, 2010).

The criteria for renal biopsy were defined as follows: (1) the patients had proteinuria of 20 mg/m²/hour or greater and haematuria or (2) the patients had proteinuria of less than 20 mg/m²/hour and recurrent macrohematuria (Kawasaki et al., 2010). According to another recent review a renal biopsy has been recommended in the following situations: (1) acute renal impairment/nephritic syndrome at presentation; (2) nephrotic syndrome with normal renal function persisting at 4 weeks; (3) nephrotic range proteinuria (urine protein/creatinine ratio, >250 mg/mmol) at 4–6 weeks (if not improving spontaneously); (4) persistent proteinuria-urine protein/creatinine ratio >100 mg/mmol for more than 3 months. Consider biopsy particularly if the diagnosis is not clear (McCarthy & Tizard, 2010).

Renal involvement in Henoch-Schönlein purpura is quantified by means of a kidney biopsy (Fig. 2), which may demonstrate positive mesangial staining and positive anti-IgA antisera on immunofluorescence, with glomerular changes graded chiefly according to the Henoch-Schönlein purpura nephritis classification described in the International Study of Kidney Disease in Children (Rai et al., 1999; Sheno, Bradbury, et al. 2007; Ronkainen et al., 2006). The grading of renal histology has been considered as an important marker of outcome (Farine et al., 1986). The classification provided by the Study of Kidney Disease in Children included grade I: minimal alterations; grade II: mesangial proliferation; grade III: focal or diffuse proliferation or sclerosis with <50% crescents; grade IV: focal or diffuse mesangial proliferation or sclerosis with 50–75% crescents; grade V: focal or diffuse mesangial proliferation or sclerosis with >75% crescents; grade VI: membranoproliferative-like lesions (Counahan et al., 1977).

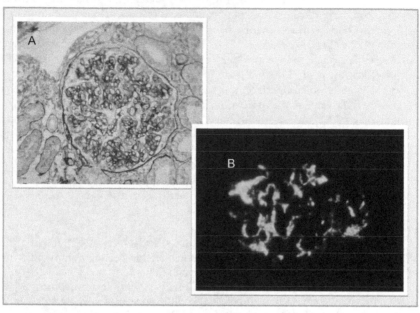

Fig. 2. Methenamine-silver stain of a glomerular of a patient with Henoch-Schönlein purpura nephritis showing diffuse mesangial and focal endocapillary proliferation (panel A). The immunofluorescence studies showed intense IgA positivity (3+) (panel B); complement C3 staining was also mildly positive (1+).

5. Risk factors

5.1 Renal involvement in Henoch-Schönlein purpura

Some authors attempted to identify prognostic factors for a child with Henoch-Schönlein purpura to develop nephritis by using univariate and multivariate analysis models. The independent risk factors for Henoch-Schönlein purpura nephritis were persistent purpura, severe abdominal symptoms and age above 4 or 7 or 10 years. Other independent risk factors were relapse or decreased serum factor XIII activity (Kaku et al., 1998; Sano et al., 2002; Rigante et al., 2005; Shin, Park, et al., 2006; Ronkainen et al., 2006). Persistent purpura, severe abdominal symptoms and an older age were confirmed as the most significant risk factors for later nephropathy (Bogdanovic, 2009). A prospective study showed that age over 8 years at onset (OR 2.7), abdominal pain (OR 2.1) and a recurrence of Henoch-Schönlein purpura disease (OR 3.1) were independent risk factors for developing nephritis(Jauhola et al., 2010).

5.2 Long-term renal impairment

Severe renal involvement at onset of Henoch-Schönlein purpura is in general predictive of a poor renal outcome. The independent predictors of a poor renal outcome were severe initial presentations with renal failure, nephritic, nephrotic syndrome or mixed syndrome and the percentage of glomeruli with crescents (Mir et al., 2007). Some few children with mild renal symptoms at onset have a poor long-term outcome. Thus, long-term follow-up is mandatory also for these patients (Algoet & Proesmans, 2003; Goldstein et al., 1992).

6. Follow-up

A clinical pathway was recommended if there is evidence of haematuria, proteinuria, renal impairment or hypertension in patients with Henoch-Schönlein purpura (Tizard & Hamilton-Ayres, 2008). Prospectively and systematically collected data suggested that weekly urine dipstick tests should be continued for 2 months from the onset of Henoch-Schönlein purpura. Beyond that point frequent routine follow-up is neither cost-effective nor necessary in patients with no urine abnormalities during follow-up. However, the length of follow-up time should be increased at least up to 6 months individually in the case of Henoch-Schönlein purpura recurrence and in those developing nephritis (Jauhola et al., 2010).

7. Prevention of Henoch-Schönlein purpura nephritis

Intervention to shorten the duration of Henoch-Schönlein purpura and prevent relapses may be helpful in preventing the development of nephritis. However, no therapy has yet been shown to decrease the duration of Henoch-Schönlein purpura, prevent recurrences, or prevent the development of nephritis (Saulsbury, 2009).

Studies reported on patients with Henoch-Schönlein purpura lacking clinical signs of nephropathy at admission were treated with prednisone at doses ranging from 1.0 to 2.5 mg/kg/day over a period of 7–21 days. Early prednisone treatment did not succeed in reducing the risk of further renal complication from Henoch-Schönlein purpura. Although prednisone is effective in alleviating the abdominal pain and joint pain associated with Henoch-Schönlein purpura, it did not short the duration of the disease, prevented the recurrences, or prevented the development of nephritis (Ronkainen et al., 2006). The relatively small subgroup of Henoch-Schönlein purpura patients who may benefit from corticosteroids included those who present with renal involvement and probably those with severe abdominal symptoms requiring medical attention (Mollica et al., 1992; Saulsbury, 1999; Narchi, 2005).

In general, the prophylactic treatment with prednisone at 2 mg/kg/day in Henoch-Schönlein purpura must be considered of value if (1) there is a quicker resolution of abdominal pain, considering the cost and potential damage from prolonged treatment; (2) the treatment performed during the acute phase reduce the rates of abdominal surgery for exploration or actual intestinal injury; (3) the avoidance of several late-onset medical conditions, including hypertension, preeclampsia, and persistent nail-fold capillary changes, suggesting a chronic vasculitis (Gibson et al., 2008). Such measure at this time has not been demonstrated. However, 2– 4 weeks of prednisone administration at doses ranging from 1.0 to 2.5 mg/kg per day over a period of 7–21 days or intravenous methylprednisolone prophylaxis (5 mg/kg four to six times per day for 3–5 days) failed to prevent renal involvement in Henoch-Schönlein purpura after 0.5–1 years (Zaffanello et al., 2009).

Dapsone, an antileprotic drug, has been used at 1–2 mg/kg/day daily in a few patients with prolonged in Henoch-Schönlein purpura, improving the time of purpuric rash, but it has not been studied in a rigorous fashion in children with nephritis (Iqbal & Evans, 2005).

The clinical course of patients in a report suggested that colchicines, an ancient anti-inflammatory drug, may be effective treatment at dosages of 1.2 mg/day in children with prolonged Henoch-Schönlein purpura possibly preventing the development of nephritis (Saulsbury, 2009). Therefore, at the current time insufficient data are available to support a recommendation for prophylaxis.

8. Conventional treatment

Conventional therapies were defined as drugs or procedures that act as immune modulators.

8.1 Treatment of mild form of Henoch-Schönlein purpura nephritis

Patients with mild renal symptoms have showed lower proportion of poor outcome than those with severe renal symptoms. In particular, patients with isolated hematuria showed a good prognosis, but 18% of patients with mild proteinuria at onset showed a poor outcome (Edström Halling et al., 2010). For this reason patients would be followed until full clinical resolution of renal symptoms. Since the level of proteinuria at onset does not seem to be a reliable predictor of outcome, the persistence of mild proteinuria in the long-term follow-up (one year) may require renal biopsy. Finally, the treatment of mild clinical form must be weighed according to International Study of Kidney Disease in Children grading score (see 8.2. and 8.3. sections).

8.2 Treatment of moderately severe Henoch-Schönlein purpura nephritis

Patients affected by moderately-severe proteinurias were treated with prednisone, intravenous gamma globulins and tonsillectomy, while pulse methylprednisolon and cyclophosphamide were introduced according to the degree of severity of renal histology.
Three Henoch-Schönlein purpura nephritis patients treated by means of intravenous (2 g/kg/month) and intramuscular gamma globulins (0.35 ml/kg every 15 days) showed improved degrees of proteinuria and acuity index at renal biopsy (Rostoker et al., 1994; Rostoker et al., 1995). The administration of the angiotensin converting enzyme inhibitor (enalapril 10 mg/day) combined with fish oil led to a significant reduction in protein excretion rate after a few weeks of treatment in case series (Dixit et al., 2004). Additionally, tonsillectomy proved to be effective in five patients affected by Henoch-Schönlein purpura nephritis (Sanai & Kudoh, 1996) as well as in 16 children with Henoch-Schönlein purpura nephritis in combination with intravenous pulse methylprednisolon at a dose of 1 gram/1.73 m^2 of body surface area (three to four cycles), prednisone (2 mg/kg/day) and cyclophosphamide (2 mg/kg/day) (Inoue et al., 2007).
Data obtained from the literature are insufficient to support the use of specific treatments, such as intravenous gamma globulins and angiotensin converting enzyme inhibitors, in moderate-severe Henoch-Schönlein purpura nephritis, based on case series (Zaffanello et al., 2009).

8.3 Treatment of rapidly progressive or crescentic Henoch-Schönlein purpura nephritis

Predictors of treatment with immunosuppression drugs were higher albuminurias and urine immunoglobulin G, and lower glomerular filtration rate at onset and a higher International Study of Kidney Disease in Children grading score in the biopsy. Unfortunately, no significant difference in outcome was found between the treated and untreated patients with crescents. Neither was there any significant difference in glomerular filtration rate between treated and untreated patients (Edström Halling et al., 2010).

Several studies have reported that patients with severe Henoch-Schönlein purpura nephritis may benefit from an intravenous pulse of methylprednisolone (Kawasaki et al., 2003; Niaudet & Habib, 1998; Edström Halling et al., 2010), cyclosporine A (Ronkainen et al., 2003), cyclophosphamide (Kawasaki et al., 2004; Tarshish et al., 2004; Shenoy et al., 2007; Kawasaki et al., 2004; Edström Halling et al., 2010), urokinase pulse therapy (Kawasaki et al., 2003; Zaffanello et al., 2007), azathioprine (Zaffanello et al., 2007; Foster et al., 2000), and plasma exchange therapy (Scharer et al., 1999). All severe cases almost received angiotensin converting enzyme inhibitors and/or angiotensin II receptor blockers combined with immunosuppressant drugs (Edström Halling et al., 2010).

Some protocols of treatment for Henoch-Schönlein purpura nephritis included the prescription of a single specific immunosuppressive treatment; other included two or multiple immunosuppressive drugs.

8.3.1 Steroids

Steroids included prednisolone or methylprednisolone at 30 mg/kg/day for 3 consecutive days or dexamethasone at 5 mg/kg/day (Kawasaki et al., 2003; Niaudet & Habib, 1998). Fifty-six patients with renal lesions graded as IIIb or higher were treated with intravenous/oral steroids, along with dipyridamole and anticoagulant warfarin. The acuity index decreased at second biopsy, whereas the chronicity index did not differ significantly (Kawasaki et al., 2003).

8.3.2 Cyclosporine A

Single treatment included cyclosporine A performed for 6 months - 2 years (Ronkainen et al., 2003).

Cyclosporine A, at the initial dose of 4–8 mg/kg/day, with blood level kept at 150–200 µg/L, and at the maintenance dose of 1–5 mg/kg/day, with blood level kept at 80–100 µg/L, proved to be effective in some case series with biopsy-proven steroid-resistant Henoch-Schönlein purpura nephritis. In particular, the treatment was effective in reducing the nephrotic proteinuria range after an average of 2 months in seven patients. Stable remission after a mean follow-up of 6 years was achieved in four subjects (Ronkainen et al., 2003). Treatment with cyclosporine A was effective in one patient with renal crescents following the failure of pulse steroid, oral prednisone and an 8 months course of azathioprine at 2 mg/kg/day (Shin et al., 2006). In seven patients, treatment with pulse or oral prednisone and cyclosporine A with or without angiotensin converting enzyme inhibitor cilazapril displayed a marked efficacy in reversing nephrotic-range proteinuria and reducing histological grading post-treatment (Shin et al., 2005). In another study involving a group of 82 children with varying degrees of renal manifestation and histology (Mir et al., 2007), the majority received steroid treatment while only a few were treated with angiotensin converting enzyme inhibitor or cyclophosphamide in combination with steroids. Despite treatment, the long-term prognosis worsened markedly in those children manifesting severe clinical presentation.

8.3.3 Cyclophosphamide

Single treatments included cyclophosphamide performed for 8-12 weeks (Tarshish et al., 2004; Zaffanello et al., 2007).

A case series of patients with biopsy-proven Henoch-Schönlein purpura nephritis displayed varying degrees of response to cyclophosphamide at 2-2.5 mg/kg/day. Several patients in whom the initial renal biopsy had revealed ≥80% crescentic glomeruli received cyclophosphamide in combination with pulse of methylprednisolone and/or long-term oral prednisone. The combined treatment was effective in aiding clinical recovery, maintaining normal renal function and reducing grade histology. Unfortunately, the lack of control patients and the small number of patients treated or short follow-up period hamper the drawing of firm conclusions (Zaffanello et al., 2007; Zaffanello et al., 2009).

Long-term outcome of patients treated with daily cyclophosphamide expressed as end-stage renal disease did not differ with controls (Tarshish et al., 2004), indicating failure at level II of evidence. In a retrospective investigation, 21 children with crescents in 40% of glomeruli who were treated with an association of azathioprine at 1-2 mg/kg/day and steroids displayed an effective clinical outcome. Unfortunately, the considerable variability of the histological patterns complicated any interpretation of the results obtained (Bergstein et al., 1998; Foster et al., 2000). Moreover, nine patients with severe histologically graded lesions were prescribed aggressive therapy with azathioprine and steroids, leading to marked clinical improvement. Regrettably, histological outcome was not reported, thus hindering the drawing of sustainable conclusions (Singh et al., 2002). Lastly, ten children treated with steroids and azathioprine were compared to ten patients receiving steroids alone. The initial biopsy revealed histological lesions comparable to those observed at follow-up, although mesangial IgA depositions were reduced in the majority of patients (Shin et al., 2005). However, the small number of patients studied led to difficulties in interpreting results.

8.3.4 Mycophenolate mofetil
Mycophenolate mofetil at 900-1,200 mg/m^2/day was tested in patients with vasculitis and connective tissue disease involving the kidney, one of whom was affected by Henoch-Schönlein purpura nephritis. This drug was administered subsequent to the failure of treatment with steroids and azathioprine (Filler et al., 2003). However, two patients featuring a prolonged course of nephritis were first prescribed steroids and azathioprine with the subsequent addition of mycophenolate mofetil (Algoet & Proesmans, 2003). Once again, due to the exceedingly low number of patients treated, no firm conclusions could be drawn.

8.3.5 Single or combined treatment
Other protocols were performed with double immunosuppressant therapy, including steroid–cyclophosphamide (Oner et al., 1995; Iijima et al., 1998; Flynn et al., 2001; Tanaka et al., 2003; Kawasaki et al., 2004; Mir et al., 2007), steroid combined with azathioprine for 8-15 months (Bergstein et al., 1998; Foster et al., 2000; Singh et al., 2002; Shin et al., 2005; Zaffanello et al., 2007), and steroid– cyclosporine A or steroid – (angiotensin converting enzyme inhibitors) – cyclosporine A (Shin et al., 2005; Shin et al., 2006; Shin et al., 2007).

Triple immunosuppressant therapy was carried out using steroid– cyclophosphamide – azathioprine (Shenoy et al., 2007) and steroid– azathioprine –mycophenolate mofetil (Algoet et al., 2003; Zaffanello et al, 2007).

8.3.6 Evidence based treatment
The majority of reports provide scarce support to the various treatment options identified in cases of severe childhood Henoch-Schönlein purpura nephritis (Zaffanello et al., 2009). As the Henoch-Schönlein purpura nephritis and IgA nephropathy have identical pathogenesis and renal lesions, for which current evidence supports the use of immunosuppressive drugs

in patients with severe disease (Samuels et al., 2003; Cheng et al., 2009), the treatment protocols with proven significant benefit in IgA nephropathy should be used in children having Henoch-Schönlein purpura nephritis of comparable severity (Bogdanovic, 2009). A recent, single-centre, retrospective review looking at treatment of severe Henoch-Schönlein purpura nephropathy and IgA nephropathy demonstrated that therapy with differing combinations of steroids, cyclophosphamide, angiotensin converting enzyme inhibitors and angiotensin receptor blockers produced a good outcome in 54% of children with severe (>stage III) histological changes on initial renal biopsy (Edström Halling et al., 2009). For this reason, many physicians prescribe similar treatments in Henoch-Schönlein purpura patients with nephritis, despite the lack of disease-specific data, although IgA nephritis lesions however, tend to have a less severe inflammatory component and clinical trials on IgA nephropathy often include adult patients, while Henoch-Schönlein purpura nephropathy is primarily a disease that develops in children (Zaffanello et al., 2010).

Moreover, several patients with moderately severe Henoch-Schönlein purpura nephritis (histological grade I–III and serum albumin >2.5 g/dl) were treated with angiotensin-converting enzyme inhibitors and/or angiotensin receptor blockers. Patients with Henoch-Schönlein purpura nephritis exceeding grade III or serum albumin ≤ 2.5 g/dl received combination therapy comprising prednisolone at 2 mg/kg/day, given in three divided doses (maximum dose, 80 mg/day) for the first 4 weeks, followed by prednisolone at 2 mg/kg given as a single dose every other morning for 8 weeks, immunosuppressant azathioprine at 2 mg/kg/day as a single dose (maximum dose 100 mg) or mizoribine at 5 mg/kg/day as a single dose (maximum dose 300 mg) maintained for 6 months, and warfarin at 1 mg/day given as a single dose each morning. The warfarin dose was then adjusted to give a thrombo-test result of 20–50%, and dipyridamole started at 3 mg/kg/day given in three divided doses, increased to 6 mg/kg/day (maximum dose, 300 mg/day) maintained for 8 weeks if the patient experienced no adverse effects, such as headache. The resolution of proteinuria, without renal dysfunction, was 50% at 5.2 months, 80% at 8.5 months, and 90% at 11.1 months (Ninchoji et al., 2011).

8.4 Plasma exchange

Patients featuring rapid progression of Henoch-Schönlein purpura nephritis, despite the treatment with immunosuppressive medications (steroids, azatioprine and cyclophosphamide), were treated with plasma exchange. Among these children, 36% developed end-stage renal disease between 1 and 7 years after the initiation of treatment (Gianviti et al., 1996). The other children showed a reduction of glomerular filtration rate and crescents > 50% of glomeruli and continued plasma exchange treatment (Hattori et al., 1999). A case series of eight children with a rapidly progressive course of disease treated with plasma exchange, the beneficial effects produced were only transient, and, despite repeated plasma exchange, the subjects progressed to end-stage renal disease after 1–4 years (Scharer et al., 1999). In case series study, children with extensive crescent formation underwent plasma exchange followed by multiple drug therapy, including steroids, pulse urokinase and cyclophosphamide. The patients manifested a decrease in acuity index and percentage of glomeruli with crescents, whereas the chronicity index remained unchanged (Kawasaki et al., 2004). Plasma exchange was recently performed in patients with a histology grading of at least III at renal biopsy. At follow-up, only one child treated later in the course of the disease underwent a kidney transplant. At the end of the study, the investigators reported that the early performing of plasma exchange may delay the rate of progression of cellular crescents to the fibrotic stage and end-stage renal disease (Shenoy et al., 2007).

Plasma exchange in patients with Henoch-Schönlein purpura nephritis, either alone or in combination with immunosuppressant, cannot currently be recommended due to the paucity of data available (Zaffanello & Fanos, 2009).

8.5 Adjuvant treatment

Adjuvant therapies were defined as any secondary treatment used in addition to the primary or conventional treatments that increased the likelihood of cure (eg, intravenous immunoglobulins, anticoagulants, enzymes and vitamins). Results on moderate urinary abnormalities and severe Henoch-Schönlein purpura nephritis are reported separately because the renal implications, clinical monitoring, and conventional treatment modalities differ in terms of outcome measures (Zaffanello et al., 2009).

8.5.1 Moderate urinary abnormalities

Adjuvant treatment in children with isolated proteinuria with or without nephrotic syndrome has been reviewed (Zaffanello et al., 2009).

Two studies (Rostoker et al., 1995; de Almeida et al., 2007) reported the usefulness of 3 months treatment with intravenous immunoglobulins (2 g/kg/month) followed by intramuscular immunoglobulins (0.35 mL/kg) twice a month for 8 months in treating nephritis with significant proteinuria. Both the severity of proteinuria and the acuity index significantly improved in the majority of these patients with renal histology of stage III and normal renal function. In patients with severe gastrointestinal involvement who did not respond to methylprednisolone, were administered intravenous immunoglobulins at 2 g/kg in a single dose (Rostoker et al., 1998; Aries et al., 2005). Finally, the efficacy of intravenous immunoglobulins (2 g/kg, infused over 10–12 hours) in inhibiting the progression of the disease has been tested although only in unstructured case series.

Intravenous administration of Factor XIII concentrate from 30 to 50 U/kg for 3 days was associated with significant improvements in the severity of proteinuria and hematuria compared with non-treated group (Erdoğan et al., 2003).

In children aged 3 to 15 years with Henoch-Schönlein purpura nephritis, tocopherol 300 mg/day was to be administered for 6-17 weeks (Kaku et al., 1998). Oxidative damage and worsening of the clinical course were observed despite significant increases in mean plasma vitamin E concentration. In 5 children with biopsy-proven Henoch-Schönlein purpura nephritis, treatment with an angiotensin-converting enzyme inhibitor (enalapril) for hypertension and adjuvant treatment with fish oil 1 g twice a day as an antioxidant was associated with significantly decreased severity of proteinuria, decreased blood pressure, and stable serum creatinine concentration and glomerular filtration rate. The limitation of this study was the small sample size and the confounding antiproteinuric effect of the angiotensin-converting enzyme inhibitor (Dixit et al., 2004; Chiurchiu et al., 2005).

A systematic review reported no clear benefit of the use of dipyridamole (3-6 mg/kg/day for 8 weeks) and heparin (adjusted to maintain activated partial thromboplastin time between 60 and 80 seconds for 4 weeks) in treating Henoch-Schönlein purpura nephritis, with limitations being the small number of studies, small sample size, and poor methodology of the studies (Chartapisak et al., 2009).

8.5.2 Severe Henoch-Schönlein purpura nephritis

Adjuvant treatments of severe Henoch-Schönlein purpura nephritis with crescent formations in children have been studies from a systematic review (Zaffanello et al., 2009).

The patients with severe Henoch-Schönlein purpura described in these articles had nephrotic syndrome, Henoch-Schönlein purpura nephritis, rapidly progressive glomerulonephritis, and/or kidney failure. Histology of kidney biopsies found a significant proportion with crescent formations (International Study of Kidney Disease in Children grade IV–V). These patients were at high risk for kidney failure despite aggressive treatment with cocktails that included adjuvant anticoagulants or antiplatelet agents such as heparin (Iijima et al., 1998), warfarin (Kaku et al., 1998; Iijima et al., 1998; Kawasaki et al., 2004) dipyridamole (Oner et al., 1995; Kaku et al., 1998; Iijima et al., 1998; Mir et al., 2007) and acetylsalicylic acid (Mir et al., 2007). Treatments associated conventional with adjuvant therapy including three days intravenous pulse of methylprednisolone and/or long-term oral prednisolone administration for 6 months (Oner et al., 1995; Kawasaki et al, 2003; Kawasaki et al., 2004; Mir et al., 2007). Intravenous steroids were used alone (Kawasaki et al., 2003) or in combination with (or to replace) cyclophosphamide(Oner et al., 1995), or comparable steroid pulse therapy was used with cyclophosphamide (Kawasaki et al., 2004; Mir et al., 2007) and Cyclosporine A (Mir et al., 2007). Oral steroid therapy was used alone or in combination with cyclophosphamide (Iijima et al., 1998; Tanaka et al., 2003; Shekelle et al., 1999).

In a case series of 12 children aged 6 to 14 years with Henoch-Schönlein purpura, quadruple therapy with cyclophosphamide for 2 months, intravenous pulse methylprednisolone for 3 days, oral prednisone for 3 months, and adjuvant oral dipyridamole for 6 months, glomerular filtration rate normalized in 11 patients and 7 patients had complete remission (Oner et al., 1995). In a case series of 14 children followed up for a mean (standard deviation) of 7.5 (0.9) years, combination treatment consisted of prednisone for 12 weeks, cyclophosphamide for 8 weeks, and adjuvant intravenous heparin for 4 weeks followed by warfarin 1 mg/day for 4 weeks, and dipyridamole for 8 weeks . The histologic abnormalities of the kidney significantly improved in the meantime (Iijima et al., 1998).

In 2 clinical trials, cyclosporine A was used for the treatment of severe Henoch-Schönlein purpura nephritis in children, either alone (Ronkainen J, 2003) or in combination with steroids and adjuvant dipyridamole (Mir et al., 2007). In particular, a retrospective, nonrandomized study in 82 children, prednisone or pulse methylprednisolone and cyclophosphamide and cyclosporine were given; asetil salicylic acid or dipyridamole were given as adjuvant therapy, although their dosing were not reported as well. In 35% of nephrotic patients and 62% of nephritic patients showed complete remission after 6 months and long-term course (Mir et al., 2007). In a case series of 13 patients with renal histology grade IIIb or IVb, prednisone was administered for 26 weeks and cyclophosphamide was administered for 8 weeks (Tanaka et al., 2003). Adjuvant therapy was dipyridamole 5 mg/kg/day (maximum, 300 mg/day). At study end, acuity index was significantly decreased, chronologic index was unchanged, and renal histology grade was improved significantly (Tanaka et al., 2003).

In a controlled study, 26 in 37 children with severe Henoch-Schönlein purpura nephritis, triple therapy with oral cyclophosphamide for 12 weeks, pulse methylprednisolone for 3 days, and intravenous pulse urokinase at 5000 U/kg/day (maximum, 180,000 U) for 7 consecutive days was effective. Thus, after 6 months, severity of proteinuria and mesangial IgA deposition were significantly reduced (Kawasaki et al., 2003; Kawasaki et al., 2004).

Observations were reported in retrospective case series, and the literature lacks reports of substantial clinical trials. Because the literature search did not find any well-structured studies reporting benefits of the use of antiplatelet agents or heparin in children with

Henoch-Schönlein purpura nephritis, the use of such therapy is not recommended at this time since lack of evidence from well structured clinical trials (Zaffanello et al., 2009).

9. Prognosis

9.1 Prognostic factors and clinical findings

Age at onset has not been shown to be a predictor of poor outcome (Ronkainen et al., 2002; Coppo et al., 1997; Counahan et al., 1977; Edström Halling et al., 2010). In the long-term, the morbidities of Henoch-Schönlein purpura are predominantly attributed to the intensity of renal involvement at presentation. Anymore, the majority of patients that first manifest nephropathy during childhood will not reach end stage renal disease before adulthood (Wyatt & Hogg, 2001).

Female had a markedly greater risk of a poor long-term outcome (Edström Halling et al., 2010).

Patients with isolated hematuria showed a good prognosis (Narchi, 2005), with some exceptions (Goldstein et al, 1992). Most children with Henoch-Schönlein purpura nephritis who present only with hematuria and/or low-grade proteinuria at onset have good probabilities of recovery (Mir et al., 2007). Only patients showing normal urinalysis for 6 months may be discharged from follow-up. In view of the possibility of late deterioration in those with mild renal involvement, long-term albeit annual follow-up was recommended (Narchi, 2005). It has been calculated that 18% of patients with mild proteinuria at onset progress towards poor outcome (Ronkainen et al., 2002; Butani & Morgenstern, 2007; Edström Halling et al., 2010).

Of children who at onset displayed mild symptoms, 72% achieved a complete recovery, compared to 47% of those with severe symptoms. Of children who had mild symptoms at onset, 15% had a poor outcome compared to 41% of those with severe symptoms (Edström Halling et al., 2010).

Henoch-Schönlein purpura nephritis patients with nephritic/nephritic syndrome and massive proteinuria (Niaudet & Habib, 1998) are considered to have severe disease (Kawasaki et al., 2003; Niaudet & Habib, 1998). Therefore, no significant difference in outcome was found between patients with nephrotic versus non-nephrotic proteinuria at onset. Of patients with nephrotic or nephritic-nephrotic features, 68% had a good outcome and specifically 59% of them achieved complete recovery. Level of urinary albumins/creatinine ratio at 1 year above or below 144 mg/mmol discriminated between poor and good outcome with a sensitivity of 95% and specificity of 40%, positive predictive value 82%, negative predictive value 73% (Edström Halling et al., 2010).

Patients with a poor outcome had lower Glomerular Filtration Rate than patients with a good outcome. An initial renal insufficiency was a predictor of poor renal outcome in Henoch-Schönlein purpura nephritis (Edström Halling et al., 2010).

There was no difference in outcome between patients who were normotensive and those who were hypertensive at the first investigation (Edström Halling et al., 2010).

9.2 Prognostic factors and biopsy findings

International Study of Kidney Disease in Children grading score and proteinuria at the 1-year follow-up were the best discriminators of a good and poor outcome (Edström Halling et al., 2010).

Kawasaki (Kawasaki et al., 2003) classified Henoch-Schönlein purpura nephritis patients with International Study of Kidney Disease in Children grade IIIb or higher as having severe disease. Shenoy (Shenoy et al., 2007) concluded that most children with Henoch-Schönlein purpura nephritis grade IIIb or higher on initial biopsy had persistent renal abnormalities at long-term follow-up. The risks for long-term renal impairment are highest in children who present and/or with more than 50% of glomeruli (grade IV or above) occupied by large crescents or sclerosing lesions (Bogdanovic, 2009) because they showed higher probabilities for development of progressive renal disease, renal failure, or end-stage renal disease after long-term follow-up (Iijima et al., 1998; Kawasaki et al., 2004; Niaudet & Habib, 1998).

Patients with segmental glomerulosclerosis had a poorer outcome than those without segmental glomerulosclerosis. The comparison of patients with crescents to those without or those with global glomerulosclerosis to those without revealed no difference in outcome. Patients with poor outcome had a higher degree of mesangial matrix expansion, mesangial proliferation, interstitial inflammation and interstitial fibrosis than did those with a good outcome. Crescents were not a factor of poor prognosis, but the majority of the patients with crescents were treated, which may have improved the course of the disease (Edström Halling et al., 2010).

10. Conclusion

At this time, randomized controlled trials are needed to demonstrate whether the present management with conventional and adjuvant treatments improve truly renal survival of patients with Henoch-Schönlein purpura nephritis. Anymore, the choice of the treatment must depend on both the histological and clinical severity of the Henoch-Schönlein purpura nephritis. In particular, recommendations include a combination therapy for clinically and histologically severe Henoch-Schönlein purpura nephritis, which is unnecessary for moderate Henoch-Schönlein purpura nephritis.

11. References

Algoet, C., Proesmans, W. (2003). Renal biopsy 2–9 years after Henoch Schonlein purpura. *Pediatric Nephrology*, Vol.18, No.5, pp.471–3, ISSN 0931041X.

Allen, A.C., Willis, F.R., Beattie, T.J., Feehally, J. Abnormal IgA glycosylation in Henoch-Schönlein purpura restricted to patients with clinical nephritis. *Nephrology Dialysis Transplantation*, Vol.13, No4, pp.930–934, ISSN 09310509.

Aries, P.M., Hellmich, B., Gross, W.L. (2005). Intravenous immunoglobulin therapy in vasculitis: Speculation or evidence? *Clinical Reviews in Allergy and Immunology*, Vol.29, No.3, pp.237–245, ISSN 10800549.

Assadi, F. (2009). Childhood Henoch-Schonlein nephritis: a multivariate analysis of clinical features and renal morphology at disease onset. *Iranian Journal of Kidney Diseases*, Vol.3, No.1, pp.17-21, ISSN 17358582.

Bergstein, J., Leiser, J., Andreoli, S.P. (1998). Response of crescentic Henoch–Schönlein purpura nephritis to corticosteroid and azathioprine therapy. *Clinical Nephrology*, Vol. 49,No. 1, pp.9–14, ISSN 03010430.

Bogdanovic, R,. (2009). Henoch-Schonlein purpura nephritis in children: risk factors, prevention and treatment. *Acta Paediatrica, International Journal of Paediatrics*, Vol. 98, No. 12, pp. 1882-1889, ISSN 08035253.

Butani, L., Morgenstern, B.Z. (2007). Long-term outcome in children after Henoch-Schonlein purpura nephritis. *Clinical Pediatrics*, Vol. 46, No. 6, pp. 505–511, ISSN 00099228.

Chartapisak, W., Opastiraku, S., Willis, N.S., Craig, J.C., Hodson, E.M. (2009). Prevention and treatment of renal disease in Henoch-Schönlein purpura: A systematic review. *Archives of Disease in Childhood*, Vol. 94, No. 2, pp. 132–137, ISSN 00039888.

Cheng, J., Zhang, X., Zhang, W., He, Q., Tao, X., Chen, J. (2009). Efficacy and safety of glucocorticoids therapy for IgA nephropathy: a meta-analysisof randomized controlled trials. *American Journal of Nephrology*, Vol.30, No.4, pp. 315–322, ISSN 02508095.

Chiurchiu, C., Remuzzi, G., Ruggenenti, P. (2005). Angiotensin-converting enzyme inhibition and renal protection in nondiabetic patients: The data of the meta-analyses. *Journal of the American Society of Nephrology*, Vol.16, pp. S58–S63, ISSN 10466673.

Coppo, R., Andrulli, S., Amore, A., Gianoglio, B., Conti, G., Peruzzi, L., Locatelli, F., Cagnoli, L. (2006). Predictors of outcome in Henoch-Schonlein nephritis in children and adults. *American Journal of Kidney Diseases*, Vol.47, No.6, pp.993–1003, ISSN 02726386.

Coppo, R., Mazzucco, G., Cagnoli, L., Lupo, A., Schena, F.P. (1997). Long-term prognosis of Henoch-Scho" nlein nephritis in adults and children. Italian Group of Renal Immunopathology Collaborative Study on Henoch-Scho"enlein purpura. *Nephrology Dialysis Transplantation*, Vol. 12, No. 11, pp. 2277–83, ISSN 09310509.

Counahan, R., Winterborn, M.H., White, R.H., Heaton, J.M., Meadow, S.R., Bluett, N.H., Swetschin, H., Cameron, J.S., Chantler, C. (1977). Prognosis of Henoch-Schönlein nephritis in children. *British medical journal*, Vol.2, pp.11 – 14, ISSN 00071447.

Davin, J.C., Weening, J.J. (2003). Diagnosis of Henoch-Schönlein purpura: renal or skin biopsy? *Pediatric Nephrology*, Vol.18, No.12, pp. 1201–1203, ISSN 0931041X.

de Almeida, J.L., Campos, L.M., Paim, L.B., Leone, C., Koch, V.H., Silva, C.A. (2007. Renal involvement in Henoch-Schönlein purpura: A multivariate analysis of initial prognostic factors. *Jornal de Pediatria*, Vol.83, No.3, pp.259–266, ISSN 00217557.

Dixit, M.P., Dixit, N.M., Scott, K. (2004). Managing Henoch–Schönlein purpura in children with fish oil and ACE inhibitor therapy. *Nephrology (Carlton)*, Vol. 9, No. 6, pp.381–386, ISSN 13205358.

Edström Halling, S., Söderberg, M.P., Berg, U.B. (2010). Predictors of outcome in Henoch–Schönlein nephritis. *Pediatric Nephrology*, Vol.25, pp.1101–1108, ISSN 0931041X.

Edström Halling, S., Söderberg. M.P., Berg, U.B. (2009). Treatment of severe Henoch–Schönlein and immunoglobulin A nephritis. A single center experience. *Pediatric Nephrology*, Vol.24, No. 1, pp.91–97, ISSN 0931041X.

Erdoğan, O., Oner, A., Aydin, A., Işimer, A., Demircin, G., Bülbül, M. (2003). Effect of vitamin E treatment on the oxidative damage occurring in Henoch-Schönlein purpura. *Acta Paediatrica, International Journal of Paediatrics*, Vol.92, pp. 546–550, ISSN 08035253.

Evans, D.J., Williams, D.G., Peters, D.K., Sissons, J.G., Boulton-Jones, J.M., Ogg, C.S., Cameron, J.S., Hoffbrand, B.I. (1973). Glomerular deposition of properdin in

Henoch-Schönlein syndrome and idiopathic focal nephritis. *British Medical Journal*, Vol.3, pp.326–328, ISSN 00071447 .

Falkner, B., Daniels, S.R., Flynn, J.T., Gidding, S., Green, L.A., Ingelfinger, J.R., Lauer, R.M., Morgenstern, B.Z., Portman, R.J., Prineas, R.J., Rocchini, A.P., Rosner, B., Sinaiko, A.R., Stettler, N., Urbina, E., Roccella, E.J., Hoke, T., Hunt, C.E., Pearson, G., Karimbakas, J., Horton, A. (2004). The fourth report on the diagnosis, evaluation, and treatment of high blood pressure in children and adolescents. *Pediatrics*, Vol.114, No.2, pp. 555-76, ISSN 00314005.

Farine, M., Poucell, S., Geary, D.L., Baumal, R. (1986). Prognostic significance of urinary findings and renal biopsies in children with Henoch–Schönlein nephritis. *Clinical Pediatrics (Phila)*, Vol.25, pp.257–259, ISSN 00099228.

Filler, G., Hansen, M., LeBlanc, C., Lepage, N., Franke, D., Mai, I., Feber, J. (2003). Pharmacokinetics of mycophenolate mofetil for autoimmune disease in children. *Pediatric Nephrology*, Vol. 18, pp. 445–449, ISSN 0931041X.

Flynn, J.T., Smoyer, W.E., Bunchman, T.E., Kershaw, D.B., Sedman, A.B. (2001). Treatment of Henoch–Schonlein purpura glomerulonephritisin children with high-dose corticosteroids plus oral cyclophosphamide. *American Journal of Nephrology*, Vol.21, pp.128–133, ISSN 02508095.

Foster, B.J., Bernard, C., Drummond, K.N., Sharma, A.K. (2000). Effective therapy for severe Henoch-Schonlein purpura nephritis with prednisone and azathioprine: a clinical and histopathologic study. *Journal of Pediatrics*, Vol. 136, pp.370-375, ISSN 00223476.

Gardner-Medwin, J.M., Dolezalova, P., Cummins, C., Southwood, T.R. (2002). Incidence of Henoch–Schönlein purpura, Kawasaki disease, and rare vasculitides in children of different ethnic origins. *Lancet*, Vol. 360, pp.1197-1202, ISSN 01406736.

Gianviti, A., Trompeter, R.S., Barratt, T.M., Lythgoe, M.F., Dillon, M.J. (1996). Retrospective study of plasma exchange in patients with idiopathic rapidly progressive glomerulonephritis and vasculitis. *Archives of Disease in Childhood*, Vol. 75, pp. 186–190, ISSN 00039888.

Gibson, K.L., Amamoo, M.A., Primack, W.A. (2008). Corticosteroid Therapy for Henoch Schönlein Purpura. *Pediatrics*, Vol.121, pp.870-871, ISSN 00314005.

Goldstein, A.R., White, R.H., Akuse, R., Chantler, C. (1992). Long-term follow-up of childhood Henoch-Schoenlein nephritis. *Lancet*, Vol. 339, pp.280-2, ISSN 01406736.

Hattori, M., Ito, K., Konomoto, T., Kawaguchi, H., Yoshioka, T., Khono, M. (1999). Plasmapheresis as the sole therapy for rapidly progressive Henoch–Schönlein purpura nephritis in children. *American Journal of Kidney Diseases*, Vol. 33, pp.427–433, ISSN 02726386.

Hung, S.P., Yang, Y.H., Lin, Y.T., Wang, L.C., Lee, J.H., Chiang, B.L. (2009). Clinical manifestations and outcomes of Henoch-Schönlein purpura: comparison between adults and children. *Pediatrics and Neonatology*, Vol.50, No.4, pp.162–168, ISSN 18759572.

Iijima, K., Ito-Kariya, S., Nakamura, H., Yoshikawa, N. (1998). Multiple combined therapy for severe Henoch-Schonlein nephritis in children. *Pediatric Nephrology*, Vol.12, pp. 244-248, ISSN 0931041X.

Inoue, C.N., Chiba, Y., Morimoto, T., Nishio, T., Kondo, Y., Adachi, M., Matsutani, S. (2007). Tonsillectomy in the treatment of pediatric Henoch–Schönlein nephritis. *Clinical Nephrology*, Vol.67, pp. 298–305, ISSN 03010430.

Iqbal, H., Evans, A. (2005). Dapsone therapy for Henoch-Schönlein purpura: a case series. *Archives of Disease in Childhood*, Vol.90, pp.985-986, ISSN 00039888.

Jauhola, O., Ronkainen, J., Koskimies, O., Ala-Houhala, M., Arikoski, P., Höltt, T., Jahnukainen, T., Rajantie, J., Örmälä, T., Turtinen, J., Nuutinen, M. (2010). Renal manifestations of Henoch-Schönlein purpura in a 6-month prospective study of 223 children. *Archives of Disease in Childhood*, Vol.95, pp.877-882, ISSN 00039888.

Kaku, Y. Nohara, K., Honda, S. (1998). Renal involvement in Henoch–Schönlein purpura: a multivariate analysis of prognostic factors. *Kidney International*, Vol.53, pp.1755-1759, ISSN 00852538.

Kawasaki, Y., Suyama, K., Yugeta, E., Katayose, M., Suzuki, S., Sakuma, H., Nemoto, K., Tsukagoshi, A., Nagasawa, K., Hosoya, M. (2010). The incidence and severity of Henoch-Schoenlein purpura nephritis over a 22-year period in Fukushima Prefecture, Japan. *International Urology and Nephrology*, Vol.42, pp.1023-1029, ISSN 03011623.

Kawasaki, Y., Suzuki, J., Murai, M., Takahashi, A., Isome, M., Nozawa, R., Suzuki, S., Suzuki, H. (2004). Plasmapheresis therapy for rapidly progressive Henoch–Schönlein nephritis. *Pediatric Nephrology*, Vol.19, No.920-923, ISSN 0931041X.

Kawasaki, Y., Suzuki, J., Nozawa, R., Suzuki, S., Suzuki, H. (2003). Efficacy of methylprednisolone and urokinase pulse therapy for severe Henoch-Schonlein nephritis. *Pediatrics*, Vol.111, pp.785-789, ISSN 00314005.

Kawasaki, Y., Suzuki, J., Suzuki, H. (2004). Efficacy of methylprednisolone and urokinase pulse therapy combined with or without cyclophosphamide in severe Henoch-Schoenlein nephritis: a clinical and histopathological study. *Nephrology Dialysis Transplantation*, Vol.19, pp.858-864, ISSN 09310509.

Lai, K.N., To, W.Y., Li, P.K., Leung, J.C. (1996). Increased binding of polymeric lambda-IgA to cultured human mesangial cells in IgA nephropathy. *Kidney International*, Vol.49, pp.839-845, ISSN 00852538.

Lau, K.K., Suzuki, H., Novak, J., Wyatt, R.J. (2010). Pathogenesis of Henoch-Schönlein purpura nephritis. *Pediatric Nephrology*, Vol.25, No.1, pp.19-26, ISSN 0931041X.

Levinsky, R.J., Barratt, T.M. (1979). IgA immune complexes in Henoch-Schönlein purpura. *Lancet*, Vol.2, pp.1100-1103, ISSN 01406736.

McCarthy, H.J., Tizard, E.J. (2010). Diagnosis and management of Henoch–Schönlein purpura. *European Journal of Pediatrics*, Vol.169, pp.643-650, ISSN 03406199.

Meadow, S.R., Glasgow, E.F., White, R.H., Moncrieff, M.W., Cameron, J.S., Ogg, C.S. (1972). Schönlein-Henoch nephritis . *The Quarterly journal of medicine*, Vol.41, pp.241-258, ISSN 00335622.

Meulders, Q., Pirson, Y., Cosyns, J.P., Squifflet, J.P., van Ypersele de, Strihou, C. (1994). Course of Henoch-Schönlein nephritis after renal transplantation. Report on ten patients and review of the literature. *Transplantation*, Vol.58, pp.1179-1186, ISSN 00411337.

Mir, S., Yavascan, O., Mutlubas, F., Yeniay, B., Sonmez, F. (2007). Clinical outcome in children with Henoch-Schönlein nephritis. *Pediatric Nephrology*, Vol.22, pp.64-70, ISSN 0931041X.

Mollica, F., Li Volti, S., Garozzo, R., Russo, G. (1992). Effectiveness of early prednisone treatment in preventing the development of nephropathy in anaphylactoid purpura. *European Journal of Pediatrics*, Vol.151, No.2, pp.140-4, ISSN 03406199.

Motoyama, O., Iitaka, K. (2005). Henoch-Schönlein purpura with hypocomplementemia in children. *Pediatrics international : official journal of the Japan Pediatric Society*, Vol.47, pp.39–42, ISSN 13288067.

Moura, I.C., Arcos-Fajardo, M., Sadaka, C., Leroy, V., Benhamou, M., Novak, J., Vrtovsnik, F., Haddad, E., Chintalacharuvu, K.R., Monteiro, R.C. (2004). Glycosylation and size of IgA1 are essential for interaction with mesangial transferrin receptor in IgA nephropathy. *Journal of the American Society of Nephrology*, Vol.15, pp.622–634, ISSN 10466673.

Narchi, H. (2005). Risk of long term renal impairment and duration of follow up recommended for Henoch-Schönlein purpura with normal or minimal urinary findings: a systematic review. *Archives of Disease in Childhood*, Vol.90, pp.916-920, ISSN 00039888.

Niaudet, P., Habib, R. (1998). Methylprednisolone pulse therapy in the treatment of severe forms of Schonlein-Henoch purpura nephritis. *Pediatric Nephrology*, Vol.12, pp.238-243, ISSN 0931041X.

Ninchoji, T., Kaito, H., Nozu, K., Hashimura, Y., Kanda, K., Kamioka, I., Shima, Y., Hamahira, K., Nakanishi, K., Tanaka, R., Yoshikawa, N., Iijima, K., Matsuo, M. (2011). Treatment strategies for Henoch-Schönlein purpura nephritis by histological and clinical severity. *Pediatric Nephrology*, Vol.26, No.4, pp.563-9, ISSN 0931041X.

Novak, J., Moldoveanu, Z., Renfrow, M.B., Yanagihara, T., Suzuki, H., Raska, M., Hall, S., Brown, R., Huang, W.Q., Goepfert, A., Kilian, M., Poulsen, K., Tomana, M., Wyatt, R.J., Julian, B.A., Mestecky, J. (2007). IgA nephropathy and Henoch-Schoenlein purpura nephritis: aberrant glycosylation of IgA1, formation of IgA1-containing immune complexes, and activation of mesangial cells. *Contributions to Nephrology*, Vol.157, pp.134–138, ISSN 03025144.

Oner, A., Tinaztepe, K., Erdogan, O. (1995). The effect of triple therapy on rapidly progressive type of Henoch-Schonlein nephritis. *Pediatric Nephrology*, Vol.9, pp.6-10, ISSN 0931041X.

Ozen, S., Ruperto, N., Dillon, M.J., Bagga, A., Barron, K., Davin, J.C., Kawasaki, T., Lindsley, C., Petty, R.E., Prieur, A.M., Ravelli, A., Woo, P. (2006). EULAR/PReS endorsed consensus criteria for the classification of childhood vasculitides. *Annals of the Rheumatic Diseases*, Vol.65, No.7, pp.936-41, ISSN 00034967.

Pillebout, E., Thervet, E., Hill, G., Alberti, C., Vanhille, P., Nochy, D. (2002). Henoch-Schönlein purpura in adults: outcome and prognostic factors. *Journal of the American Society of Nephrology*, Vol.13, pp.1271–8, ISSN 10466673.

Rai, A., Nast, C., Adler, S. (1999). Henoch–Schönlein purpura nephritis. *Journal of the American Society of Nephrology*, Vol.10, pp.2637-2644, ISSN 10466673.

Rigante, D., Candelli, M., Federico, G., Bartolozzi, F., Porri, M.G., Stabile, A. (2005). Predictive factors of renal involvement or relapsing disease in children with Henoch Schönlein purpura. *Rheumatology International*, Vol.25, pp.45-48, ISSN 01728172.

Ronkainen, J., Ala-Houhala, M., Autio-Harmainen, H., Jahnukainen, T., Koskimies, O., Merenmies, J., Mustonen, J., Ormala, T., Turtinen, J., Nuutinen, M. (2006). Long-term outcome 19 years after childhood IgA nephritis: a retrospective cohort study. *Pediatric Nephrology*, Vol.21, pp.1266-1273, ISSN 0931041X.

Ronkainen, J., Autio-Harmainen, H., Nuutinen, M. (2003). Cyclosporin A for the treatment of severe Henoch-Schonlein glomerulonephritis. *Pediatric Nephrology*, Vol.18, pp.1138-1142, ISSN 0931041X.

Ronkainen, J., Koskimies, O., Ala-Houhala, M., Antikainen, M., Merenmies, J., Rajantie, J., Örmälä, T., Turtinen, J., Nuutinen, M. (2006). Early prednisone therapy in Henoch-Schönlein purpura: a randomized, double-blind, placebo-controlled trial. *Journal of Pediatrics*, Vol.149, pp.241-247, ISSN 00223476.

Ronkainen, J., Nuutinen, M., Koskimies, O. (2002). The adult kidney 24 years after childhood Henoch-Schönlein purpura: a retrospective cohort study. *Lancet*, Vol.360, pp.666 – 70, ISSN 01406736.

Rostoker, G., Desvaux-Belghiti, D., Pilatte, Y., Petit-Phar, M., Philippon, C., Deforges, L., Terzidis, H., Intrator, L., André, C., Adnot, S., Bonin, P., Bierling, P., Remy, P., Lagrue, G., Lang, P., Weil, B. (1995). Immunomodulation with low-dose immunoglobulins for moderate Immunomodulation with low-dose immunoglobulins for moderate results of a prospective uncontrolled trial. *Nephron*, Vol.69, pp.327–334, ISSN 00282766.

Rostoker, G., Desvaux-Belghiti, D., Pilatte, Y., Petit-Phar, M.,Philippon, C., Deforges, L., Terzidis, H., Intrator, L., André, C., Adnot, S., Bonin, P., Bierling, P., Remy, P., Lagrue, G., Lang, P., Weil, B. (1994). High-dose immunoglobulin therapy for severe IgA nephropathy and Henoch–Schönlein purpura. *Annals of Internal Medicine*, Vol. 120, pp.476–484, ISSN 00034819.

Rostoker, G., Rymer, J.C., Bagnard, G., Petit-Phar, M., Griuncelli, M., Pilatte, Y. (1998). Imbalances in serum proinflammatory cytokines and their soluble receptors: A putative role in the progression of idiopathic IgA nephropathy (IgAN) and Henoch-Schönlein purpura nephritis, and a potential target of immunoglobulin therapy? *Clinical and Experimental Immunology*, Vol.114, pp.468–476, ISSN 00099104.

Rostoker, G. (2001). Schonlein-Henoch purpura in children and adults: diagnosis, pathophysiology and management. *Biodrugs*, Vol.15, pp.99–138, ISSN 11738804.

Samuels, J.A., Strippoli, G.F., Craig, J.C., Schena, F.P., Molony, D.A. (2003). Immunosuppressive agents for treating IgA nephropathy. *Cochrane Database Syst Rev*, No.4, CD003965, ISSN 1469493X (electronic).

Sanai, A., Kudoh, F. (1996). Effects of tonsillectomy in children with IgA nephropathy, purpura nephritis, or other chronic glomeruloIgA nephropathy, purpura nephritis, or other chronic glomerulonephritides. *Acta Otolaryngologica. Supplementum*, Vol.523, pp.172–174, ISSN 0365-5237.

Sano, H., Izumida, M., Shimizu, H., Ogawa, Y. (2002). Risk factors of renal involvement and significant proteinuria in Henoch–Schönlein purpura. *European Journal of Pediatrics*, Vol.161, pp.196–201, ISSN 0340-6199.

Saulsbury, F.T. (2007). Clinical update: Henoch-Schönlein purpura. *Lancet*, Vol.369, pp.976–978, ISSN 01406736.

Saulsbury, F.T. (2001). Henoch-Schönlein purpura. *Curr Opin Rheumatol*, Vol.13, No.1, pp.35-40, ISSN 10408711.

Saulsbury, F.T. (1999). Henoch-Schönlein purpura: report of 100 patients and review of the literature. *Medicine*, Vol.78, pp.395-409, ISSN 00257974.

Saulsbury, F.T. (2009). Successful treatment of prolonged Henoch-Schönlein purpura with colchicine. *Clinical Pediatrics*, Vol.48, pp.866-868, ISSN 00099228.

Scharer, K., Krmar, R., Querfeld, U., Ruder, H., Waldherr, R., Schaefer, F. (1999). Clinical outcome of Schonlein-Henoch purpura nephritis in children. *Pediatric Nephrology*, Vol.13, pp.816-823, ISSN 0931041X.

Schmitt, R., Carlsson, F., Mörgelin, M., Tati, R., Lindahl, G., Karpman, D. (2010). Tissue deposits of IgA-binding streptococcal M proteins in IgA nephropathy and Henoch-Schonlein purpura. *American Journal of Pathology*, Vol. 176, No.2, pp.608-18, ISSN 00029440.

Shekelle, P.G., Woolf, S.H., Eccles, M., Grimshaw, J. (1999). Clinical guidelines: Developing guidelines. *British Medical Journal*, Vol.318, pp.593-596, ISSN 09598146.

Shenoy, M., Bradbury, M.G., Lewis, M.A., Webb, N.J. (2007). Outcome of Henoch-Schonlein purpura nephritis treated with long-term immunosuppression. *Pediatric Nephrology*, Vol.22, pp.1717-1722, ISSN 0931041X.

Shenoy, M., Ognjanovic, M.V., Coulthard, M.G. (2007). Treating severe Henoch–Schönlein and IgA nephritis with plasmapheresis alone. *Pediatric Nephrology*. Vol.22, pp.1167-1171, ISSN 0931041X.

Shin, J.I., Kim, J.H., Lee, J.S., Kim, P.K., Jeong, H.J. (2007). Methylprednisolone and cyclosporin therapy in a patient with nephroticproteinuria. *Indian Journal of Pediatrics*, Vol.74, pp.593-594, ISSN 0973-7693.

Shin, J.I., Park, J.M., Kim, J.H., Lee, J.S., Jeong, H.J. (2006). Factors affecting histological regression of crescentic Henoch–Schönlein nephritis in children. *Pediatric Nephrology*, Vol.21, pp.54-59, ISSN 0931041X.

Shin, J.I., Park, J.M., Lee, J.S., Kim, J.H., Kim, P.K., Jeong, H.J. (2006). Successful use of cyclosporin A in severe Schönlein–Henoch nephritis resistant to both methylprednisolone pulse and azathioprine. *Clinical Rheumatology*, Vol.25, pp.759-760, ISSN 07703198.

Shin, J.I., Park, J.M., Shin, Y.H., Hwang, D.H., Kim, J.H., Lee, J.S. (2006). Predictive factors for nephritis, relapse, and significant proteinuria in childhood Henoch-Schönlein purpura. *Scandinavian Journal of Rheumatology*, Vol.35, pp.56-60, ISSN 03009742.

Shin, J.I., Park, J.M., Shin, Y.H., Kim, J.H., Kim, P.K., Lee, J.S., Jeong, H.J. (2005). Cyclosporin A therapy for severe Henoch–Schönlein nephritis with nephrotic syndrome. *Pediatric Nephrology*, Vol.20, pp.1093-1097, ISSN 0931041X.

Shin, J.I., Park, J.M., Shin, Y.H., Kim, J.H., Lee, J.S., Kim, P.K., Jeong, H.J. (2005). Can azathioprine and steroids alter the progression of severe Henoch–Schönlein nephritis in children? *Pediatric Nephrology*, Vol.20, pp.1087-1092, ISSN 0931041X.

Singh, S., Devidayal, Kumar, L., Joshi, K., Minz, R.W., Datta, U. (2002). Severe Henoch–Schönlein nephritis: resolution with azathioprine and steroids. *Rheumatology International*, Vol.22, pp.133-137, ISSN 01728172.

Soler, M.J., Mir, M., Rodriguez, E., Orfila, A., Munne, A., Vázquez, S., Lloveras, J., Puig, J.M. (2005). Recurrence of IgA nephropathy and Henoch-Schönlein purpura after kidney transplantation: risk factors and graft survival. *Transplantation Proceedings*, Vol.37, pp.3705-3709, ISSN 00411345.

Soylemezoglu, O., Ozkaya, O., Ozen, S., Bakkaloglu, A., Dusunsel, R., Peru, H., Cetinyurek, A., Yildiz, N., Donmez, O., Buyan, N., Mir, S.,Arisoy, N., Gur-Guven, A., Alpay, H., Ekim, M., Aksu, N., Soylu, A., Gok, F., Poyrazoglu, H., Sonmez, F. (2009). Turkish Pediatric Vasculitis Study Group.Henoch-Schonlein nephritis: a nationwide study. *Nephron - Clinical Practice*, Vol.112, No.3, pp.c199-204, ISSN 16602110.

Stewart, M., Savage, J.M., Bell, B., McCord, B. (1988). Long term renal prognosis of Henoch-Scho¨ nlein purpura in an unselected childhood population. *European Journal of Pediatrics*, Vol.147, pp.113–5, ISSN 03406199.

Suzuki, H., Moldoveanu, Z., Hall, S., Brown, R., Vu, H.L., Novak, L., Julian, B.A., Tomana, M., Wyatt, R.J., Edberg, J.C., Alarcón, G.S., Kimberly, R.P., Tomino, Y., Mestecky, J., Novak, J. (2008). IgA1-secreting cell lines from patients with IgA nephropathy produce aberrantly glycosylated IgA1. *The Journal of Clinical Investigation*, 2008 Vol.118, No.2, pp.629-39. ISSN 00219738.

Suzuki, H., Suzuki Y., Narita, I., Aizawa, M., Kihara, M., Yamanaka, T., Kanou, T., Tsukaguchi, H., Novak, J., Horikoshi, S., Tomino, Y. (2008). Toll-like receptor 9 affects severity of IgA nephropathy. *Journal of the American Society of Nephrology*, Vol.19, No.12, pp. 2384-2395, ISSN 10466673.

Tanaka, H., Suzuki, K., Nakahata, T., Ito, E., Waga, S. (2003). Early treatment with oral immunosuppressants in severe proteinuric purpura nephritis. *Pediatric Nephrology*, Vol.18, pp.347–350, ISSN 0931041X.

Tarshish, P., Bernstein, J., Edelmann, C.M., Jr. (2004). Henoch-Schonlein purpura nephritis: course of disease and efficacy of cyclophosphamide. *Pediatric Nephrology*, Vol.19, pp.51-56, ISSN 0931041X.

Tizard, E.J., Hamilton-Ayres, M.J. (2008). Henoch Schonlein purpura. *Archives of Disease in Childhood Educ Pract Ed*, Vol. 93, No.1, pp.1-8, ISSN 17430585.

Trapani, S., Micheli, A., Grisolia, F., Resti, M., Chiappini, E., Falcini, F., De Martino, M. (2005). Henoch-Schonlein purpura in childhood: epidemiological and clinical lanalysis of 150 cases over a 5-year period and review of literature. *Seminars in Arthritis and Rheumatism*, Vol.35, pp.143-153, ISSN 00490172.

Waldo, F.B. (1988). Is Henoch-Schönlein purpura the systemic form of IgA nephropathy? *American Journal of Kidney Diseases*, Vol.12, pp.373–377, ISSN 02726386.

Wyatt, R.J., Hogg, R.J. (2001). Evidence-based assessment of treatment options for children with IgA nephropathies. *Pediatric Nephrology*, Vol.16, pp.156–167, ISSN 0931041X.

Wyatt. R.J., Kanayama, Y., Julian, B.A., Negoro, N., Sugimoto, S., Hudson, E.C., Curd, J.G. (1987). Complement activation in IgA nephropathy. *Kidney International*, Vol.31, pp.1019–1023, ISSN 00852538.

Yang, Y.H., Hung, C.F., Hsu, C.R., Wang, L.C., Chuang, Y.H., Lin, Y.T., Chiang, B.L. (2005). A nationwide survey on epidemiological characteristics of childhood Henoch-Schönlein purpura in Taiwan. *Rheumatology*, Vol.44, pp.618−22, ISSN 14620324.

Zaffanello, M., Brugnara, M., Franchini, M. (2007). Therapy for children with henoch-schonlein purpura nephritis: a systematic review. *ScientificWorldJournal*, Vol.7, pp.20-30, ISSN 1537-744X.

Zaffanello, M., Brugnara, M., Franchini, M., Fanos, V. (2009). Adjuvant Treatments in Henoch-Schönlein Purpura Nephritis in Children: a systematic review. *Current Therapeutic Research - Clinical and Experimental*, Vol.70, No.3, pp. 254-265, ISSN 0011393X.

Zaffanello, M., Emma, F., Weiss, P.F., Hastings, M.C., Eison, T.M. (2010). Commentaries on 'Interventions for preventing and treating kidney disease in Henoch-Schonlein Purpura'. *Evidence-Based Child Health*, Vol.5, pp.703–708, ISSN.

Zaffanello, M., Fanos, V. (2009). Treatment-based literature of Henoch–Schönlein purpura. *Pediatric Nephrology*, Vol.24, pp.1901–1911, ISSN 0931041X.

4

Mixed Hematopoietic Chimerism Allows Cure of Autoimmune Glomerulonephritis: Its Potential and Risks

Emiko Takeuchi

Kitasato University School of Medicine
Japan

1. Introduction

Patients with severe autoimmune lupus glomerulonephritis that is resistant to immunosuppressive therapy need alternative treatment. Recently, bone marrow transplantation (BMT) has been proposed as a potential therapy for refractory autoimmune disease. BMT involves the administration of hematopoietic stem cells, which are self- renewing and capable of giving rise to all mature hematopoietic cell types and possibly some non-hematopoietic cell types. The etiologic and pathogenic bases of many autoimmune diseases ultimately reside in the self-renewing hematopoietic stem cell population. Therefore, the effects of BMT as a treatment for and/or preventive measure against these autoimmune diseases have been investigated extensively (Sykes&Nicolic, 2005). Studies in animal models have shown that the transfer of hematopoietic stem cells can reverse the autoimmune state. The induction of fully allogeneic bone marrow (BM) chimerism, however, is fraught with difficulties. Each of the various methods of inducing fully allogeneic BM chimerism through hematopoietic cell transplantation (HCT) requires a different set of conditions, such as host T cell depletion, donor myeloablation, major histocompatibility complex (MHC) fully matched donor BM, or lethal dose of total body irradiation (TBI). Meeting these conditions is usually a burden on the recipient. Moreover, fully allogeneic BM chimerism is always associated with risks of graft versus host disease (GVHD) and immunodeficiency, which make it less practical for clinical application.

Accordingly, the induction of mixed allogeneic BM chimerism has been proposed as a treatment for autoimmune disease. Mixed chimerism refers to a state in which allogeneic donor hematopoietic cells coexist with recipient cells in host bone marrow.

In this paper, the advantages of inducing mixed BM chimerism are summarized and a process for inducing peripheral/central tolerance is introduced. Several mechanistic pathways which are thought to be involved in reversing the autoimmune state are then described. Based on our original data, we propose one possible mechanism in which newly developed donor T cells, which have been positively selected in the host thymus and restricted host MHC, are able to regulate auto-reactive B cells through T cell receptor (TCR)/MHC interaction. Finally, we discuss the potential risks associated with fully MHC-mismatched allogeneic mixed chimerism. This information will help to determine the role that HCT can play in the treatment of autoimmune glomerulonephritis.

2. Bone marrow mixed chimerism

2.1 What is the advantage of mixed chimerism?

Mixed chimerism refers to a state in which allogeneic donor hematopoietic cells coexist with recipient cells in host bone marrow, whereas fully allogeneic chimerism refers to a state in which donor hematopoietic cells completely replace recipient cells.

It is known that fully allogeneic chimeras transplanted from a donor with fully mismatched MHC usually reject donor BM, or experience severe GVHD. Even if donor BM cells were safely engrafted in host BM, the resulting fully MHC-mismatched chimeras would develop immunodeficiency. In fully allogeneic chimeras, all mature T cells are supposed to be restricted to the host MHC type, irrespective of their own genetic background. This occurs because thymocytes, the precursors of mature T cells, are positively selected for weak reactivity to the self-peptide/MHC complex in the host thymus; this positive selection is mediated only by thymic cortical epithelial cells and not by bone marrow-derived cells. Therefore, in the periphery, all TCRs have certain affinity to host MHC molecules but not to donor MHC molecules. Thus, if the donor MHC is fully mismatched with the host MHC, there are no peripheral T cells which can interact with peripheral B cells differentiated from donor hematopoietic stem cells which generate donor-type MHC. This is the cause of deficiency in humoral immunity in fully MHC-mismatched allogeneic chimerism (Janeway et al., 2001).

In mixed chimerism, on the other hand, TCR/MHC interactions are at least partially maintained, because B cells differentiated from recipient hematopoietic stem cells are still being generated. Moreover, during intrathymic development, thymocytes that have high affinity to self MHC molecules are deleted from the repertoire in a process known as negative selection. Thymocytes from both the recipient and the donor mature on the thymic epithelium expressing MHC molecules with the recipient haplotype. Nevertheless, the repertoire of T cells, which react with high affinity to MHC molecules with the donor haplotype, eliminated in mixed chimera. This implies that bone marrow-derived cells must be able to induce negative selection. Actually, negative selection in the thymus can be mediated by several different cells. The most important of these are the BM-derived dendritic cells and macrophages. In mixed chimera, the dendritic cells and macrophages differentiated from both donor and host hematopoietic stem cells are located in the thymus, where they eliminate T cells with strong reactivity to self-peptides on both donor and host MHC; thus donor- and host-specific tolerance to each other is established.

To summarize, mixed chimerism offers several advantages over full chimerism as a means of treating autoimmune disease:

1. Mixed chimeras exhibit superior immune-competence across complete MHC barriers. Mixed chimeras possess certain populations of antigen presenting cells (APCs) and B cells which express host-type MHC molecules in the periphery, whereas mixed chimeras exhibit normal humoral and cellular immune responses.
2. In mixed chimeras, dendritic cells and macrophages differentiated from both the recipient and the donor hematopoietic stem cells locate to the thymus where they delete both host-reactive and donor-reactive T cells through negative selection, resulting in a

peripheral T cell repertoire that is tolerant toward both donor and host cells. Therefore, GVHD, one of the most important complications of allogeneic BMT, is not seen in mixed chimeras.

3. Mixed chimerism can be achieved through non-myeloablative regimens, which are generally less toxic than the myeloablative regimens necessary to induce full BM chimerism (this point will be discussed in detail in the next section).

2.2 How is mixed chimerism induced?

As explained above, once specific tolerance is established, the state of mixed chimerism is thought to be stable. The difficulty in establishing stable mixed chimerism lies in blocking the first attack of host peripheral T cells on donor bone marrow stem cells until "tolerized" T cells are renewed in the host thymus. Because host T cells play a dominant role in the rejection of allografts, several methods of deleting host T cells through the injection of various lymphocyte-deleting antibodies along with either total body irradiation or immunosuppressive drugs have been attempted (Tomita et al, 1996. Nikolic et al, 2000). These regimens enabled BM engraftment but were a burden on recipients and frequently made them susceptible to infection. The toxicity of the necessary conditioning regimens has precluded the use of this approach in clinical transplantation.

Another method of inducing allogeneic tolerance involves the temporary inhibition of co-stimulatory interaction between APCs and T cells by injecting blocking antibodies. This method works because T cell activation without proper co-stimulation can induce a state of antigen-specific non-responsiveness (Fig.1).

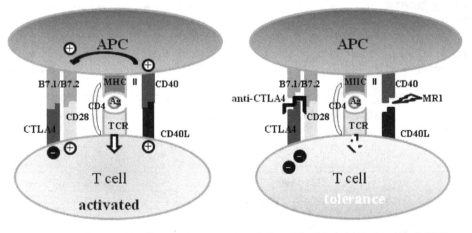

Fig. 1. Activation of naïve T cells requires co-stimulation. Binding of the peptide/MHC complex by the TCR and the CD4 or CD8 co-receptor transmits the first signal to the T cell. Activation of naïve T cells requires a second signal, namely, the ligation of B7 molecules (B7.1/B7.2) and CD28, which stimulates the clonal expansion of naïve T cells. Binding of CD40L by CD40 plays a central role effector function in the full differentiation of T cells. This ligation also activates APCs to express B7 molecules (left). Stimulation of CTLA4 with anti-CTLA4 Ab and/or Blocking CD40/CD40L by MR1 induces antigen-specific T cell tolerance (right).

Recently, Takeuchi et al. have shown that administration of MHC-mismatched donor bone marrow to mice receiving 3Gy TBI one day before BMT and a single injection of Hamster- anti-mouse CD40L monoclonal antibody (MR1, hybridoma) intraperitoneally (i.p.) with BMT permitted the induction of permanent mixed chimerism and tolerance without T cell depletion (Y. Takeuchi et al., 2004). This regimen is quite simple and less toxic than the alternatives, because 3Gy TBI is nonlethal and does not require MHC matching. Therefore we have adopted this regimen for treatment of autoimmune disease in systemic lupus erythematosus (SLE) model mice ("BXSB"mice) and investigated the effect of induction of fully MHC-mismatched bone marrow mixed chimerism (E. Takeuchi & Y. Takeuchi, 2007).

3. Treatment of autoimmune glomerulonephritis in BXSB lupus mice

3.1 BM mixed chimerism can be induced in BXSB mice

BXSB mice spontaneously develop autoimmune disease with features similar to human SLE. The disease is associated with auto-antibodies to self-antigens (Ags) including double strand (ds) DNA, single strand (ss) DNA, anti-platelet antibodies (Abs) and anti-erythrocyte Abs, with accompanying splenomegaly and lymphadenopathy. Immune complex-mediated nephropathy is the hallmark disease associated with the BXSB genotype. Histopathological changes are evident by 10 weeks of age, leading to end-stage renal disease and 70% mortality by 40 weeks of age. We sought to determine whether the simple regimen described above was also effective for the induction of long-term mixed chimerism in BXSB mice. Twenty million normal bone marrow cells from MHC-matched (B6/GFP: H-2^b) or -mismatched (BALB/c: H-2^d) donors were injected with 2.0mg MR1 (i.p.) to seven-week old BXSB mice (H-2^b) that had received a nonlethal dose of 4Gy TBI one day prior to BMT. We increased the TBI dose for BXSB mice from 3 to 4Gy because BXSB mice are more resistant to engraftment than normal recipients are. This regimen allowed the induction of multi-lineage mixed chimerism in 70-90% of host BXSB mice.

As shown in Table 1 and Fig.2, long-term stable chimerism was observed in MHC-mismatched chimeric mice. No clinical signs of GVHD were seen during the observation period.

	CD4 T cell	CD8 T cell	B cell	macrophage
20wks after BMT	73.9 ± 11.3	46.9 ± 10.8	51.0 ± 11.8	94.9 ± 4.02
40wks after BMT	78.1 ± 13.1	56.1 ± 17.6	68.6 ± 14.4	85.2 ± 7.75

Table 1. The percentage of donor cells among PBL of chimeric mice. (n=9)

To confirm the establishment of donor-specific tolerance, chimeric BXSB mice also received skin grafts from a BM donor and a third party (C3H/HeN, H-2^k) one day after BMT. All chimeric BXSB mice accepted the donor skin, but rejected the third-party skin grafts within 20 days (Fig.3), indicating that chimeric BXSB mice acquired donor-specific tolerance without immune-deficiencies (E. Takeuchi, 2011).

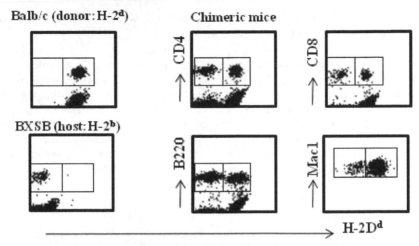

Fig. 2. An example of chimerism in peripheral blood lymphocytes (PBL).
The percentage of BALB/c (H-2D^d) donor cells present among PBL of various lineages was analyzed through two-color FACS. These data were obtained 24 weeks after BMT.

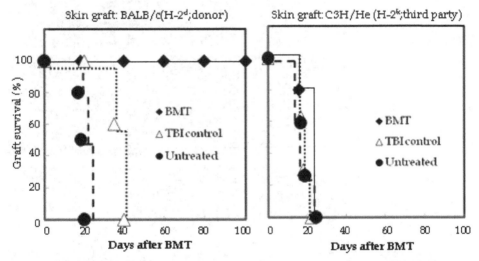

Fig. 3. Donor-specific skin graft tolerance. Donor and third-party skin was grafted 1 day post-BMT. Chimeric mice receiving MHC-mismatched BALB/c BM (◆BMT: n=9) accepted BALB/c skin grafts permanently, while third-party skin was rejected. Mice treated with TBI and anti-CD40L Ab (△: n=5) and mice receiving no treatment (●:n=5) rejected both donor and third-party skin.

These results indicate that, with regard to reciprocal tolerant between donor and host, T cells in stable mixed chimeric mice do not reject additional tissue grafts transplanted from the same donor. In lupus patients who suffer from renal disorders, and who are treated by means of kidney transplantation, the induction of specific immunologic tolerance to donor antigens would prevent both chronic graft rejection and the side effects associated with chronic, nonspecific immunosuppressive therapy.

3.2 Induction of mixed chimerism suppressed lupus nephritis in BXSB mice

Even when transplanted kidneys are engrafted stably, when pre-existing lupus goes untreated, renal disorder will eventually recur. It is also known, however, that the induction of mixed chimerism reverses the autoimmune state. To evaluate the effect of inducing MHC-matched or MHC-mismatched mixed chimerism, individual kidneys were harvested from experimental mice and tissue sections were stained with periodic acid-Schiff (PAS) for histopathologic examination. None of the donor mouse strains were prone to autoimmune disease (Fig.4A). In both the fully MHC-matched and the fully MHC-mismatched chimeric mice groups, lupus glomerulonephritis was significantly ameliorated compared with that in untreated BXSB mice, as revealed by pathological analysis conducted more than 40 weeks after BMT (Figs.4D and E).

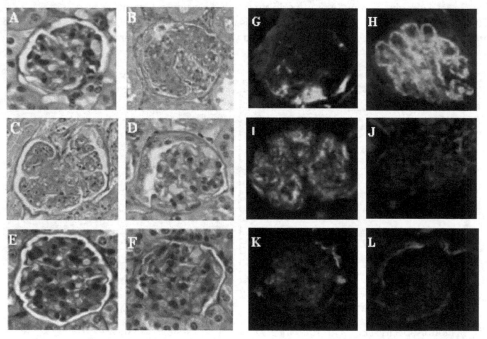

Fig. 4. Kidney sections stained with PAS (left panel) and IF with anti-mouse complement C3 (right panel). Kidneys were harvested from normal control mice or 47-50-week-old (40-43 weeks after BMT) BXSB mice with or without the indicated treatments. C57BL/6 control mice (A and G), untreated BXSB mice (B and H), irradiated BXSB mice (C and I), BALB/c BMT chimeric mice (D and J), GFP/B6 BMT chimeric mice (E and K), BALB/c×GFP/B6 F1 BMT chimeric mice (F and L).

Both untreated (Fig.4B) and irradiated BXSB mice (Fig.4C) exhibited severe glomerulonephritis with PAS-positive deposits. BXSB mice that had received TBI+MR1 exhibited histopathology similar to BXSB mice that had received only TBI (data not shown). For semiquantitative histologic analyses, more than 30 glomeruli from each kidney section were examined. Glomerulonephritis was scored on a scale of 0-4, based on the intensity and extent of histopathological changes [0; no glomerular lesions. 1; minimal thickening of the mesangium. 2; noticeable increase in both mesangeal and glomerular capillary cellularity. 3; same as 2 with the addition of superimposed inflammatory exudates and capsular adhesions. 4; obliteration of the glomerular architecture (>70% of glomeruli)]. Mean renal scores of both MHC-matched and –mismatched chimeric mice were significantly better than those of untreated or irradiated control BXSB mice (BALB/c BMT: 0.97 ± 0.74, GFP/B6 BMT: 0.07 ± 0.26 vs. untreated BXSB: 2.96 ± 0.72, TBI: 1.85 ± 0.77, TBI+MR1: 2.47 ± 3.4, >30 glomeruli from each kidney section in three mice of each group were evaluated. $p<0.05$). We also evaluated immune-complex mediated glomerulonephritis through immunofluorescence (IF) staining with anti-mouse complement C3 in 30 glomeruli per renal section (Fig.4. right panels). Untreated mice and irradiated mice exhibited the peripheral loop pattern (Figs. 4H and I), while almost all glomeruli in the sections from chimeric mice showed negative staining (Figs. 4J and K). Because the cause of death in BXSB mice is most often renal failure, the improvement of their glomerulonephritis may have contributed to the prolongation of their life-spans. These results indicate that the induction of mixed chimerism significantly inhibited the development of lupus-like disease.

It should be noted, however, that the induction of mixed chimerism in BXSB mice could not completely eliminate auto-reactive host lymphocytes because our regimen retains certain stem cells and lymphocytes belonging to the host. This naturally leads to the question of how donor cells reverse the host autoimmune state, which is discussed in the next section.

4. How does BM chimerism reverse the autoimmune state?

4.1 Hypothesis
We and several other groups have shown that the induction of bone marrow mixed chimerism is an effective treatment for and/or means of prevention against the development of autoimmune disease. Previous studies have debated the mechanisms that may be responsible for the reversal of the autoimmune state in BM chimerism, but the mechanism of the exclusion of self-reactive lymphocytes has not yet been conclusively identified. Preceding studies have argued about the mechanisms underlying the reversal of the autoimmune state in BM chimerism. In several studies which reversed destructive autoimmune type I diabetes (NOD mice with induced mixed chimerism), the suppression of autoimmune disease was attributed to reciprocal clonal deletion or to anergy induction of T lymphocytes of recipient and donor origin (Mathieu et al., 1997. Nikolic et al., 2004). Other mechanisms have also been proposed, including induction of peripheral anergy, a change in the Th1/Th2 profile, correction of abnormal secretion of cytokines and positive selection of regulatory T cells in the thymus. Among proposed hypotheses, we have focused on the role of cognate TCR/MHC interactions in the pathogenesis of autoimmune disease in BXSB mice (E. Takeuchi et al., 2011)

4.2 The induction of MHC-mismatched chimerism does not suppress anti-DNA Abs
During the development of their lupus-like autoimmune disease, BXSB mice are known to produce auto-antibodies to self-antigens including dsDNA. We measured serum anti-

dsDNA antibody (anti-DNA Ab) levels by means of ELISA to evaluate whether auto-reactive Abs were eliminated by the induction of mixed chimerism. Actually, the anti-DNA Ab levels in both MHC-matched and MHC-mismatched chimeric mice were lower than those in untreated or irradiated BXSB mice. Meanwhile, anti-DNA Ab levels in fully MHC-matched mixed chimeric mice (GFP/B6 BMT) were not statistically different from those in normal control B6 mice, but those in fully MHC-mismatched mixed chimeric mice (BALB/c BMT) were significantly higher than those in normal controls. This tendency was even more pronounced when anti-DNA IgM levels in the above groups were compared. There were no significant differences in anti-DNA IgM levels between MHC-mismatched chimeric mice and untreated or TBI+MR1 mice, even though total anti-DNA levels were much lower in chimeric mice than in other groups.

These data indicated that anti-DNA Ab producing cells were still present in the BXSB chimeric mice, though they stopped switching iso-types from IgM to IgG in MHC-mismatched chimera. Only in MHC-matched chimeric mice could the expansion of anti-DNA Ab production be suppressed down to a normal level; the induction of fully MHC-mismatched chimerism did not completely suppress or eliminate anti-DNA-producing B cells.

4.3 Selective suppression of auto-reactive antibodies in chimeric mice

In order to distinguish the contributions of donor-type and host-type B cells to anti-dsDNA antibody production, we determined IgM allotypes [IgMa: BALB/c (donor), IgMb: BXSB (host)] in the serum of fully MHC-mismatched (BALB/c→BXSB) chimeric mice 20 weeks after BMT. At this point, the percentage of allogeneic donor B cells in the chimeric mice was 51.0±11.8%, indicating that allogeneic donor and host B cells had contributed equally to the immune response. Surprisingly, however, we found that the majority of the anti-DNA IgM was IgMa (allogeneic donor-type), whereas IgMb (host-type) anti-DNA antibody production was suppressed (Fig. 5A).

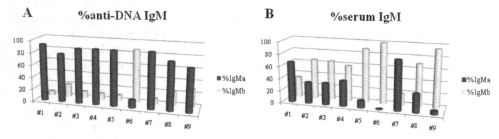

Fig. 5. The ratio of host-type IgM to donor-type IgM. (A) Serum anti-DNA IgM in BALB/c BMT BXSB was measured in each sample by means of ELISA. The percentages of anti-DNA IgMa (donor-type IgM: dark bar) and IgMb (host-type IgM: light bar) add up to the total anti-DNA IgM. (B) Total IgM in each BALB/c BM-transplanted BXSB mouse was measured individually. The percentages of serum IgMa (donor-type IgM: dark bar) and IgMb (host-type IgM: light bar) add up to the total IgM.

The majority of the total serum IgM, on the other hand, was host-type IgMb (Fig. 5B), suggesting that the production of "normal" serum Ig is dependent on host MHC-restricted T cells. Total serum IgM levels in fully MHC-mismatched chimeric mice were not significantly different from those in other groups (data not shown). These results indicated that normal B cells derived from donor BALB/c mice, rather than genetically lupus-prone host-type B cells, were responsible for anti-DNA antibody production in these chimeric BXSB mice. Thus the regulation of auto-antibody production appears to be under MHC-restriction of the host type. Additionally, to confirm which set of B cells (donor-type or host-type) could react with foreign antigens, sheep red blood cells (SRBC) were administered intraperitoneally to five BALB/c chimeric BXSB mice. Three days after immunization, serum anti-SRBC Ab was detected through flow cytometry. All chimeric mice produced antibodies that were reactive with SRBC. As expected, almost all of the detected anti-SRBC Ab was IgMb (host-type), not IgMa (allogeneic donor-type) (data not shown). In mixed chimeras, all peripheral T cells are supposed to be restricted to host MHC, because of positive selection in the host thymus. T cells in fully MHC-mismatched chimeric mice should therefore be capable of cognate interaction with host-type B cells but not with donor-type B cells. Accordingly, only host-type B cells were activated by antigens through cognate interaction with helper T cells. Donor-type B cells remained "silent" because they could not interact properly with T cells. Interestingly, however, our results indicated the possibility that not only "proper" activation against foreign antigens, but also suppression of auto-reactive antibody production were regulated through TCR/MHC cognate interactions.

4.4 Do T cells survey auto-reactive antibody production?

Based on these data, we drew the following conclusions: 1. Allogeneic BM chimerism ameliorates autoimmune disease, but fully MHC-mismatched chimerism fails to suppress the production of anti-DNA antibodies. 2. In MHC-mismatched mixed chimeras, anti-DNA antibodies are produced by donor-type B cells rather than host-type B cells. 3. In MHC-mismatched chimera, TCRs are restricted to host-type MHC. Accordingly, T cells can recognize only host B cells but not donor B cells. To tie theses conclusions together, we propose a possible T cell surveillance system of mixed chimerism, as depicted in Fig.6.

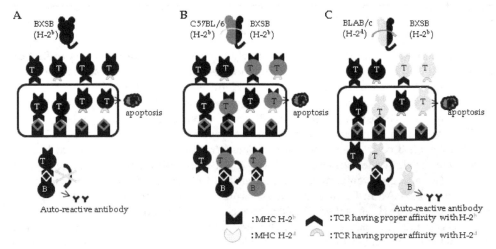

Fig. 6. The proposed of T cell surveillance model.

T cell precursors derived from BM differentiate to mature T cells in the host thymus. Through a process known as positive selection, all T cell populations can interact with self-MHC with proper affinity. Since these processes are performed by MHC molecules expressed on thymic epithelial cells, the TCR repertoire in mixed chimera is restricted to host MHC. We and others speculate that under genetically normal conditions, T cell-mediated trimming of autoantibody production may occur through cognate interactions between TCR and MHC+peptide presented on B cells (Rathmell et al., 1995, Shinohara et al., 1997). In the case of the BXSB mouse, it is known that T cells have certain defects which might play an important role in the pathogenesis of autoimmunity (Wofsy, 1986). We also speculate that the pivotal defect of BXSB may be a genetic defect in this surveillance function of T cells (Fig.6A). In the case of fully MHC-matched chimerism, T cells derived from donor BM can take this place of defective host T cells. Auto-reactive B cells derived from both donor and host BM can be regulated or trimmed by donor T cells through TCR/MHC interactions (Fig.6B). In MHC-mismatched chimerism, immature T cells are positively selected on the basis of their weak reactivity with self-peptides presented exclusively on $H-2^b$ MHC molecules, since thymic epithelial cells express only host MHC. Therefore, in the periphery, all T cells recognize antigens presented by APCs on $H-2^b$ MHC molecules (BXSB: host type MHC). Yet, B cells expressing $H-2^d$ MHC (BALB/c: donor type MHC) are still generated from donor BM stem cells as this process is genetically determined. T cells developing in the BXSB thymus should be incapable of cognate interactions with these "wrong" MHC molecules expressed on donor B cells. We speculate that the failure of cognate interaction with T cells might be the reason why auto-reactive antibody levels rose in MHC fully-mismatched chimeric mice (Fig.6C).

The present study did not address the question of how anti-self B cells were initially triggered. We also induced fully MHC-mismatched BM chimerism in normal B6 mice (BALB/c→B6) as opposed to lupus BXSB mice. The anti-DNA Ab levels seen in BALB/c→B6 chimeric mice were slightly higher than those in normal B6 mice, but, much lower than those seen in BALB/c→BXSB chimeric mice (data not shown). This means that the induction of fully MHC-mismatched chimerism in normal mice may carry a risk of autoantibody production, though uncertain factors in host BXSB mice drives a non-physiological priming of B cells.

4.5 BMT from haplo-identical donor effectively suppressed auto-antibody production

If there is indeed a host-type MHC restriction in the suppression of auto-reactive antibody production, BMT from a donor with partially identical MHC that is sufficient to maintain cognate interaction should be equally as effective as BMT from a fully MHC-matched GFP/B6 mouse. To test this hypothesis, BM cells taken from BALB/c ($H-2^d$) × GFP/B6 ($H-2^b$) F1 mice with haplo-identical MHC ($H-2^{b/d}$) were transplanted to BXSB ($H-2^b$) mice. In this case, all B cells, even those differentiated from donor BM, contained at least one $H-2^b$ allele. As shown in Figs.4F and L, lupus glomerulonephritis in F1 chimeric mice was alleviated to a degree comparable to that seen in MHC-matched GFP/B6 chimeric mice. Serum anti-DNA Ab in F1 chimeric mouse group was decreased to level comparable to that seen in fully MHC-matched GFP/B6 chimeric mice (data not shown).

The survival rates in both the GFP/B6 chimeric mouse group and the F1 chimeric mouse group, which were higher than that in the BALB/c chimeric mouse group, indicated that BMT from F1 mice is also effective as a treatment for lupus-like disease in BXSB mice (B6

BMT: 100%, F1 BMT: 80%, vs BALB/c BMT: 70%, TBI+MR1: 60%, TBI: 20%, untreated: 20% survival, 50weeks after BMT). These results suggest that the maintenance of TCR/MHC cognate interaction with all B cells is important in regulating auto-reactive Ab production, and that reconstitution of the T cell surveillance system may reverse the autoimmune state of lupus-like disease in the BXSB mouse. Moreover, our results indicate one possibility for clinical application: BMT between parent and child, both parent→child and child→parent, may be able to reverse the autoimmune state of SLE effectively.

5. Clinical application and unknown risks of mixed chimerism

This paper has demonstrated that the maintenance of TCR/MHC interaction with all B cells is important in regulating auto-reactive Ab production. However, we and several other groups have reported that the induction of fully MHC-mismatched chimerism is certainly effective as a treatment for autoimmunity. How does the induction of fully MHC-mismatched mixed chimerism suppress autoimmune disease? One answer to this question is demonstrated by the results of an immunohistochemical experiment in which we staind for several isotypes of immunoglobulin.

As depicted in Table 2, linear staining patterns with IgG and/or IgM were definitely observed on the glomeruli of kidney sections taken from MHC-mismatched chimeric mice; the same sections were negative for C3 depositions, however. Linear staining with both IgG and C3 was observed on the glomeruli taken from untreated mice.

treatment		C3	IgG	IgG1	IgG2a	IgG3	IgM
Untreated	1	+	-	-	-	-	-
	2	+	M	-	-	M	M
	3	+	-	-	M	-	M
	4	+	+	-	-	+	+
	5	+	+	+	M	-	+
BALB/c BMT	1	M	+	-	-	-	+
	2	-	-	-	-	-	+
	3	-	-	-	-	-	
	4	-	+	-	-	-	+
	5	-	-	-	-	-	+

+: linear staining, -: negative staining M: mesangeal staining

Table 2. Immunofluorescence staining with several isotype Ig of glomeruli.

This indicates that antibodies deposited in fully MHC-mismatched chimeric mice, mainly IgM, did not activate the complements effectively. As a result, lupus glomerulonephritis is milder in chimeric mice than in untreated mice. We presume that class-switching from IgM to other isotypes does not occur on donor anti-dsDNA IgM-producing B cells, since TCR/MHC cognate interactions were disrupted.

Given that T cells could neither activate nor suppress B cells, B cells are expected to be inactive or "silent". In fact, we have confirmed that, when fully MHC-mismatched chimeric mice are immunized with foreign antigen (sheep red blood cells, SRBC), antigen-specific antibodies (anti-SRBC IgM) are mainly produced by host B cells (as mentioned in 4.3). In rare cases, however, especially when immunization with the same antigen is repeated several times, donor B cells accidentally respond and produce specific antibodies. A T cell that is specific for one peptide on an MHC molecule may cross-react with peptides presented by other allogeneic MHC molecules. By these accidental interactions, donor B cells are activated and start to produce specific antibodies. During activation and proliferation, B cells undergo variable-region somatic hypermutation and change their antigen affinity, resulting in the generation of variant immunoglobulins, some of which are thought to bind to the original foreign antigen with higher affinity. However, the potential disadvantage of this process is that some of the antibodies could be auto-reactive.

To test this hypothesis, we induced an auto-cross-reactive antibody (Ab) by introducing a foreign antigen with a homolog to an auto-antigen into a BXSB lupus mouse strain of mixed chimerism with several combinations of donor BM. The titer of auto-cross reactive foreign Ab plateaued at low levels in normal mice and MHC-matched/haplo-identical chimeric mice, but rose higher in BXSB and fully MHC-mismatched chimeric mice (unpublished data). These results indicate that the induction of fully MHC-mismatched chimerism may carry a risk of secondary auto-antibody production.

Under normal conditions, these auto-reactive B cells may be anergic. In lupus patients, however, non-physiological factors may prime auto-reactive B cells. For example, it has been reported that circulating B cell activating factor (BAFF) is elevated in the serum of human patients with lupus, and that the overexpression of BAFF in mice promotes TLR-induced production of auto-antibodies through a T cell independent process (Groom et al., 2007). Under autoimmune conditions, normal B cell may have the potential to run off the rails. The maintenance of TCR/MHC interaction may be a "rein" by which immune-response is controlled in chimeras.

Because several mechanisms have been suggested as drivers of autoimmune disease, further study is necessary to identify each mechanism's role. Nevertheless, our results showing the specific suppression of auto-reactive antibody production suggest the existence of a surveillance system that trims auto-reactive B cells after priming. The reconstitution of this surveillance system through the induction of BM mixed chimerism can be an effective treatment for lupus disease. Moreover, the induction of BM mixed chimerism with haplo-identical donor BM, which maintains cognate T/B interaction with both donor and host cells, can be equally effective as fully MHC-matched donor BM. These results may support the clinical application of BMT as a treatment for lupus disease.

6. Conclusions

Induction of BM mixed chimerism can be useful for treatment of refractory lupus glomerulonephritis. Elucidation the mechanism through which mixed chimerism reverses the autoimmune state is necessary for clinical application.

In this paper, we suggested the existence of T cell surveillance system through TCR/MHC interaction. Through TCR/MHC interaction, T cell-mediated trimming of auto-antibody production may occur under normal condition. The induction of bone marrow mixed chimerism may reverse the auto-immune state through reconstruction of the T cell surveillance system and the maintenance of TCR/MHC interaction with all B cells is important in regulating auto-antibody production.

7. References

Groom, J.R., Fletcher, C.A., Walters, S.N., Grey, S.T., Watt, S.V., Sweet, M.J., & Mackay, F. (2007) BAFF and MyD88 signals promote a lupus like disease independent of T cells. *J Exp Med,* 204, 1959-1971

Janeway, C.A., Travers, P., Walport, M., & Shlomchik, M. (2001) *Immunobiology: The immune system in health and disease,* 5th edition, Garland Publishing, NY. 08153 3624 X.

Mathieu, C., Casteels, K., Bouillon, R., & Wear, M. (1997) Protection against autoimmune diabetes in mixed bone marrow chimeras. *J Immunol,* 158, 1453-1457

Nikolic, B., Takeuchi, Y., Leykin, I., Fudaba, Y., Smith, R.N., & Sykes, M. (2004) Mixed hematopoietic chimerism allows cure of autoimmune diabetes through allogeneic tolerance and reversal of autoimmunity. *Diabetes,* 53, 376-383

Nikolic, B., Zhao, G., Swenson, K., & Sykes M. (2000) A novel application of cyclosporine A in nonmyeloablative pretransplant host conditioning for allogeneic BMT. *Blood,* 96, 1166-1172

Rathmell, J.C., Cooke, M.P., Ho, W.Y., Grein, J., Townsend, S.E., Davis, M.M., & Goodnow, C.C. (1995) CD95 (Fas)-dependent elimination of self-reactive B cells upon interaction with CD4+ T cells. *Nature,* 376, 181-184

Shinohara, N. Komano, H., Lee, M.H., Tachibana, M., & Iwata, M. (1997) CD4+T cells, positive selection, and surveillance of autoantibody production. *The Immunologist,* 5, 121-126

Sykes, M., & Nikolic, B. (2005) Treatment of severe autoimmune disease by stem cell transplantation. *Nature,* 435, 620-627

Takeuchi, E. (2011) Allogenic mixed chimerism prevented autoimmune thrombocytopenia in BXSB lupus mice receiving donor BMT with nonlymphoablative conditioning of low-dose TBI and anti-CD40L mAb. *Kitasato Med J,* 41, 50-56

Takeuchi, E., Shinohara, N., & Takeuchi, Y. (2011) Cognate interaction plays a key role in the surveillance of autoreactive B cells in induced mixed bone marrow chimerism in BXSB lupus mice. *Autoimmunity* [Epub ahead of print]

Takeuchi, E., & Takeuchi, Y. (2007) Allogeneic mixed chimerism induced by nonlymphoablative regimen including donor BMT with low-dose TBI and anti-CD40L cured proliferative glomerulonephritis in lupus mice. *Ann NY Acad Sci,* 1110, 362-367

Takeuchi, Y., Ito, H., Kurtz, J., Wekerle, T., Ho, L., & Sykes, M. (2004) Earlier low-dose TBI or DST overcomes CD8+ T-cell-mediated alloresistance to allogeneic marrow in recipients of anti-CD40L. *Am J Transplant,* 4(1), 31-40

Tomita, Y., Abrar, K., & Sykes, M. (1996) Mechanism by which additional monoclonal antibody (mAB) injections overcome the requirement for thymic irradiation to achieve mixed chimerism in mice receiving bone marrow transplantation after conditioning with anti-T cell mABs and 3Gy whole body irradiation. *Transplantation,* 61(3), 477-485

Wofsy, D. (1986) Administration of monoclonal anti-T cell antibodies retards murine lupus in BXSB mice. *J Immunol,* 136, 4554-4560

5

Differential Diagnosis of the Pulmonary-Renal Syndrome

Martin Kimmel, Niko Braun and Mark Dominik Alscher
Department of Internal Medicine, Division of Nephrology,
Robert-Bosch-Hospital, Stuttgart
Germany

1. Introduction

The pulmonary-renal syndrome involves the combination of diffuse alveolar hemorrhage and a rapid progressive glomerulonephritis (RPGN). It is usually a systemic vasculitis that can led through a vast vasculitic process to life-threatening injury to the involved organs lung and kidney [Niles 1996, Salant 1987, Boyce 1986, Gallagher 2002 & De Groot 2005].
In the differential diagnosis other diseases of acute renal and lung injury with alveolar hemorrhage without RPGN have to be discussed.

2. Pulmonary-renal syndrome

The *diffuse alveolar hemorrhage* is defined by the triad of hemoptysis, diffuse alveolar infiltrates and low hematocrit. However, the clinical presentation is variable (slight cough, progressive dyspnea, manifest hemoptysis) and these symptoms don`t have to occur simultaneously [Hauber 2007]. Slowly protracted courses through to fulminant organ failure are described.
A *rapid-progressive glomerulonephritis (RPGN)* is manifested by a rapidly progressive renal function loss (a few days to few weeks) and the presence of a nephritic sediment with deformed erythrocytes of a glomerular origin and possibly red cell casts.

2.1 Pathophysiology

The underlying cause of a pulmonary-renal syndrome is usually a systemic vasculitis of the small pulmonary and renal vessels. These vasculitides have a heterogeneous pathogenesis - there are three different pathophysiological mechanisms of injury [Niles 1996, Salant 1987 & De Groot 2005]:
1. mediated by anti-neutrophil-cytoplasmic antibodies (ANCA),
2. immune-complex mediated vasculitis of small vessels or
3. by antibodies against the glomerular basement membrane (Goodpasture   Syndrome).

In the kidney a *RPGN* is caused by damage of the capillaries and basal membranes with leakage of erythrocytes, followed by an influx of macrophages, fibrinogen and the formation of extracapillary cell proliferation (so called crescents) [Salant 1987].
In the lungs, a *diffuse alveolar hemorrhage* is caused by a pulmonary capillaritis [Hauber 2007]. In the case of ANCA-associated systemic vasculitis the detection of ANCA is possible in ~ 80% of patients. Besides the correlation of ANCA titers with disease activity, there is

evidence of a pathogenetic role of ANCA. Myeloperoxidase (MPO) and proteinase 3 (Pr3) are detected in the cytoplasm of non-stimulated neutrophils. It is assumed that cytokines (e.g. TNF, interleukins) raise the expression of Pr3 and MPO on the cell surface of granulocytes and thus a reaction of these antigens with ANCA is possible. This process leads to activation of granulocytes and release of adhesion molecules to the interaction of leukocytes with vascular endothelial cells. Finally cell necrosis and apoptosis contribute to vascular inflammation process [Bosch 2006].

2.2 Diagnosis
2.2.1 Basic steps
As with any systemic vasculitis the diagnosis of pulmonary-renal syndrome is made in three steps:
1.   *Adequate evaluation and networking* of existing and past patient's symptoms.
2.   *Establishing the diagnosis* by laboratory, technical and biopsy examinations.
3.   Differential diagnosis of vasculitis.

2.2.2 Imaging
The value of imaging refers to the extent of pulmonary capillaritis resulting in *diffuse alveolar hemorrhage*: in a conventional X-ray or in a computer tomography of the chest confluent or mixed interstitial-alveolar infiltrates are found (Fig. 1).

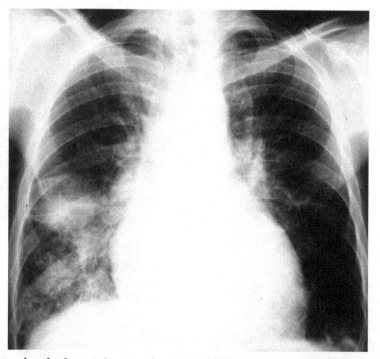

Fig. 1. Diffuse alveolar hemorrhage in chest x-ray in Wegener's granulomatosis.

In a RPGN sonographically enlarged kidneys presents with a wide parenchym area.

2.2.3 Serology

Antibodies against the glomerular basement membrane (GBM) can be found typically in the rare Goodpasture's syndrome (Tab. 1).

The above briefly described heterogeneous pathogenesis of small vessels vasculitis results in the immunological classification considering serological / immunological parameters such as anti-neutrophil-cytoplasmic antibodies (ANCA) by immunfluorescence-optical findings (perinuclear or cytoplasmtic fluorescence) or ELISA against the target antigen proteinase 3 or myeloperoxidase (Tab. 1) [Bosch 2006]. In addition, the eosinophils, IgE and the extended autoimmunserology: anti-nuclear factor (ANA), anti-ds-DNA, C3, C4 and cryoglobulins can be determined.

Disease	Proteinase-3-Antibody	Myeloperoxidase (MPO-)-Antibody	ANCA negative	Anti-GBM-Ab
Wegener`s Granulomatosis	70 %	20 %	10 %	<10%
Microscopic Polyangiitis	30 %	60 %	10 %	<10%
Churg-Strauss-Syndrome	10 %	60 %	30 %	<10%
Goodpasture Syndrome	<10%	<30%	70%	95%

Table 1. ANCA-Sensitivity.

The rapid availability of these antibodies has improved the time to establish an early diagnosis, which is prognostically relevant [Saxena 1995].

2.2.4 Renal biopsy

The diagnosis of RPGN is done by renal biopsy: in light microscopy there is a glomerulonephritis with crescent formation in the Bowman's capsule compartment (extracapillary proliferation) in more than 50% of the glomeruli. The further work is carried out by immunohistochemistry and electron microscopy.

In immunohistology, the type of immunoglobulins and the deposition pattern (capillary, mesangial, granular, linear along the glomerular basement membrane) differ. Only in Goodpasture syndrome, linear deposits are found along the glomerular basement membrane. In case of an ANCA triggered form immune deposits are missing (pauci-immune RPGN). In contrast, in immune-complex vaculitis there can be found a different picture, usually with granular deposition of IgG, IgM, IgA or complement.

2.2.5 Bronchoscopy

The diagnosis of *diffuse alveolar hemorrhage* includes the clinical picture and a brochoscopy with a bronchoalveolar lavage and the microscopic detection of siderophages. Especially in the case of diffuse infiltrates in imaging without hemopytsis a bronchoscopy can be helpful and a definite diagnosis can be established [Hauber 2007].

3. Differential diagnosis of the pulmonary-renal syndrome

As already stated the pulmonary-renal syndrome is usally caused by a systemic small vessels vasculitis (Tab. 2), these can be categorized [Niles 1996, Salant 1987, De Groot 2005, Jennette 1994 & Falk 1997]:
- morphological criteria (size of the infesting vessels, presence or absence of granulomas),
- etiological criteria (idiopathic or secondary forms) and
- immunological criteria (ANCA-associated vasculitis, immune-complex vasculitis or caused by anti-basement antibodies).

3.1 ANCA-associated small vessel vasculitis
The Chapel Hill Consensus Conference classification defines [Jennette 1994]:
1. Wegener's granulomatosis,
2. microscopic polyangiitis and
3. Churg-Strauss syndrome.

Renal involvement is present in many systemic diseases, especially in the small vessel vasculitis – pointed out by Gallo in the New England Journal of Medicine: "The kidney is often a window on systemic disease" [Gallo 1991].

The suspicion of a pulmonary-renal syndrome in an ANCA-associated systemic vasculitis can often be taken from a careful history and thorough clinical examination with detection of other vasculitic signs (eye inflammation, intractable rhinitis / sinusitis, skin rashes, arthralgia, myalgia or polyneuropathy) (Fig. 2).

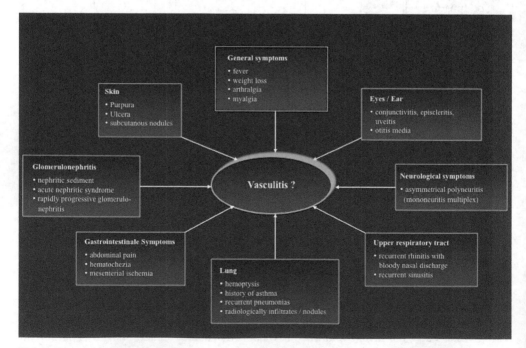

Fig. 2. General symptoms and signs of organ involvement in systemic small vessels vasculitis.

	ANCA-vasculitis				
	WG	**MP**	**CSS**	**GP**	**SLE**
Clinical presentation					
Vasculitic general symptoms	+	+	+	-	+
Granulomatous inflammation	+	-	+	-	-
Eye involvement	+	(+)	(+)	-	(+)
Recurrent asthma bronchiale	-	-	+	-	-
Pulmonary-renal syndrome possible	+	+	(+)	+	(+)
Skin (purpura, necrosis)	+	+	+	-	+
Gastrointestinal symptoms	(+)	(+)	(+)	-	(+)
	WG	**MP**	**CSS**	**GP**	**SLE**
Laboratory workup					
ANCA	80 - 90 %	80 - 90 %	50 - 70 %		
Pr3-antibody	~ 70 %	~ 30 %	~ 10 %	< 30 %	-
MPO-antibody	~ 20 %	~ 60 %	~ 60 %		
Eosinophilia	-	-	+	-	-
Reduced complement levels	-	-	-	-	+
Anti-ds-DNA	-	-	-	-	+
Anti-GBM-Ab	-	-	-	95%	-
Histology/Immunohistology					
Leucocytoclastic vasculitis	+	+	+	-	+
Granulomatous inflammation	+	-	+	-	-
Eosinophil granulomatous inflammation	-	-	+	-	-
Kidney Biopsy					
Light microscopy	necrotising intra- and extracapillary proliferative GN			necrotising intra- and extracapillary proliferative GN	Lupus-nephritis
Immunohistology	pauci-immune GN without immune-complex deposits			linear IgG-deposits in the glomerular basement membrane	granular deposits of IgG, IgM, IgA and complement factors

WG = Wegener's Granulomatosis. MP = microscopic polyangiitis. CSS = Churg-Strauss syndrome. GP = Goodpasture's Syndrome SLE = systemic lupus erythematosus. ANCA = antineutrophil cytoplasmic antibodies. PR-3 = proteinase-3. MPO = myeloperoxidase. IC = immune complex. GBM = Glomerular basement membrane. ds = double strand.

Table 2. The most important differential diagnoses of pulmonary-renal syndrome with clinical features, laboratory and histological findings.

3.1.1 Wegener's granulomatosis

Wegener's granulomatosis is a necrotizing vasculitis of the small and medium-sized vessels, associated with granulomas inflammation of the upper and lower respiratory tract and the frequent finding of glomerulonephritis. In active disease in about 90% of cases c-ANCA are directed against proteinase 3 (Tab. 1 and 2). Figure 3 shows the predominant symptoms in image and Figure 4 in number (at onset and during disease) [Hoffmann 1992].

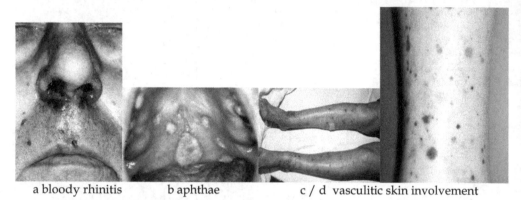

a bloody rhinitis   b aphthae   c / d vasculitic skin involvement

Fig. 3. Wegener's granulomatosis.

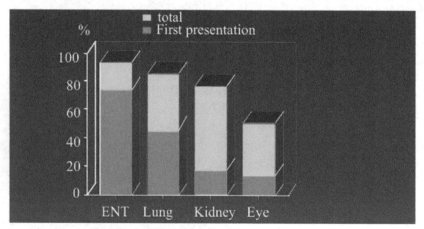

Fig. 4. Organ involvement in Wegener's granulomatosis.

3.1.2 Microscopic polyangiitis

Microscopic polyangiitis is characterized by a necrotizing vasculitis of small vessels with minimal or missing immune deposits and an inflammation of the pulmonary capillaries. Typically, there are p-ANCA directed against myeloperoxidase (Tab. 1 and 2) [Jennette 1994 & Falk 1997]. Wegener`s granulomatosis and Microscopic polyangiitis shows comparable organ involvement, but the symptoms of the upper respiratory tract are usally milder in Microscopic polyangiitis, because there is no granulomatous inflammation. Compared to Wegener's granulomatosis disease recurrence is rare in patients with Microscopic polyangiitis.

3.1.3 Churg-Strauss syndrome

The Churg-Strauss syndrome is characterized by recurrent asthma attacks and allergic rhinitis, an intermittently or permanently detectable eosinophilia (> $1500/mm^3$) and necrotizing granulomas and / or necrotizing arteritis with a Wegner's granulomatosis-like presentation. The serological diagnosis is less clear: c-ANCA or anti-PR3-Ab detected only rarely, p-ANCA and anti-MPO-Ab can be detected in up to 60% of cases (Tab. 1 and 2) [Hoffmann 1992].

The Churg-Strauss syndrome can be distinguished clinically (asthma attacks, eosinophilia) from Wegener`s granulomatosis or Microscopic polyangiits. Renal involvement is seen in approximately 25% of patients.

3.2 Goodpasture syndrome

The Goodpasture's syndrome is a rare disease with an incidence of 0.1-1 per million per year and affects mainly caucasian males. It is characterized by hemoptysis and / or radiological evidence of pulmonary infiltrates and a RPGN, which usually develops after hemoptysis. There is the very reliable detection of anti-GBM antibody, the identified antigen is the C-terminal end of the alpha-3-chain of type IV collagen. The immunohistological workup of the renal biopsy shows linear IgG deposits in the glomerular basement membranes (Tab. 1 and 2) [Goodpasture 1919, Salama 2001, Pusey 2003 & Hudson 2003].

Compared to the ANCA-associated small vessel vasculitidies (Wegener`s Granulomatosis, Microscopic polyangiitis and Churg-Strauss syndrome) there are no other, general vasculitic symptoms in patients with Goodpasture syndrome.

3.3 Immune-complex vasculitis of small vessels

Immune-complex vasculitidies like
1.   systemic lupus erythematosus,
2.   cryoglobulinemic vasculitis and
3.   Purpura Schoenlein-Hennoch [Markus 1989]
are important differential diagnostic considerations of the pulmonary-renal syndrome.

They can be distinguished by the previously described extended-serological diagnostic workup.

3.4 Further differential diagnoses

If this diagnostic workup is unremarkable, there are several more differential diagnosis:
1.   antiphospholipid syndrome with vasculitis and / or pulmonary embolism
2.   mixed connective tissue diseases (systemic sclerosis, polymyositis)
3.   thrombotic thrombozypenic purpura.
4.   infectious diseases involving kidney and lung (e.g Hanta-virus, cytomegalie-virus, Legionella, Mycoplasma, Leptospirosis, tuberculosis, sepsis)

Moreover, a primary renal disease can lead to a pulmonary disease and mimic the image of a pulmonary-renal syndrome:
1.   acute renal failure with pulmonary edema and uremic hemoptysis
2.   thromboembolism in nephrotic syndrome: renal vein thrombosis and/ or pulmonary embolism
3.   immunosuppression in renal disease and a pneumonia.

Conversely, a primary pulmonary disease can lead to renal disease and can mimic the image of pulmonary-renal syndrome:

1. Infection of the respiratory tract with prerenal renal failure and / or postinfectious glomerulonephritis or hematuria in IgA nephropathy
2. Lung cancer with immune-complex nephritis.

4. Conclusions

Since early treatment with the mentioned diseases is critical, the diagnosis has to be established quickly - the fast antibody-diagnostic and diagnostic imaging have a central role.

5. Acknowledgment

This work was supported by the Robert-Bosch Foundation.

6. References

Niles JL et al. The syndrome of lung hemorrhage and nephritis is usually an ANCA-associated condition. *Arch Intern Med* 1996; 156: 440-445.

Salant, DJ. Immunopathogenesis of crescentic glomerulonephritis and lung purpura. *Kidney Int* 1987; 32: 408-425.

Boyce NW, Holdsworth SR. Pulmonary manifestations of the clinical syndrome of acute glomerulonephritis and lung hemorrhage. *Am J Kidney Dis* 1986; 8: 31-36.

Gallagher H, Kwan JT, Jayne DR. Pulmonary renal syndrome: A 4-year, single-center experience. *Am J Kidney Dis* 2002; 39: 42-47.

De Groot K, Schnabel A. *Internist* (Berl). 2005; 46: 769-781.

Hauber HP, Zabel P. Lunge und Autoimmunerkrankungen – Klinik und Diagnostik. *Dtsch Med Wochenschr* 2007; 132: 1633-1638.

Bosch X, Guilabert A, Font J. Antineutrophil cytoplasmic antibodies. *Lancet* 2006; 368: 404-418.

Saxena et al., Circulating autoantibodies as serological markers in the differential diagnosis of pulmonary renal syndrome. *J Intern Med* 1995; 238: 143-152.

Jennette JC et al. Nomenclature of systemic vasculitides: Proposal of an international consensus conference. *Arthritis Rheum* 1994; 37, 187-192.

Falk RJ, Jennette JC. ANCA small-vessel vasculitis. *J Am Soc Nephrol* 1997; 314-322.

Gallo G. Renal complications of B-cell dyscrasias. *N Engl J Med* 1991; 324: 1889- 1990.

Hoffmann GS et al. Wegener granulomatosis: an analysis of 158 patients. *Ann Intern Med.* 1992;116: 488-498.

Masi AT et al. The American College of Rheumatology 1990 criteria for the classification of the Churg-Strauss syndrome (allergic granulomatosis and angiitis). *Arthritis Rheum* 1990; 33: 1094-1100.

Goodpasture EW. The significance of certain pulmonary lesions in relation to the aetiology of pneumonia. *Am J Med Sci* 1919; 158: 863-870.

Salama AD et al. Goodpastures`s disease. *Lancet* 2001; 358: 917-920.

Pusey CD. Anti-glomerular basement membrane disease. *Kidney Int* 2003; 64: 1535-1550.

Hudson BG et al. Alport`s syndrome, Goodpasture`s syndrome, and type IV collagen. *N Engl J Med 2003*; 348: 2543-2556.

Markus HS, Clark JV. Pulmonary hemorrhage in Henoch-Schönlein purpura. *Thorax* 1989; 44: 525-526.

6

RPGN - Clinical Features, Treatment and Prognosis

Mitra Naseri
Mashhad University of Medical Sciences,
Islamic Republic of Iran

1. Introduction

Rapidly progressive glomerulonephritis (RPGN) is one of the nephrology emergencies which needs special attention. RPGN is a clinical description which determines by symptoms and signs of glomerulonephritis (GN); edema, hypertension and gross hematuria, and evidence of acute renal failure(severe decrease in glomerular filtration rate presents as oliguria or anuria, and increased serum levels of BUN and creatinine). Definite diagnosis of the disorder is based on kidney biopsy's findings. Early diagnosis and appropriate treatment plays a critical role in renal saving and preventing permanent glomerular damage.

This chapter will focus on clinical manifestations, therapeutic protocols and prognostic factors in patients with different subtypes of RPGN.

Rapidly progressive glomerulonephritis (RPGN) is defined as a syndrome with abrupt or insidious onset of hematuria, proteinuria, anemia, and rapidly progressing acute renal failure(ARF), and special findings on light microscopy examination of kidney biopsy's specimen; crescentic lesions which usually involved most glomerular architectures (Hirayama, et al., 2008; Rutgersetal., 2004). It also characterized by rapid loss of renal function (GFR<50% within 3 months)with histological findings of crescent lesions which usually involves>50 % of glomeruli (Couser, 1988).

RPGN can be primary or secondary. Secondary forms occur in any form of severe glomerulonephritis including membranoproliferative GN, IgA nephropathy, post infectious GN, and systemic lupus erythematous (SLE). Primary RPGN is an autoimmune disease which is divided into three immunopathologic categories:(Rutgerset al., 2004; Haas .& Eustace, 2004):

Type 1 RPGN: glomerulonephritis with antibodies directed against the glomerular basement membrane (GBM) (anti-GBM mediated GN)

Type II RPGN: immune-complex induced glomerulonephritis

Type III RPGN: Antineutrophil cytoplasmic antibody associated glomerulonephritis (ANCA-associated glomerulonephritis or pauci-immune GN)

RPGN type 1 and 2 are responsible for 10-20 % and 40 % of all cases respectively. **RPGN type 2** can be found in different forms of systemic disease such as post infectious GN(PSGN), Ig-A nephropathy, Henoch–Schönlein purpura (HSP), SLE, membranous GN(MGN) or membrano- proliferative GN(MPGN). A few cases of idiopathic immune-complex-mediated RPGN have been reported (Jindal, 1999).

Interestingly different forms of RPGN share similar clinical features including hematuria, proteinuria, edema, hypertension and symptoms of ARF .patients with Anti –GBM anti - body or pauci-immune RPGN (ANCA-associated vasculitis) may have pulmonary hemorrhage and hemoptysis (Jindal, 1999). In pauci-immune RPGN the initial symptoms are non-specific; often fatigue, fever, night sweats and artheralgias are first clinical manifestations (Jindal, 1999).

2. Histopathology characteristics of RPGN and laboratory findings

Variable clinical manifestations and non-specific histologic changes complicate diagnosis and classification of vasculitis .To confirm the diagnosis light microscopy and immuno - fluorescence examinations of kidney biopsy shouldbe accompanied by appropriate serologic tests, includingANCA (Vizjak et al., 2003).

2.1 Light microscopy findings

Histopathologically, RPGN is characterized by avasculitis which involves glomerular capillaries, and results in formation of cellular crescents within most glomeruli (Hricik et al., 1998). The hallmark histologic lesions are crescents; a morphologic expression of severe glomerular injury. In severe glomerular injury rupture of the glomerular capillaries allows inflammatory mediators to spill into Bowman's space, resulting in epithelial cell proliferation and invasion of monocyte and macrophage to Bowman's space (Couser, 1988; Jennette & Falk, 1998; Jennette &Thomas, 2001). Crescents are divided into cellular, fibro cellular or fibrous types. Halmarks of irreversible glomerular or tubulointerstitial injuries are glomerular sclerosis, fibrous or fibro cellular crescents, and interstitial fibrosis.The lesions usually are seen in various stages of activity or resolution.Necrotizing inflammation in small cortical arteries is reported in 10 % of biopsy specimens .Inflammation of medullary vasa rectae with papillary necrosis is another finding that may be found(Lionakiet al., 2007).

In acute pauci-immune glomerulonephritis(RPGN type III) fibrinoid necrosis accompanies crescents. These lesions occur at the same frequency irrespective of the presence or absence of associated vasculitis (DAgati et al., 1986). Acute lesions range from focal segmental fibrinoid necrosis affecting less than 10 %of glomeruli to severe diffuse necrotizing and crescentic glomerulonephritis that may injure all glomeruli.Periglomerular granulomatous inflammation may occur, but is not specific for pauci-immune glomerulonephritis (Lionakiet al., 2007).

3. Histopathology characteristics on immunoflurecent microscopy

Anti-GBM glomerulonephritis characterized by linear staining for IgG and usually C3 along the glomerular capillary. Immune complex-mediated glomerulonephritis, which is found in severe forms of various types of glomerulonephritis such as PSGN, IgA nephropathy, and lupus nephritis, characterized by granular glomerular staining for one or more immuno-globulins and/or complement components, and pauci-immune glomerulonephritis characterized by mild or absent glomerular tuft staining for immunoglobulins and/or complement (Rutgerset al., 2004) .

Anti-neutrophil cytoplasmic antibodies(ANCAs) associated glomerulonephritis are usually pauci immune; however, immunofluorescence microscopy often reveals a low level of staining (less than +2, in the 0–4 scale (Harriset al., 1998). **Figure 1** presents histologic findings in light and immunoflurecent microscopy.

3.1 Electron microscopy findings
On electron microscopy examination absence of electron-dense immune complex deposits (type I RPGN), multiple electron-dense deposits (type II RPGN), and few or no electron-dense deposits (typeIII RPGN) are main findings **(figure 2)**(Haas, M.&Eustace, 2004).

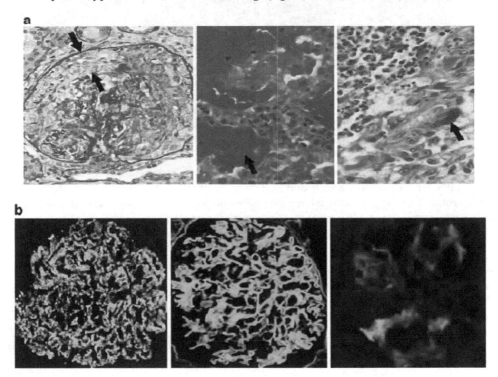

Fig. 1. Histopathologic findings in light and immunoflurecent microscopy (Lionakiet al., 2007) **a/left**; light microscopic demonstration of ANCA-associated necrotizing GN (with a crescent), arrows; (alveolar capillaritis with intra-alveolar hemorrhage); arrow; **middle** (and pulmonary necrotizing granulomatous inflammation with a multinucleated giant cell) arrow; **right** **b/middle**; Immunofluorescence microscopy can separate crescentic glomerulonephritis into anti-GBM with linear IgG staining, (**left**) immune complex with granular staining, (**right**); or pauci-immune categories with little or no immunoglobulin staining

4. Anti-neutrophil cytoplasmic and anti-GBM antibodies

Anti-neutrophil cytoplasmic antibodies(ANCAs)are characteristic markers of small vessel vasculitides; Wegener'sgranulomatosis(WG), Microscopic polyangiitis(MPA), Churg-Strauss Syndrome(CSS), and idiopathic pauci-immune necrotizing glomerulonephritis for them the term ANCA associated vasculitides(AAV) has long being used(Jennette et al., 1989).

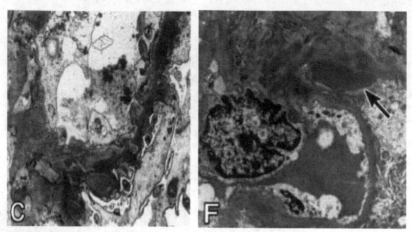

Fig. 2. Electron microscopy findings (Haas, M. &Eustace, 2004)
C: Electron microscopy showing multiple sub-epithelial electron-dense deposits, some appearing partially resorbed, with extension of the glomerular basement membrane (GBM) around the deposits (uranyl acetate and lead citrate stain, original magnification ×6300)
F: Electron microscopy showing a large subepithelial deposit in a "notch" area (arrow), as well as mesangial deposits (uranylacetate and lead citrate stain, original magnification×3800).

The standard approach for detection of ANCA is indirect immunofluorescence (IIF) technique followed by antigen-specific quantitative assays .Myeloperoxidase (MPO) and proteinase3 (PR3) are major ANCA antigens (Falk .&Jennette, 1988; Goldschmeding et al., 1989; Niles et al., 1989).

In patients with RPGN, there are two major sub classes of ANCA, namely perinuclear (p -ANCA) and cytoplasmic (c -ANCA) (Guillevinet al., 1999) .The main epitope of p-ANCA is myeloperoxidase(MPO), and that of c-ANCA is proteinase-3 (PR3) (Asarodet al., 2000). MPO-ANCAis a useful serum marker for MPA and idiopathic pauci-immune crescentic GN, and PR3-ANCA is regarded as a serum marker for Wegener's granulomatosis and MPA (Asarodet al., 2000). Majority (approximately80- 85%) of cases of pauci-immune crescentic glomerulonephritis are ANCA positive(Haueret al., 2002;Jennette, 2003). Greater than 95% of cytoplasmic ANCA are PR3-ANCA and >95 %of perinuclear ANCA are MPO-ANCA (Lionakiet al., 2007). The c and p-ANCAs are mostly directed against the azurophilic granule proteins proteinase 3 (PR3)and myeloperoxidase (MPO), respectively .Detection of c and especially p-ANCAs are not equivalent to the presence of PR3-and MPO-ANCA. It is recommended to detect ANCA by an antigen-specific ELISA (Savigeet al., 2000; Cohen Tervaert et al., 1991).

Anti-GBM antibodies which are directed to the non-collagenous part ofthe α 3 chain of type IV collagen, can also be evaluated byboth IIF and ELISA(Rutgerset al., 2004) .The ANCA-GBM dot-blot is a qualitative assay that uses nitrocellulose strips on which purified antigens are blotted at preset spots .MPO and PR3 antigens that are used in these tests are produced from human leukocytes .The GBM-ANCA dot-blot assay has been revealed reactivities that had not been detected by ELISA(**Table 1**) (Rutgers et al., 2004).

	MPO-ANCA	PR3-ANCA	Anti-GBM antibodies
Sensitivity	80–86%[a]	92–95%[a]	100%
Specificity	100%	100%	91–94%[a]
Inter-observer effect	5%	1%	8–24%[b]

Table 1. Characteristics of the GBM-ANCA Dot-Blot Assay (Rutgerset al., 2004)

5. RPGN, Pulmonary–renal syndrome (PRS), and ANCA-associated vasculitis (AAVs)

The ANCA-associated vasculitis(WG, MPA, and CSS) are a group of rare autoimmune conditions characterized by the development of necrotizing vasculitis .They share a number of clinical features and are therefore treated using similar treatment protocols.

The AAVs are rare with an annual incidence of 20/million in Europe, with WG as the most common and CSS the least frequent (Ntatsaki et al., 2010).In far-east, MPA is more common than WG .It's thought that they arise from interaction between an environmental factor and a genetically predisposing agent(Ntatsaki et al., 2011).

Pulmonary–renal syndrome (PRS) is defined as combination of diffuse alveolar hemorrhage (DAH) and glomerulonephritis(Savageet al., 1997;Seo& Stone, 2004;Jennette& Falk, 2003).

This syndrome is caused by different diseases, including various forms of primary systemic vasculitis especially WG and MPA, ANCA-associated systemic vasculitis(AAV), Good pasture's syndrome, SLE, and infection-associated or drug induced glomerulonephritis (Westmanm et al., 1997;Brusselle, 2007).

Immunologic injuries or non-immunologic mechanisms are involved in pathogenesis of PRS .Immunologic mechanisms such as production of anti-GBM antibodies, ANCA, immune complexes mediated injuries and non-immunologic mechanisms such as thrombotic microangiopathy(Rondeauet al., 1989)have been suggested .Pulmonary involvement in the majority of cases is the result of small-vessel vasculitis that involves arterioles, venules and alveolar capillaries (necrotic pulmonary capillaritis). These lesions are clinically expressed with DAH(Levy. &Winearls, 1994). In the majority of cases the underlying renal pathology is a form of focal proliferative glomerulonephritis (Jayne et al., 2000), with fibrinoid necrosis, as well as micro vascular thrombi, and extensive crescent formation accompanies glomerular tuft disease (Walters et al., 2010).

According to results of ANCA pulmonary renal syndrome can be categorized into two sub-groups:

1. ANCA-positive Pulmonary–renal syndrome
2. ANCA-negative Pulmonary–renal syndrome

Circulating ANCAs are detected in the majority of pulmonary–renal syndromes(The Wegener's Granulomatosis Etanercept Trial [WGET] Research Group2005; Dickersinet al., 1994.)Three major systemic vasculitis syndromes are associated with positive ANCAs consists of Wegener's granulomatosis, microscopic polyangiitis and Churg–Strauss syndrome (The Wegener's Granulomatosis Etanercept Trial[WGET]Research Group, 2005), and idiopathic pulmonary–renal syndrome(Bolton&turgill, 1989).

Majority of cases of pulmonary-renal syndromes are related to ANCA associated vasculitis (Brusselle, 2007).Pulmonary–renal syndrome in ANCA-negative systemic vasculitis is very rare and has been reported in Behçet's disease, HSP, IgA nephropathy and in mixed cryo–globulinaemia and rarely in thrombotic thrombocytopenic purpura(TTP)(Naseri & Zabolinejad, 2008).

ANCA-positive Pulmonary–renal syndrome : More than 80 %of patients with necrotizing pauci immune small-vessel vasculitis have circulating ANCA (Jennette .&Falk, 1997). The main clinicopathological expressions of AAV are WG, MPA, CSS and renal-limited vasculitis (RLV). The highest incidence is for WG in northern Europe (Haugebergm etal., 1998; Watts et al., 2000, 2008; Laneet al., 2000; Reinhold-Keller et al., 2005), while the incidence of MPA/RLV is higher in Japan (Fujimotoet al., 2006).

Wegener's granulomatosis (WG): Friedrich Wegener in 1939 was the firsti nvestigator to recognize a group of diseases characterized by extra vascular necrotizing granulomatous inflammation of the respiratory tract with vasculitis and/or glomerulonephritis (Schultz &Tozman, 1995). In 1983, Fauci et al reported details of 85 patients with Wegener's granulomatosis followed over a 21-year period. Their diagnosis was based on upper and lower respiratory tract complications, renal disease, and variable involvement of other organs with disseminated vasculitis .Tissue biopsies confirmed the characteristic clinical findings (Fauciet al., 1983).Pathologically Wegener's granulomatosis was characterized by small-vessel necrotizing vasculitis and granulomatous inflammation involving mostly the upper and lower respiratory tracts and the kidneys (Sugimoto et al., 2007).

Diffuse alveolar hemorrhage is the most serious complication in small-vessel vasculitis. Respiratory symptoms including cough and hemoptysis.CXR or chest CT-scan may reveal diffuse lung infiltrate.Clinical manifestations, pathologic and serologic findings play important role in the diagnosis of WG. 75- 90 %of patients with active disease have PR3-ANCAs (Langford, 2005;, Ozaki, 2007). The role of PR3-ANCA in the pathogenesis of the disease is not clear, but in vitro evidence suggests that PR3-ANCA can directly or indirectly damage endothelial cells (Preston et al., 2002).With the recognition of association between ANCAs and Wegener'sgranulomatosis, the concept of Wegener's granulomatosishas been modified and recently a less restrictive definition has been proposed, termed "Wegener's vasculitis." This term includes ANCA-positive patients with clinical presentations of WG such as sinusitis, pulmonary infiltrates, nephritis, and documented necrotizing vasculitis, but without biopsy-proven granulomatousin flammation. Both classic Wegener's granulomatosis and Wegner's vasculitis are different manifestations of the same disease process.The term "Wegener'ssyndrome "is a more generic term suggested by the working classification of ANCA-associated vasculitides(Tervaert, &Stegeman, 2003).

Diagnostic criteria have been reported by the research group of intractable vasculitis, ministry ofHealth, Labor, and Welfare {MHLW} of Japan for definite diagnosis of AAV including WG (**Table 2**) (Ozaki, 2007).Necrotizing granulomatous lesions commonly affect the ear, nose and throat (E), lung (L), and kidney(K).Systemic symptoms in WG are classified as the following :

1. E Symptoms: nasal symptoms; purulent rhinorrhea, epistaxis, and a saddle nose, eye symptoms; ophthalmic pain, visual disturbance, and exophthalmia, ear symptoms; otalgia and otitis media, and throat symptoms; pharyngeal ulcer, hoarseness, and laryngeal obstruction.

2.   lung (L)symptoms: bloody sputa, cough, and dyspnea
3.   Kidney(K)symptoms :hematuria, proteinuria, rapidly progressive renal failure, edema, and hypertension

---

1. Symptoms
   (1) E symptoms
      Nose (purulent rhinorrhea, epistaxis, and saddle nose)
      Eyes (ophthalmic pain, visual disturbance, and exophthalmia)
      Ears (otalgia and otitis media)
      Throat (pharyngeal ulcer, hoarseness, and laryngeal obstruction)
   (2) L symptoms
      Bloody sputa, cough, and dyspnea
   (3) K symptoms
      Hematuria, proteinuria, rapidly progressive renal failure, edema, and hypertension
   (4) Others due to vasculitis
      (a) General symptoms: fever (38°C or higher, 2 weeks or longer), weight loss (6 kg or more for 6 months)
      (b) Local symptoms: purpura, polyarthritis/polyarthralgia, episcleritis, mononeuritis multiplex, ischemic heart disease, gastrointestinal bleeding, and pleuritis
2. Histological findings
   (1) Necrotizing granulomatous vasculitis with giant cells at the sites of E, L, and/or K
   (2) Necrotizing crescentic glomerulonephritis without immune deposits
   (3) Necrotizing granulomatous vasculitis of arterioles, capillaries, and venules
3. Laboratory findings
   (1) Positive PR3-ANCA (or C-ANCA by an indirect immunofluorescence)
<Diagnosis>
1. Definite WG
   (1) Positive for 3 or more of the symptoms, including E, L, and K symptoms
   (2) Positive for 2 or more of the symptoms, and positive for either of the histological findings
   (3) Positive for 1 or more of the symptoms, positive for either of the histological findings, and positive PR3-ANCA/C-ANCA
2. Probable WG
   (1) Positive for 2 or more of the symptoms
   (2) Positive for 1 of the symptoms, and positive for either of the histological findings
   (3) Positive for 1 of the symptoms, and positive PR3-ANCA/C-ANCA

Table 2. Diagnostic criteria for Wegener's granulomatosis (Ozaki, 2007)

Biopsies of the nasal mucosa, lung, and kidney reveal necrotizing granulomatous vasculitis and necrotizing crescentic glomerulonephritis without immune deposits(Ozaki, 2007). WG with E, L, and K involvement is classified as the generalized form, while when there is no kidney involvement, E only, L only, or E +L, the term of limited form is used. The therapeutic strategies are different for each forms (Ozaki, 2007).

Microscopic polyangiitis (MPA)

Renal and pulmonary symptoms are characteristic in MPA, and interstitial pneumonitis and pulmonary hemorrhage are common clinical features .MPO-ANCA is positive in 50-75% of patients and biopsy of the lung and kidney reveals necrotizing vasculitis of arterioles, capillaries, and venules with few immune deposits necrotizing and crescentic GN (Ozaki; 2007). Granulomatous inflammation and asthma are not seen in MPA (Jennette &Falk, 1997).

Table 3 presents diagnostic criteria for microscopic polyangiitis(Ozaki, 2007).

Allergic granulomatous angiitis (AGA) or Churg-Strauss syndrome(CSS)

Churg and Strauss was firstly described allergic granulomatous angiitis(Churg, & Strauss, 1951). The disease is characterized by presence of asthma, eosinophilia, and necrotizing granulomatous inflammation .Clinical manifestations of small-vessel vasculitis; palpable purpura of the lower extremities, mononeuritis multiplex, abdominal pain, and gastro - intestinal bleeding develop several years after the onset of asthma.Positive MPO-ANCA are seen and skin biopsy shows necrotizing vasculitis of small vessels with massive eosinophilic infiltration and extravascular granulomatosis(Ozaki, 2007). **Table 4** presents diagnostic criteria for CSS(Ozaki, 2007).

---

1. Symptoms
   (1) Rapidly progressive glomerulonephritis
   (2) Pulmonary hemorrhage
   (3) Other organ symptoms:
       Purpura, subcutaneous hemorrhage, gastrointestinal bleeding, and mononeuritis multiplex
2. Histological findings
   (1) Necrotizing vasculitis of arterioles, capillaries, and ve- nules, and perivascular infiltration of inflammatory cells
3. Laboratory findings
   (1) Positive MPO-ANCA
   (2) Positive CRP
   (3) Proteinuria, hematuria, elevation of BUN and serum creatinine
<Diagnosis>
1. Definite MPA
   (1) Positive for 2 or more of the symptoms, and positive histological findings
   (2) Positive for 2 or more of the symptoms including the symptoms (1) and (2), and positive MPO-ANCA
2. Probable MPA
   (1) Positive for 3 of the symptoms
   (2) Positive for 1 of the symptoms, and positive MPO- ANCA

Table 3. Diagnostic criteria for microscopic polyangiitis(Ozaki, 2007)

SLE and AAV

Systemic lupus erythromatosis is an autoimmune disorder .Variety of autoantibodies are present in SLE patients including ANCA which have been reported in 3-69 %of cases(Molnaretal., 2002;Edgar et al., 1995; Pradhan et al., 2004).Some studies(Chinet al., 2000; Nishiyaet al., 1997) have reported p-ANCA in 37.3-42 %of patients with lupus nephritis, mainly those who have diffuse proliferative GN(DPGN), and minority of patients without renal involvement. In Pradhan et al's study predominant ANCA pattern was p-ANCAwhile c-ANCApattern was not found in any patient(Pradhan et al., 2004).Their study revealed that ANCA can be used as a serological marker to differentiate vasculitides in lupus nephritis cases from SLE without nephritis.

1. Symptoms

   (1) Bronchial asthma and/or allergic rhinitis

   (2) Eosinophilia

   (3) Symptoms due to vasculitis

     (a) General symptoms: fever (38°C or higher, 2 weeks or longer), weight loss (6 kg or more for 6 months)

     (b) Local symptoms: mononeuritis multiplex, gastrointestinal bleeding, purpura, polyarthritis/polyarthralgia, and myalgi (muscle weakness)

2. Characteristic clinical course

   (1) Symptoms (1) and (2) precede the development of (3)

3. Histological findings

   (1) Granulomatous or necrotizing vasculitis of small vessels with marked infiltration of eosinophils

   (2) Extravascular granulomas

<Diagnosis>

1. Definite

   (1) Positive for 1 or more of the symptoms (1) and (2), and positive for either of the histological findings (Definite AGA)

   (2) Positive for 3 of the symptoms, and the characteristic clinical course (Definite Churg-Strauss syndrome)

2. Probable

   (1) Positive for 1 of the symptoms, and positive for either of the histological findings (Probable AGA)

   (2) Positive for 3 of the symptoms, but not the characteristic clinical course (Probable Churg-Strauss syndrome)

Table 4. Diagnostic criteria for Churg-Strauss syndrome (Ozaki, 2007)

Organ involvement	ANCA serology			Other autoantibodies				
	anti-MPO (12/59)	anti-LF (10/59)	anti-CG (8/59)	ANA (59/59)	anti-dsDNA (45/59)	anti-ssDNA (40/59)	anti-nRNP (38/59)	anti-Sm (16/59)
Skin (50)	4	0	1	48	42	40	38	16
Renal (41)	12	10	8	34	29	28	28	12
DPGN with crescents (21)	5	3	4	19	16	17	15	3
FPGN with crescents (14) *	5	3	2	12	10	10	9	4
RPGN with crescents (4)	2	4	1	2	2	1	2	3
MPGN with crescents (2)	0	0	1	1	1	0	2	2
Joint (35) **	0	6	3	26	18	20	35	12
Serositis (16)	0	6	2	14	14	12	10	10
Haematological (8)	0	0	2	4	4	5	2	2
GI tract (8)	0	0	2	6	6	4	2	2
CNS (8)	0	0	3	3	3	4	2	2

Table 5. Correlation of organ involvement with ANCA serology and other autoantibodies in SLE patients(Pradhan et al., 2004)

Atypical or X-ANCA has been reported among SLE patients by Savige et al, This antibody showing specificities tocathepsin G and lactoferrin (Savige et al., 1996). **Table 5** shows correlation of organ involvement with ANCA serology and other autoantibodies in SLE patients (Pradhan et al., 2004).

6. Treatment of RPGN

Untreated RPGN typically progresses to end-stage renal disease over a period of weeks to a few months. Early diagnosis and initiation of appropriate therapy is essential to minimize the degree of irreversible renal injuries. The therapy of most patients involves pulse methyl-prednisolone followed by daily oral prednisone, oral or intravenous (IV) cyclophosphamide, and in some cases plasmapheresis. Empiric therapywith IV methylprednisolone should be begun in patients with severe disease with adding of plasmapheresisespecially if the patient has hemoptysis (Appel et al., 2010), If a renal biopsy performs soon after initiating empiric therapy the histological abnormalities will not alter.

6.1 Treatment of ANCA associated vasculitis (AAV)

Pauci-immune crescentic glomerulonephritis is a severe form of glomerular inflammation, which if left untreated, usually progresses to end-stage renal failure in weeks or months, AAV is responsible for 80 %of cases(Sakaiet al., 2002).The evidence based studies for the management of the AAV is well established and the strategy of induction, consolidation and maintenance therapy is accepted. Guidelines have been designed by both the British Society for Rheumatology (Lapraiket al., 2007) and European league against rheumatism (Mukhtyaret al., 2009) on the management of the AAVs. The AAVs are conventionally treated with a strategy of remission induction followed by maintenance therapy using glucocorticoids combined with cyclophosphamide during induction and azathioprine (AZA) for maintenance (Ntatsaki et al., 2011). Current standard treatment is combination of cyclophosphamide and steroids, but the optimal doses, routes of administration, and duration of therapy remain poorly defined (Hotta, et al., 2005). As immunosuppressive therapies increases the risk of infection, therefore one of the most important aspect of successful treatment srategies should be sufficient attenuation of inflammation without serious immunosuppression which leading to life-threatening infection.

Corticosteroids

For the induction of remission corticosteroid regimen is recommended which includea daily intravenous pulse of methylprednisolone (15 mg /kg)for 3 days, followed by oral prednisone (1mg/kg/day) for 3 weeks, which then tapered progressively (Pagnouxet al., 2008). In pauci-immuneRPGN and MPA usefulness of combination of methylprednisolone pulse therapy for 3 days, oral corticosteroid of 1mg/kg/day for 1 month, and cyclophos -phamide of 2 mg/ kg/day for 6 to 12 months has been confirmed in several studies (Salama, et al., 2002; J indal, 1999; Hoffman, 1997; Guillevin et al., 1991).

Cyclophosphamide(CYC)

Different therapeutic agents have been used in treatment of AAV.Standard therapy for AAV is treatment with combination of cyclophosphamide and prednisolone(Pagnouxet al., 2008). After induction with daily oral or pulse intravenous cyclophosphamide therapy, relapse rates of 15% at 12 months(Haubitzet al,. 1998), and 38% at 30 months(Guillevinet al., 1997) have been reported.In long-time follow-up 50 %of patients experience relapse within 5 years (Hoffman et al., 1992).Treatment with cyclophosphamide is effective, but also very toxic (Hoffmanet al., 1992).Repeated treatment with cyclophosphamide increases adverse effects. To avoid cyclophosphamide -related toxicity, alternative induction treatments are needed (Stassen et al., 2007).

Mycophenolate mofetil (MMF): MMF is considered as a potent immuno suppressive drug with favorable side effects, so it has been considered as an alternative to cyclophosphamide treatment in patients with AAV (Stassen et al., 2007;Pesavento et al., 1999; Haidinger et al., 2000; Joy et al., 2005;Koukoulaki, & Jayne, 2006). MMF is a drug which usually is well tolerated. In patients with auto-immune diseases such as SLE, MMF is effective in inducing remission with short-term efficacy which is comparable with cyclophosphamide (Chanet al., 2000, 2005; Ong et al., 2005; Ginzler etal., 2005). Induction treatment with MMF and oral steroids consisted of oral MMF 1000 mg twice daily and oral prednisolone 1 mg/kg once daily (maximum 60 mg). If patients are still in remission after 1 year, MMF is tapered by 500 mg every 3 months and Prednisolone is tapered after 6 weeks by 10 mg every2 weeks until a dose of 30 mg was reached, and by 5 mg every2 weeks until 10 mg. Next, the dose is reduced2.5 mg every month (Stassen et al., 2007). Stassen et al reported that combination of oral steroids and MMF induced complete and partial remission in 78% and 19 %of patients respectively(Stassen et al., 2007), Therefore they suggested oral steroids with MMF in patients with relapses of AAV intolerant to cyclophosphamide therapy.Bone marrow suppression is an uncommon side effect of MMF treatment which can result in anemia, leucocytopenia or thrombocytopenia in a number of patients .Fortunately this side effect responds to temporary dose reduction in nearly all patients(Stassen et al., 2007).

Methotrexate(MTX)

For remission maintenance in patients who are intolerant of AZA or relapse while taking it other alternative agents such as MTX or MMF have been recommended (Ntatsaki et al., 2011). Methotrexate is an alternative drug for cyclophosphamide which is currently studied (De Grootet al., 2005; Sneller et al., 1995; Stoneet al., 1999). According to one randomized (De Groot et al., 2005) and two uncontrolled studies (Sneller et al., 1995; Stoneet al., 1999) MTX effectively induced remission in 90 %and 71–74 %of patients respectively, but relapses occurred more frequently than when cyclophosphamide was used (70%vs. 47%)(De Groot et al., 2005). MTX is excreted by kidney, therefore should be used with caution in those with renal impairment (Ntatsaki et al., 2011; M etzler et al., 2007).

Groot et al conducted an unblended, randomized, controlled trial study todetermine whether MTX could replace treatment with cyclophosphamide and oral corticosteroids(De Grootet al., 2005).They found that MTX can replacecyclophosphamide for initial treatment of early AAV, but it was less effective for induction of remission in patients with extensive disease or those with pulmonaryinvolvement .In addition the relapse was more common in patients who treated with MTX than those who received cyclophosphamide.Patients were randomized to receive either MTX 7.5 mg/week increasing to 20 mg/week at 8 weeks or LEF loading dose 100 mg/day for 3 days, followed by20 mg /day until Week 4, then 30 mg/day for 2 years .Their study showed no differences in efficacy or safety between two treatments. Pagnoux et al(Pagnouxet al 2008)compared AZA with MTX in maintaining remission in WG and MPA patients who had achieved remission with intravenous pulse of cyclophos - phamide. They found no significant difference in adverse events and relapses rates either during the 12-month treatment phase or subsequent follow-up between two groups.

Intravenous immunoglobulins(IVIG)

ANCAs can induce cytokine-primed neutrophils undergo degranulation and respiratory bursts during which they release toxic oxygen species and lytic enzymes (Falk et al., 1990). Anti-idiotype antibodies with inhibitory effects on ANCA in vitro have been found in a pooled human gamma globulin preparation (Pall et al., 1994.)Evidence showed that IVIG acts in different phases of theimmune response including neutralization of circulating pathogenic antibodies, Fc receptor modulation, blockade or suppression of antibody-dependent cell toxicity, natural killer cell function, auto antibodyproduction and complement activation, and acceleration of neutrophil apoptosis (Kazatchkine & Kaver i, 2001; Tsujimoto et al., 2002).

Beneficial effect of high-dose intravenous immunoglobulin in ANCA–associated vasculitis has been approved by different studies (Ito-Iharaet al., 2006; Tuso et al., 1992; Jayneet al., 1993; Richteret al., 1995). Ito et al evaluated IVIG monotherapy (400 mg/kg/day for 5 days)in AAV patients. Their study showed that IVIG decreased the leukocyte count, C- reactive protein level, Birmingham Vasculitis Activity Score and improved the systemic symptoms (Ito-Iharaet al., 2006). Other studies suggested that IVIG induces remission in 40–82% of patients (Richter et al., 1995; Jayne et al., 1991; Levy et al., 1999; Jayne et al., 2000). IVIG appears to have an important place in the management of ANCA-RPGN, but it's indications have not been determined. Because IVIG is an expensive drug additional studies on its cost-effectiveness and rational introduction into clinical practice are needed(Hotta et al., 2005).

Anti-B-cell therapy(Rituximab)

Beneficial effects of Rituximab which is a monoclonal antibody against anti-CD20 have been reported in several case series(Gottenberg et al., 2005; Omdal et al., 2005; Speckset al., 2001), and uncontrolled studies(Eriksson, 2005; Keogh et al., 2005a, 2005b; Smith et al., 2006).The main problem of treatment with rituximab is that relapses commonly occurred after 6–9 months(Keogh et al., 2005a, 2005b; Smith et al., 2006).

Apheresis therapies

Results of clinical trial of apheresis therapies, either plasmapheresis or cytapheresis in AAV are disappointing. These studies showed no benefit(Glöckner et al., 1988; Cole et al., 1992; Zäuneret al., 2002), benefits just in dialysis dependent patients(Pusey et al., 1991)or benefits on preserving the renal function (Furutaet al., 1998; Hasegawaet al., 2005).

Pusey et al .Found that plasma exchange is of added benefit in dialysis-dependent patients because in patients who were initially dialysis-dependent, renal function was more likely to have recovered when treated with plasma exchange plus drugs rather than drugs alone (Pusey et al., 1991).Report from the European community group suggested that adding plasma exchange to immuno suppressive therapy was not beneficial if there was severe tubular atrophy and fewer than 33 %of the glomeruli were normal(De Lind van Wijngaarden et al., 1998).

In contrast to AAV in anti-GBM RPGN, the beneficial effect of plasma exchange has been well established .It might be attributable to the direct role of anti-GBM antibody in the pathogenesis of anti-GBM antibody RPGN, while in AAV no direct role for ANCA have been established (Hotta et al., 2005). The main advantage of Apheresis therapies is that no severe infectious episodes have been noted (Nagaseet al., 1998; Sawadaet al., 2003). Japan nation wide survey of RPGN (Yamagataet al., 2004) recommends cytapheresis in patients with aggressive forms of RPGN (rapid deterioration of renal function like the PR3-ANCA-associated RPGN, or pulmonary renal syndrome complicated by severe inflammation, or relapses with high MPO-ANCA titer).

Anti-TNF-alpha

Insights into the role of Th1 cytokines in the pathogenesis of WG have led to trial therapies with antagonists of tumor necrosis factor-alpha (TNFα)and inhibitors of monocyte function, such as interleukin-10(Kamesh et al., 2002) .Etanercept(Enbrel ;soluble receptors), infliximab (Remicade;human-mouse chimeric antibody against TNF), and adalimumab (Humila; human anti-TNF antibody)are biological antagonists of TNF(Ozaki, 2007).Etanercept have been reported ineffective in maintaining remission and a higher rate of malignancy have been noted in patients who have received the drug (Wegener's granulomatosis etanercept trial [WGET] research group, 2005).In an open label study, infliximab was added to standard immuno suppressive therapy in 16 patients with acute AAV at first presentation or relapse and in 16 with persistent disease despite multiple immuno suppressive regimens, 88% of patients achieved remission within a mean of 6.4 weeks(Boothet al., 2004) .

Anti-T cell antibodies :Different studies have been reported that active systemic vasculitis is mediated in part by T cell-induced injury .This finding has led to the evaluation of anti-T cell antibodies in patients with Wegener's granulomatosis who are resistant to cytotoxic therapy (Lockwoodet al., 1993; Hagenet al., 1995; Schmittet al., 2004).

In one study, the administration of a combination of two humanized monoclonal antibodies led to long-lasting remission in four patients with different forms of refractory vasculitis (Lockwoodet al., 1993).In other study 15 patients with refractory disease received anti-thymocyte globulin(ATG)which resulted in a partial or complete remission in 9 and 4 patients, respectively (Schmittet al., 2004).The role of these experimental therapies remains to be determined.

Intravenous azathioprine

High dose intravenous azathioprine has been tested for treating a variety of immune-mediated diseases .In one report, four patients with WG who had not responded to oral cyclophosphamide were treated with monthly infusions of azathioprine) (Benensonetal., 2005).Two reached remission of disease, one of whom developed renal involvement during relapse, which responded to retreatment.

15-Deoxyspergualin

15-deoxyspergualin (gusperimus), a drug with anti-proliferative effect on antigen-stimulated B cells, has been evaluated in a small number of patients who didn't respond to cyclophosphamide or had contraindications to the use of cyclophosphamide .The administration of 15-deoxyspergual in 20 patients resulted in complete or partial remission in six and eight respectively(Bircket al., 2003).All patient experienced transient leucopenia with each treatment cycle. In another study seven patients treated with 15-deoxyspergualin and glucocorticoids, all reached complete or partial remission .The main problem was that to maintain remission prolonged treatment up to 4 years was required(Schmittet al., 2005).In addition serial monitoring of white blood count is required to avoid excessive leucopenia.

Radiation therapy

Radiation therapy has been evaluated in patients with WG and air way involvement (Eagletonet al., 1979; Neviani et al., 2002).The use of ionizing radiation for non-malignant disease is controversial .Current data do not support its use in systemic disorder like Wegener's granulomatosis (Stone et al., 2010).

Stem cell transplantation: High-dose, myeloablative chemotherapy with stem cell transplantation has been used for the treatment of refractory severe vasculitis. There are few case reports of successful treatment in patients with WG (Kötteret al., 2005). More studies are required to determine the role of stem cell transplantation in the management of resistant AAV.

Prophylaxis against Pneumocystis carinii pneumonia(PCP)

Opportunistic infections especially Pneumocystis carinii pneumonia are potentially fatal complications of immuno suppressive therapy in RPGN and AAV .The estimated incidence of PCP is approximately 6 percent(Ognibeneet al., 1995).Different approaches to prophylaxis against PCP infection during initial immunosuppressive therapy have been suggested: trimethoprim-sulfamethoxazole one single strength (80 mg/400 mg)tablet daily or one double strength tablet (160 mg/800 mg)three times per week or Atovaquone in patients who are allergic to sulfonamides or do not tolerate trimethoprim-sulfamethoxazole.During treatment with methotrexate and glucocorticoids, the addition of trimethoprim-sulfamethoxazole increases the risk of pancytopenia, therefore Atovaquone is suggested for prophylaxis in such patients..It has been recommended to continue PCP prophylaxis in maintenance immuno suppressive therapy phase until the CD4-positive T cell count exceeds 300/microL(Mansharamaniet al., 2000).patients who have received trimethoprim-sulfamethoxazole for prophylaxis during induction, should continue the prophylaxis when azathioprine is used and switch to atovaquone when methotrexate is replaced for maintenance therapy.

Some patients have low CD4-positive T cell counts for prolonged periods after the cessation of cyclophosphamide and require prolonged PCP prophylaxis; in addition glucocorticoids should be tapered to the lowest possible dose .If patients develop neutropenia when receive prophylaxis, the drug should be switched to atovaquone (Stoneet al., 2010).

Management of RPGN and AAV in pregnancy: As with active disease in non-pregnant patients, prednisone alone is relatively ineffective, and to induce remission combined therapy with cyclophosphamide is needed.The major challenges of treatment during pregnancy are potentially serious adverse effects which can occur with both MMF and cyclophosphamide. In addition, insufficient data about the safety of rituximab is available. High risk of skeletal and palatal defects, as well as malformations of the limbs and eyes has been noted in case of fetal cyclophosphamide exposure during the first trimester.Although fetal risk is much smaller during the second and third trimesters, pancytopenia and impaired fetal growth can occur .MMF fetal exposure increases the risk of miscarriage and congenital malformation such as cleft lip and palate .As a result, some consider MMF to be contraindicated in pregnancy.The safer immuno suppressive drugs that have been effective in WG and MPA include glucocorticoids, azathioprine, cyclosporine and tacrolimus. Alternatives that could be considered include cyclophosphamide or rituximab in the second or third trimester once organogenesis is complete(Stoneet al., 2010).

6.1.1 Prognosis of RPGN and ANCA associated vasculitis

RPGN If left untreated typically progresses to end-stage renal disease over a period of weeks to a few months .Patients with fewer crescents may present slowly progressive course(Baldwin et al., 1987) .Despite various immuno suppressive therapy protocols mortality of ANCA positive RPGN is still high, and the major cause of death is infectious complications(Booth et al., 2003; De Lind van Wijngaardenet al 1998).Outcome of AAV depends on patient 's age, degree of renal impairement at presentation and presence of pulmonary involvement. During the first 6 months of treatment mortality is very high as a result of aggressive course of the disease and toxic effects of early immuno suppressive treatments(Sakai et al 2002;Boothet al., 2003). Although the introduction of steroids and cyclophosphamide pulse therapy have improved the overall mortality of AAV, the 2-year mortality rate is still high (20 % in 2-year follow-up)(Booth et al., 2003;Hogan et al., 1996;Falk et al 2000;Franssen et al 2000). Serum creatinine, dialysis dependency, and percentage of non-crescentic glomeruli at diagnosis have been considered as the best predictors of disease outcome(Bajema et al., 1999; Levy et al., 2001; Slotet al.2003).The prognosis for patients with anti-GBM antibody disease is poor(Hirayama, et al., 2008), and renal survival and mortality rates of 20.9%and 23.3 %at 6 months after onset have been reported respectively. Early diagnosis and starting treatment without delay might improve the prognosis(Hirayama, et al., 2008.)A large nationwide survey of RPGN in Japan showed that mortality correlates with age, severity of renal dysfunction, presence of pulmonary involvement, and high C-reactive protein level(Sakaiet al., 2002). The mortality rate of Japanese patients was higher than in European or American patients because of the high incidence of lethal infection (Hotta et al., 2005).

Japan Nationwide Survey of RPGN noted that 6-month renal and patients' survival for PR3-ANCA-associated RPGN were 88.2 %and 92.3% respectively, while for MPO-ANCA they were 69.9 %and 74.2 %respectively(Yamagata et al., 2005).patients' survival is very low in MPA if the disease presents as pulmonary renalsyndrome (Gallagheret al., 2002 Lauque et al., 2000; Niles et al., 1996).Introduction of immuno suppressive agents considerably has improved the outcome of AAV over the past 30 years .WG and MPA if left untreated have a rapidly progressive and usually fatal course(Ntatsaki et al., 2011). Walton reported a mean survival of 5 months in patients with WG, and mortality rate of 82 % and 89 %in 1 and 2 year follow-up respectively (Walton, 1958).Standard treatments significantly have improved prognosis in WG and MPA, and some studies have reported 5-year survival rates of 81 %for MPA and 87 % for WG (Eriksson et al., 2009).in European Vasculitis Study, there was 11.1 %mortality at 1 year (Littleet al., 2010.)High age at presentation, severe renal involvement (high serum creatininelevel at presentation), pulmonary involvement, high ESR and high scores of disease activity and damage were poor prognostic factors (Holle et al., 2011).

Suzuki et al 's study confirmed that ANCA-associated vasculitis is the most serious etiologies of RPGN(Suzukiet al., 2010).In nationwide survey byYamagata and Koyama (Koyamaet al., 2009; Yamagata et al., 2005), and Suzuki's study main causes of patients' death were infectious complications, including DIC which was mainly linked to pneumonia by opportunistic pathogens(Pneumocystis carinii, Candida albicans, and cytomegalovirus).

Researchers hope they will find new immuno suppressive drugs with highest efficacy, lowest side effects and high safety during pregnancy to improve patients' survival and quality of life .It's a dream that undoubetly will be achieved in next years.

7. Conclusion

RPGN is a nephrology emergency which needs special attention.If the disease left untreated typically progresses to end-stage renal disease over a period of weeks to a few months.When there is a strong clinical suspecsion special immuno suppressive treatment should be started as soon as possible (preferably after kidney biopsy) .Despite various immuno suppressive therapy protocols mortality of ANCA positive RPGN patients is still high, also prognosis of anti-GBM antibody disease is poor.acctually treatment of RPGN and AAV are serious challenges in nephrology medicine which needs more clinical trial studies in larger groups of patients.

8. Acknowledgement

The author would like to appreciate all authors and researchers whose studies have been applied in this chapter.

9. References

Koyama, A. Yamagata, K. Makino, H. Arimura, Y. Wada, T. Nitta, K.Nihei, H. Muso, E. Taguma, Y. Shigematsu, H. Sakai, H. Tomino, Y. Matsuo, S .& Japan RPGN Registry Group (2009). A nationwide survey of rapidly progressive glomerulonephritis in Japan :etiology, prognosis and treatment. Clinical and Experimental Nephrology J, Vol.13, No.6, (Dec 2009) PP. 633-50, 1342-1751

Appel, GB. Kaplan, AA. Glassock, RJ.&Sheridan AM.(2010.)Overview of the classification and treatment of rapidly progressive crescenticglomerulonephritis, In :Up to date, Oct 2010, Available from<www.up o date. com>

Benenson, E, Fries, JW, Heilig, B, Pollok M, &Rubbert, A .(2005.)High-dose azathioprine pulse therapy as a new treatment option in patients with active Wegener's granulomatosis and lupus nephritis refractory or intolerant to cyclophosphamide . Clin Rheumatol, Vol.24, No.3, (Jun 2005), PP.251-7, 0770-3198

Birck, R .Warnatz, K .Lorenz, HM Choi, M .Haubitz, M .Grünke, M .Peter, HH ..Kalden,, JR . Göbel, U .Drexler, JM .Hotta, O.Nowack, R .&van der Woude, FJ .(2003).15-Deoxyspergualin in patients with refractory ANCA-associated systemic vasculitis : a six-month open-label trial to evaluate safety and efficacy .J Am Soc Nephrol, Vol. 14, No.2, (February 2003), PP.440-7, 1046-6673

Bolton WK .&turgill BC.(1989).Methylprednisolone therapy for acute crescentic rapidly progressive glomerulonephritis .Am J Nephrol, Vol .9, PP .368-375 .

Booth, AD. Mike, KA .Aine, B. Ellis, P.Gaskin, G. Neild, GH. Plaisance, M. Pusey, CD.Jayne, DR. & renal research group .(2003).Outcome of ANCA-associatedrenal vasculitis :a 5-year retrospective study .Am JKidney Dis, Vol.41, No.4, (Apr 2003), PP.776–84

Booth, A .Harper, L .Hammad, T. Bacon, P. Griffith, M. Levy, J. Savage, C. Pusey, C. Jayne, D.(2004).Prospective study of TNF alpha blockade with infliximab in anti-neutrophil cytoplasmic antibody-associated systemic vasculitis .J Am Soc Nephrol, Vol.15, No.3, (Mar2004) , PP.717, 1046 -6673

Chan, TM .Tse, KC. Tang, CS. Mok, MY.&Li, FK.(2005) Long-term study of mycophenolatemofetil as continuous induction and maintenance treatment for diffuseproliferative lupus nephritis .J Am Soc Nephrol, Vol .16, No, 4, (April 2005), PP .1076–84, 1046-6673

Chan, TM.Li, FK .Tang, CS. Wong, RW. Fang, GX .&Ji YL .(2000). Efficacy of myco-phenolate mofetil in patients with diffuse proliferative lupus nephritis .HongKong-Guangzhou Nephrology Study Group .N Engl J Med, Vol.343, (October2000), PP.156–62

Chin, HJ. Ahn, C. Lim, CS. Chung, HK .&Lee JG) .(2000) Clinicalimplications of anti-neutrophil cytoplasmic antibody test inlupus nephritis .Am J Nephrol, Vol. 20, No.1, (Jan 2000), PP.57-63, 0250-8095

Churg, J .& Strauss, L .(1951).Allergic granulomatosis, allergic angiitisand periarteritis nodosa, Am .J .Pathol, Vol.27, No, 2, (Apri1951,) PP, 277-301

Cole, E .Cattran, D .Magil, A. Greenwood, C. Churchill, D. Sutton, D. Clark, W .Morrin, P. Posen, G. Bernstein, K (.1992) .A prospective randomizedtrial of plasma exchange as additive therapy in idiopathic crescenticglomerulonephritis .Am J Kidney Dis, Vol.20, No.3, (Sep1992), PP .230–9

DAgati, V. Chander, P .Nash, M .& Mancilla-Jimenez, R. (1986) .Idiopathic microscopic polyarteritis nodosa :ultra structuralobservations on the renal vascular and glomerular lesions .AmJ Kidney Dis, Vol.7, No.1, (Jan1986), PP .95-110

De Groot, C .Rasmussen, N .Bacon, PA .Cohen Tervaert, JW.Feighery, C .Gregorini, G . Gross, WL.Luqmani, R .& Jayne, DRW .(2005) .Randomized Trial of Cyclophosphamide Versus Methotrexate for Induction of Remission in Early Systemic Antineutrophil Cytoplasmic Antibody–Associated Vasculitis .Arthritis & Rheumatism, Vol .52, No .8, (August 2005), pp .2461–2469, 1529-0131

De Groot, K. Rasmussen, N.Bacon, PA. Tervaert, JW. Feighery, C.&Gregorini, G, (2005.)Randomized trial of cyclophosphamide versus methotrexate for induction ofremission in early systemic antineutrophil cytoplasmic antibody-associatedvasculitis .Arthritis Rheum, Vol.52, No.8, (August 2005), PP.2461–9, 1529 -0131

De Lind van Wijngaarden, RAF. Hauer, HA.& Wolterbeek, R .(1998 .)Treatment decisions in severe ANCA-associated glomerulonephritis .J Am Soc Nephrol, Vol.16 PP.52A, 1046-6673

Dickersin, K .Scherer, R .Lefebvre, C .(1994.)Identifying relevant studies for systematic reviews .BMJ, Vol .309, No.6964, (Nov 1994), PP.1286-1291

Eagleton, LE.Rosher, RB .Hawe, A .&Bilinsky, RT .(1979).Radiation therapy and mechanical dilation of endobronchial obstruction secondary to Wegener's granulomatosis . Chest, Vol.76, No.5, (Nov 1979) , PP.609-10, 0012-3692

Eriksson, P(.2005) .Nine patients with anti-neutrophil cytoplasmic antibody-positive vasculitis successfully treated with rituximab .J Intern Med, Vol .257, No.6, (Jun2005), PP.540–8, 0954-6820

Eriksson, P. Jaconsson, L .Lindell, A .Nilsson, JA .&Skogh, T .(2009).Improved outcome in Wegener's granulomatosis andmicroscopic polyangiitis? A retrospective analysis of95 cases in two cohorts .J Intern Med, Vol.265, No.4, (Apr2009,) PP:.496-506, 0954-6820

Falk, RJ .&Jennette, JC .1988) .Anti-neutrophil cytoplasmic auto antibodies with specificity for myeloperoxidase in patientswith systemic vasculitis and idiopathic necrotizing and crescenticglomerulonephritis .N Engl J Med, Vol.318, (June 1988), PP .1651-1657

Falk, RJ. Nachman, PH .Hogen, SL .&Jennette, JC.(2000). ANCA glomerulonephritisand vasculitis :A Chapel Hill perspective .Semin Nephrol, Vol.20, No.3, (May2000), PP . 233-43

Falk, RJ .Terrell, RS.Charles, LA .&Jennette, J C .(1990).(nti-neutrophil cytoplasmic antibodies induce neutrophils to degranulate and produceoxygen radicals in vitro . Proc Natl Acad Sci USA, vol .87, No.11, (June1990), PP .4115-19

Franssen,   CFM.Stegeman,   CA   .&Kallenberg,   CG.(2000.)Antiproteinase3-and antimyeloperoxidase-associated   vasculitis .KidneyInt, Vol .57, (January 2000), PP.2195-206, 0085-2538

Furuta, T.Hotta, O. Yusa, N. Horigome, I. Chiba, S .& Taguma Y) .(1998). Lymphocyt apheresis   to   treat   rapidly   progressive   glomerulonephritis :a   randomized comparison with steroid-pulse treatment .Lancet, Vol.352, No.9123, (Jul1998), PP.203-4

Gallagher, H.Kwan, JTC .&Jayne, DR .(2002).Pulmonary renal syndrome :a 4-year, single-center experience .Am J Kidney Dis, Vol.39, No.1, (Jan 2002), PP.42-47

Ginzler, EM.Dooley, MA. Aranow, C. Kim, MY .Buyon, J .&Merrill, JT .(2005) Mycophenolate mofetil or intravenous cyclophosphamide for lupus nephritis. N Engl J Med, Vol.353, (Nov 2005), PP.2219-28

Glöckner, WM. Sieberth, HG .Wichmann, HE. Backes, E.Bambauer, R. Boesken, WH. Bohle, A. Daul, A. Graben, N .& Keller, F .(1988).Plasmaexchange and immuno suppression in rapidly progressiveglomerulonephritis :a controlled, multi-center study . ClinNephrol, Vol.29, No.1, (Jan1988), PP .1-8, 0301-0430

Goldschmeding, R. van der Schoot, CE .Ten BokkelHuinink, D.Hack, CE. Van den Ende, ME. Kallenberg, CG. von dem Borne, AE.(1989).Wegener's granulomatosis auto antibodiesidentify a novel diisopropylfluorophosphate-binding proteinin the lysosomes of normal human neutrophils .J Clin Invest, Vol .84, No.5, (Nov1989), PP :1577-1587

Gottenberg, JE.Guillevin, L. Lambotte, O. Combe, B. Allanore, Y .& Cantagrel, A.(2005).Tolerance and short term efficacy of rituximab in 43 patients with systemicautoimmune diseases .Ann Rheum Dis, Vol.64, (November 2004), PP.913-20, 0003-4967

Guillevin, L. Cohen, P .Gayraud, M.Lhote, F. Jarrousse, B .&Casassus, P .(1999).Churg-Strauss syndrome :Clinical study and long-term follow-up of 96 patients .Medicine, Vol.78, No.1 ,(Jan 1999), PP .26-37

Guillevin, L. Cordier, JF .Lhote F. Cohen, P. Jarrousse, B. Royer, I. Lesavre, P. Jacquot, C. Bindi, P. Bielefeld, P. Desson, JF. Détrée, F.Dubois, A. Hachulla, E. Hoen, B. Jacomy, D. Seigneuric, C. Lauque, D (.1997).A prospective, multicenter, randomizedtrial comparing steroids and pulse cyclophosphamide versus steroids and oral cyclophosphamide in the treatment of generalized Wegener's granulomatosis .Arthritis Rheum, Vol.40, No.12, (♀Dec1997), PP.2187-98, 1529-0131

Guillevin, L. Jarrousse, B .Lok, C. Lhote, F. Jais, JP. Le ThiHuong, Du D .&Bussel, A . (1991).Long-term follow-up after treatmentof polyarteritis nodosa and Churg-

Strauss angiitis with comparisonof steroids, plasma exchange and cyclophosphamideto steroids and plasma exchange .A prospective randomizedtrial of 71 patients .The cooperative study group for polyarteritis nodosa .J Rheum, Vol.18, No.4, (pr1991), PP .567–574, 1462-0324

Haas, M .&Eustace, J .(2004). Immune complex deposits in ANCA-associated crescentic glomerulonephritis :A study of 126 cases .Kidney International, Vol .65, (January 2004), pp .2145–2152, 0085-2538

Jennette, JC .(2003).Rapidly progressive glomerulonephritis.KidneyInt, Vol.63, PP.1164–1177, 0085-2538

Hagen, EC .De Keizer, RJ .Andrassy, K.van Boven, WP. Bruijn, JA.vanes, LA .& van der Woude FJ.(1995) Compassionate treatment of Wegener's granulomatosis with rabbit anti-thymocyte globulin .Clin Nephrol, Vol. 43No.6, (Jun 1995) , PP.351-9, 0301-0430

Haidinger, M .Neumann, I .Grutzmacher, H. Bayer, P .&Meisl, FTh.(2000). Myco phenol-late mofetil (MMF)treatment of ANCA-associated small-vessel vasculitis :a pharmoco kinetically controlled study .Clin Exp Immunol, Vol.120, No. 1, PP .72

Harris, Jennette AA .Falk, RJ .&, JC .(1998).Crescentic glomerulonephritis with a paucity of glomerular immunoglobulin localization.Am J Kidney Dis, vol.32, No.1, (Jul 1998) , PP.179–184

Hasegawa, M.Watanabe, A.Takahashi, H. Takahashi, K. Kasugai, M.Kawamura, N.Kushimoto, H. Murakami, K. Tomita, M.Nabeshima, K. Oohashi, A. Kondou, F.Ooshima H.Hiki, Y .& Sugiyama, S .(2005).Treatmentwith cytapheresis for anti-neutrophil cytoplasmic anti-body associatedrenal vasculitis and its effect on anti-inflammatoryfactors .Ther Apher Dial, Vol.9, No.4, (Aug2005), PP.297–302, 1477-9979

Haubitz, M. Schellong, S .Göbel, U. Schurek, HJ. Schaumann, D.Koch, KM. &Brunkhorst, R .(1998).Intravenous pulse administration of cyclophosphamide versus daily oral treatment in patients with antineutrophil cytoplasmicAntibody-associated vasculitis and renal involvement :a prospective, randomizedstudy .Arthritis Rheum, Vol .41, No.10, (Oct1998), PP.1835-44, 1529-0131

Hauer, HA.Bajema, IM .Van houwelingen, HC. Ferrario, F .Noël, LH .Waldherr, R .Jayne, DRW. Rasmussen, N. Bruijn, JA .& Hagen, EC .(2002).Renal histologyinANCA-associated vasculitis :Differences between diagnosticand serologic subgroups . Kidney Int Vol.61, (August 2001), PP:.80–89, 0085-2538

Hoffman, GS .(1997).Treatment of Wegener's granulomatosis :time to change the standard of care? Arthritis Rheum, Vol.40, No.12, (Dec 1997), PP .2099–2104, 1529-0131

Hoffman, GS. Kerr, GS. Leavitt, RY. Hallahan, CW .Lebovics, RS .&Travis, WD . (1992)()Wegener granulomatosis :an analysis of 158 patients .Ann Intern Med, Vol.16, No.6, (March1992), PP.488–98, 0003-4819

Hogan, SL. Nachman, PH. Wilkman, AS.Jennette, JC .& Falk, RJ .(1996).Prognostic markersin patients with antineutrophil cytoplasmic autoantibody associatedmicroscopic polyangitis and glomerulonephritis .J Am Soc Nephrol, Vol.7, No.1, (Jan 1996), PP .23–32, 1046-6673

Hogan, SL.Nachman, PH.Wilkman, AS. Jennette, JC .&Falk, RJ .(1996).Prognostic markers in patients with antineutrophil cytoplasmicautoantibody-associated microscopic polyangiitis andglomerulonephritis .J Am Soc Nephrol, Vol. 7, No.1, (Jan 1996), PP.23–32, 1046-6673

Holle, JU .Gross, WL.Latza, U.Nölle, B .Ambrosch, P .Heller, M .Fertmann, R .&Reinhold-Keller, E .(2011).Improved outcome of445 Wegener's granulomatosis patients in a Germanvasculitis centre over four decades .Arthritis Rheum, Vol.63, No.1, (Jan2011), PP .257-66, 1529-0131

Hotta, S. Ishida, A. Kimura, T.& Taguma, Y.(2005) .Improvements in treatment strategies for patients withantineutrophil cytoplasmic antibody-associated rapidlyprogressive glomerulonephritis .Therapeutic apheresis and dialysis, Vol .10, No.5, (November 2005), PP.390–395, 1744-9979

Ito-Ihara, T. Ono, T .Nogaki, F. Suyama, K. Tanaka, M. Yonemoto, S. Fukatsu, A. Kita, .T. Suzuki, K. &Muso E.(2006).Clinical efficacy of intravenousimmunoglobulin for patients with MPO-ANCA associatedrapidly progressiveglomerulonephritis . NephronClin Pract, Vol. 102, No.1, (Sep2005), PP .c35–c42, 1660-2110

Tuso, P. Moudgil, A. Hay, J. Goodman, D. Kamil, E.Koyyana, R.&Jordan, SC . (1992).Treatment of antineutrophil cytoplasmicautoantibody-positive systemic vasculitis andglomerulonephritiswith pooled intravenous gamma globulin .Am JKidney Dis, Vol.20 ,No.5, (Nov1992), PP.504–8

Jayne, DR. Davies, M. Fox, CJ. Black, CM.& Lockwood, CM .(1991).Treatment of systemicvasculitis with pooled intravenous immunoglobulin .Lancet, Vol.337, No.8750, PP.1137–9

Jayne, DR.Esnault, VL .&Lockwood CM .(1993).ANCA anti-idiotypeantibodies and the treatment of systemic vasculitis with intravenousimmunoglobulin .J Autoimmun, Vol .6, No.2, (Apr 1993), PP .207–19, 0896-8411

Jayne, DRW.Chapel, H. Adu, D. Misbah, S. O'Donoghue, D.& Scott D(2000).Intravenous immunoglobulin for ANCA-associated systemic vasculitis withpersistent disease activity .QJM, vol.93, No.7, (May2000), PP.433–9, 1460-2725

Jennette, JC .&Falk, RJ .(1998) .Pathogenesis of the vascular andglomerular damage in ANCA-positive vasculitis .Nephrol DialTransplant, Vol.13, No.1, PP.6–20, 0931-0509

Jennette, JC .&Falk, RJ .(1997).Small-vessel vasculitis .N Engl J ed., Vol .337, No.21, (November 1997), PP.1512–23

Jennette, JC. Thomas, DB(.2001).(rescentic glomerulonephritis.Nephrol Dial Transplant, Vol. 16, No.6, PP.80–82,, 0931-0509

Jennette, JC .Wilkman, AS .&Falk RJ.(1989).Anti-neutrophil cytoplasmic autoantibody-associated glomerulonephritis and vasculitis.Am J Pathol, Vol.135, No.5,)Nov 1989,(PP.921-930

Jennette, J .& Falk, R .(2003).Renal and systemic vasculitis, In :Comprehensive clinical nephrology,)second ed ,(edited by Johnson, R .Feehally, J, PP .341-357Mosby, 0723432589, Retrieved from <www.google.com>

Jindal, KK .(1999) .Management of idiopathic crescentic and diffuse proliferative glomerulonephritis :evidence-based recommendations .Kidney Int, Vol.55, No.70, PP .S33–40, 0085-2538.

Joy, MS. Hogan, SL .Jennette, JC .Falk, RJ .&Nachman, PH .(2005).A pilot study usingmycophenolate mofetil in relapsing or resistant ANCA small vessel vasculitis . Nephrol Dial Transplant, Vol.20, No.12, (Sep 2005), pp .2725–32, 0931-0509

Kamesh, L .Harper, L.&.Savage, CO .(2002) .ANCA-positive vasculitis .J Am Soc Nephrol, Vol.13, No.7, (July 2002), PP .1953, 1046-6673

Kazatchkine, MD.&Kaveri, SV.(2001).Immuno modulation of autoimmune and inflammatory diseases with intravenous immuneglobulin .N Engl J Med, Vol.345, No.10, (Sep 2001), PP.747–55

Keogh, KA. Wylam, ME.Stone, JH.& Specks, U.(2005) .Induction of remission by B lymphocyte depletion in eleven patients with refractory antineutrophil cytoplasmic antibody-associated vasculitis .Arthritis Rheum, Vol .52, No.1, (Jan2005), PP .262–8, 1529-0131

Keogh, KA. Ytterberg, SR .Fervenza, FC. Carlson, KA. Schroeder, DR .&Specks U . (2006).Rituximab for refractory Wegener's granulomatosis :report of a prospective, open-label pilot trial .Am J Respir Crit Care Med, Vol .173, No.2, (October 2005), PP .180–7

Kötter, I.Daikeler, T .Amberger, C.Tyndall, A.& Kanz, L.(2005).Autologous stem cell transplantation of treatment-resistant systemic vasculitis--a single center experience and review of the literature .Clin Nephrol, VoL .64, No.6, (Dec 2005), PP.485-9, 0301-0430

Koukoulaki, M..& Jayne, DR .(2006).Mycophenolate mofetil in anti-neutrophil cytoplasmantibodies-associated systemic vasculitis .Nephron Clin Pract, Vol.102, No.3-4, (November 2005) PP.c100–7, 1660-2110

Koyama, A.. Yamagata, K. Makino, H. Arimura, Y. Wada, T. Nitta, K.Nihei, H. Muso, E .. Taguma, Y. Shigematsu, H.Sakai, H. Tomino, Y. Matsuo, S .& Japan RPGN Registry Group) .2009.(Nationwide survey of rapidly progressive glomerulonephritis in Japan :etiology, prognosis and treatment diversity .Clinical and Experimental Nephrology J, Vol. 13, No.6,)Dec 2009), PP .633-50, 1342-1751

Lapraik, C. Watts, R .Bacon, P..Carruthers, D .Chakravarty, K. D'Cruz, D. Guillevin, L.Harper, L .Jayne, D .Luqmani, R .Mooney, J .Scott, D(.2007).BSR & BHPR guidelinesfor the management of adults with ANCA associatedvasculitis . Rheumatology, Vol.46, (April 2007,) PP1-11, 1462-0324

Lauque, D. Cadranel, J. Lazor, R. Pourrat, J. Ronco, P. Guillevin, L .&Cordier, JF . (2000).Microscopic polyangiitis with alveolarhemorrhage .A study of 29 cases and review of the literatureMedicine. Baltimore, Vol.79, No.4, (Jul2000), PP .222–233

Levy, JB.&Winearls, CG .(1994).Rapidly progressive glomerulonephritis :what should be first-line therapy? Nephron, Vol 67, No.4, PP.402-407, 0028-2766

Jayne, DR.Chapel, H .Adu, D .Misbah, S .O'Donoghue, D .Scott, D .& Lockwood CM . (2000.)Intravenous immunoglobulin for ANCA-associated systemic vasculitis with persistent disease activity .QJM, Vol.93, No.7, (Jul2000), PP.433-439

Levy, Y. Sherer, Y .George, J. Langevitz, P. Ahmed, A .& Bar-Dayan, Y .(1999) .Serologicand clinical response to treatment of systemic vasculitis and associatedautoimmune disease with intravenous immunoglobulin .Int Arch Allergy Immunol, Vol.119, No.3, (Jul 1999()PP.231–8, 1018-2438

Lionaki, S. Jennette, JC.&Falk, RJ .(2007). Anti-neutrophil cytoplasmic (ANCA) and anti-glomerularbasement membrane (GBM)auto antibodiesin necrotizing and crescentic glomerulonephritis.Semin Immunopathol, Vol.29, No .4 ,(Nov2007), PP.459–474, 1863-2297

Little, MA. Nightingale, P. Verburgh, CA.Hauser, T. De Groot, K. Savage, C. Jayne, D. Harper, L .(2010.)Earlymortality in systemic vasculitis :relative contribution ofadverse events and active vasculitis .Ann Rheum Dis, Vol.69, No.6, (Jun2010), PP. 1036-43, 0003-4967

Lockwood, CM .Thiru, S .&Isaacs, JD. Hale, G. Waldmann, H.(1993) .Long-term remission of intractable systemic vasculitis with monoclonal antibody therapy .Lancet, Vol. 341, No.8861, (Jun1993), PP.1620-2

Mansharamani, NG. Garland, R.Delaney, D .&Koziel, H .(2000).Management and outcome patterns for adult Pneumocystis carinii pneumonia, 1985 to 1995 :comparison of HIV-associated cases to other immunocompromised states .Chest, Vol.118, No.3, (Sep2000), PP.704-711, 0012-3692

Metzler, C. Miehle, N. Manger, K .Iking-Konert, C . .De Groot, K.Hellmich, B . .Gross, WL . .& Reinhold-Keller, E .(2007).Levated relapserate under oral methotrexate versus leflunomide formaintenance of remission in Wegener's granulomatosis. Rheumatology, Vol .46, No .7, (January 2007), PP .1087-91, 1462-0324

Molnar, K. Kovacs, L. Kiss, M..Husz, S. Dobozy, A .&Pokoerny, G .(2002) .Anti-neutrophil cytoplasmic antibodies in patients withsystemic lupus erythematosus .Clin Exp Dermatol, Vol. 27, No.1, (Jan2002), PP.56-61, 0307-6938

Edgar, JD. Mc Millan, SA. Bruce, IN .&Conlan SK .(1995) .An audit ofANCA in routine clinical practice .Postgrad Med J, Vol .71, N., 840(Oct1995), PP .605-12, 0032-5473

Mukhtyar, C. Guillevin, L.Cid, M. Dasgupta, B. De Groot, K. GrossW, Hauser, T . Hellmich, B. Jayne, D. Kallenberg, C G M. Merkel, P A . Raspe, H . Salvarani, C . Scott, DGI Stegeman, C. Watts, R .Westman., K .Witter, J .Yazici, H & Luqmani, R.(2009.)EULAR recommendationsfor the management of primary small and mediumvasculitis .Ann Rheum Dis, Vol.68, No.3, (March 2009),, PP .310-7, 0003-4967

Mukhtyar, C.Flossmann, O.Hellmich, B.Bacon, P.Cid, M .&Cohen-Terrvaretm, JW(.2008) . Outcomes from studies of antineutrophil cytoplasm antibody associated vasculitis : a systematic review by the European League against rheumatism systemic vasculitis task force. Ann Rheum Dis, Vol.6, No.7, (Jul2008), PP .1004-1010, 0003-4967

Nagase, K. Sawada, K .Ohnishi, K.Egashira, A. Ohkusu, K .& Shimoyama T . (1998).Complications of leukocytapheresis.Ther Apher, Vol.2, No.2, (May1998), PP . 120–4

Naseri, M .& Zabolinejad, N.(2008).ANCA-Negative Pulmonary-Renal Syndrome with Pathologic Findings Suggesting Thrombotic Thrombocytopenic Purpura.Iran J Ped, Vol.17, No.1, (March 2007), PP.63-8, 2008-2114

Neviani, CB .Carvalho Hde, A .Hossamu, C.Aisen, S.& Nadalin, W.(2002) .Radiation therapy as an option for upper airway obstruction due to Wegener's granulomatosis . Otolaryngol Head Neck Surg, Vol. 126, No.2, (Feb2002), PP.195-6, 0194-5998

Niles, JL .Bottinger, EP. Saurina, GR. Kelly, KJ. Pan, G. Collins, AB .&McCluskey, RT . (1996).The syndrome of lung hemorrhage andnephritis is usually an ANCA-associated condition .Arch InternMed, Vol.156, No.4, PP .440–445

Niles, JL. McCluskey, RT .Ahmad, MF.& Arnaout MA.(1989).Wegener's granulomatosis auto antigen is a novel serineproteinase .Blood, Vol .74, No .6, (Nov 1989), PP.1888-1893, 0006-4971

Nishiya, K. Chikazawa, H.Nishimura, S.Hisakawa, N.&Hashimoto K .(1997).Anti-neutrophil cytoplasmic antibody inpatients with systemic lupus erythematosus is unrelated toclinical features .Clin Rheumatol, Vol.16, No.1, (Jan 1997), PP.70-5, 0770-3198

Ntatsaki, E. Mooney, J .&Watts, RA) .2011 .(ANCA vasculitis :time for a change in treatment paradigm? Not yet.Rheumatology, Vol.50, No.2, (February 2011), PP.1-6, 1462-0324

Ntatsaki, E..Watts, RA .& Scott, DGI.(2010).Epidemiology ofANCA-associated vasculitis . Rheum Dis Clin North Am, Vol.36, No.3 ,(Aug2010), PP .447-61

Ognibene, FP .Shelhamer, JH.Hoffman, GS .Kerr, GS .Reda, D .Fauci, AS .& Leavitt, RY. (1995) .Pneumocystis carinii pneumonia :a major complication of immunosuppressive therapy in patients with Wegener's granulomatosis .Am J Respir Crit Care Med, Vol .151, No.3, (Mar 1995), PP .795-799

Omdal, R. Wildhagen, K. Hansen, T. Gunnarsson, R.& Kristoffersen, G .(2005) .Anti-CD20therapy of treatment-resistant Wegener's granulomatosis :favourable buttemporary response .Scand J Rheumatol, vol.34, No.3, (2005 May), PP.229–32, 0300-9742

Ong ,LM.Hooi, LS .Lim, TO. Goh, BL. Ahmad, G .&Ghazalli, R(.2005) . Randomized controlled trial of pulse intravenous cyclophosphamide versus mycophenolatemofetil in the induction therapy of proliferative lupus nephritis . Nephrology(Carlton), Vol.10, No.5, (Oct2005), PP.504–10, 1320-5358

Pagnoux, C. Mahr, A .Hamidou, MA .Boffa, JJ. Ruivard, M. Ducroix, JP. Kyndt, X. Lifermann, F. Papo, T. Lambert, M. Noach, JL. Khellaf, M. Merrien, D .Puechal, X . Vinzio, S.Cohen, P. Mouthon, L .Cordier, JF .&Guillevin, L .(2008). Azathioprine or Methotrexate Maintenancefor ANCA-Associated Vasculitis .N Engl J Med, Vol.359, No.26, (December 2008), PP.2790-803

Pagnoux, C.Mahr, A .Hamidou, MA. Boffa, JJ .Mouthon, L .Cordier, JF.Guillevin, L .&French Vasculitis Study Group .(2008).Azathioprineor methotrexate maintenance for ANCA-associatedvasculitis .N Engl J Med, Vol .359, No.26, (December 2008), PP.2790-803

Pall, AA. Varagunam, M .Adu, D, Smith, N .Richards, N T .Taylor, C M .& J Michael . (1994.)Anti-idiotypic activityagainst anti-myeloperoxidase antibodies in pooled humanimmunoglobulin .Clin Exp Immunol, Vol.95, No.2, (February1994), PP.257–62

Pesavento, T. Falkenhain, M.Rovin, B.&Hebert, L.(1999) .Mycophenolate mofetil therapy (MMF)in anti-neutrophil cytoplasmatic antibody (ANCA)vasculitis .J Am Soc Nephrol, Vol.10, PP.114A, 1046-6673

Pradhan, VD. Badakere, SS .Bichile, LS .&Almeida, AF(.2004)(Anti-neutrophil Cytoplasmic Antibodies (ANCA)in Systemic Lupus Erythematosus :Prevalence, clinical associations and correlation with otherauto antibodies, JAPI, Vol .52, (July 2004), PP.533-7

Pusey, CD. Rees, AJ .Evans, DJ..Peters, D K.& Lockwood, C M(.1991.(Plasma exchange in focalnecrotizing glomerulonephritis without anti-GBM antibodies. Kidney Int, Vol.40, (May 1991), PP .757–63, 0085-2538

Richter, C. Schnabel, A. Csernok, E .De Groot, K. Reinhold-Keller, E.& Gross, WL .(1995) . Treatment of anti-neutrophil cytoplasmic antibody (ANCA)- associated systemic

Vasculitis with high-dose intravenous immunoglobulin .Clin Exp Immunol, Vol.101, No.1, (July 1995), PP.2–7

Richter, C. Schnael, A. Csernok, E. De Groot, K .Reinhold-Keller, E .& Gross, W L .(1995) . Treatment   of   antineutrophilcytoplasmic   antibody   (ANCA)associated systemicvasculitis with high-dose intravenous immunoglobulin .Clin Exp Immunol, Vol.101, No.1, (July 1995), PP.2-7

Rondeau, E.Levy, M .Dosquet, P .Ruedin, P .Mougenot, B .Kanfer, A.& Sraer, JD. (1989 .) Plasma   exchange   and   immunosuppression   for   rapidly   progressive glomerulonephritis :prognosis and complications .Nephrol Dial Transplant, Vol.4, No.3, PP. 4:196-200, 0931-0509

Sakai, H .Kurokawa, K .Koyama, A. Arimura, Y. Kida, H. Shigematsu, H. Suzuki, S. Nihei, H. Makino, H. Ueda, N.Kawamura, T. Gejyo, F.Saito, T.Harada, T. Hiki, Y .& Yoshida, M.(2002) .Guideline for management ofrapidly progressive glomerulonephritis in Japan .Jpn J Nephrol, Vol.44, No .2, (Mar 2002), PP.55–82, o385—2385

Salama, AD .Dougan, T .Levy, JB .Cook HT.Morgan, SH .Naudeer, S .Maidment, G .George, AJT.Evans, D .Lightstone, L .& Pusey, CD.(2002).Goodpasture's Disease in the Absence of Circulating Anti–Glomerular Basement Membrane Antibodies as Detected by Standard Techniques .American Journal of Kidney Diseases, Vol. 39, No, (June 2002), pp .1162-1167

Savage, CO .Harper, L .&Adu, D .(1997.)Primary systemic vasculitis .Lancet, Vol.349, No.9051, (Feb1997), PP.553-558

Savige, JA. Chang, L. Wilson, D .& Buchanan, RR .(1996).Auto antibodiesand target antigens in anti-neutrophil cytoplasmic antibody (ANCA)associated vasculitides . Rheumatol Int, Vol. 16, No .3, PP.109-14, 0172-8172

Sawada, K.Muto, TShimoyama, T. Satomi, M. Sawada, T.Nagawa, H. Hiwatashi, N . Asakura, H.. &Hibi, T. (2003).Multicenter randomizedcontrolled trial for the treatment of ulcerative colitis withleukocytapheresis column .Curr Pharm Des, Vol.9, No.4, PP .307–21, 1381-6128

Schmitt, WH .Birck, R .& Heinzel, PA.(2005.)Prolonged treatment of refractory Wegener's granulomatosis with 15-deoxyspergualin :an open study in seven patients .Nephrol Dial Transplant, Vol.20, No.6, (Jun2005), PP.1083-92, 0931-0509

Schmitt, WH .Hagen, EC.&Neumann, I. Nowack, R. Flores-Suárez, LF. van der Woude, FJ.(2004) .Treatment of refractory Wegener's granulomatosis with antithymocyte globulin (ATG) :(an open study in 15 patients .Kidney Int, Vol.65, No.4, (Apr2004), PP.1440-8, 0085-2538

Seo, P.& Stone, JH.(2004).The antineutrophil cytoplasmic antibody-associated vasculitides.Am J Med, Vol.117, No.1, (Jul2004 l(, PP.39-50

Smith, KG. Jones, RB. Burns, SM.&Jayne, DR .(2006).Long-term comparison of rituximab treatment for refractory systemic lupus erythematosus and vasculitis :remission, relapse and re-treatment .Arthritis Rheum, vol .54, No.9, (Sep2006), PP.2970–82, 1529-0131

Sneller, MC. Hoffman, GS. Talar-Williams, C. Kerr, GS .Hallahan, CW.& Fauci AS(.1995).An analysis of forty-two Wegener's granulomatosis patients treated with methotrexate and prednisone .Arthritis Rheum, Vol .38, No.5, (May1995), PP.608–13, 1529 -0131

Specks, U. Fervenza, FC. McDonald, TJ.& Hogan, MC.(2001) .Response of Wegener's granulomatosis to anti-CD20 chimeric monoclonal antibody therapy . ArthritisRheum, Vol.44, No.12, (Dec 2001), PP.2836–40, 1529-0131

Stassen, PM. Cohen Tervaert, JW .& Stegeman, CA .(2007).Induction of remission in active anti-neutrophil cytoplasmicantibody-associated vasculitis with mycophenolate mofetil inpatients who cannot be treated with cyclophosphamide .Ann Rheum Dis, Vol.66, No.6, (December2006), PP .798–802, 0003-4967

Stone, JH . Kaplan, AA . Falk, RJ. Appel, GB .& Sheridan, AM .(2010).Initial immuno suppressive therapy in Wegener's granulomatosis and microscopic polyangiitis.In : Up to date, Oct 2010, Available from :< www.up to date. com>

Stone, JH. Tun, W .&Hellman, DB .(1999.)Treatment of non-life threatening Wegener'sgranulomatosis with methotrexate and daily prednisone as the initial therapy ofchoice .J Rheumatol, vol.26, No.5, (May1999), PP .1134–9, 1462-0324

Stone, JH. Falk, RJ. Glassock, RJ. Appel, GB. & Sheridan, AM.(2010).Treatment of cyclophosphamide-resistant Wegener's granulomatosis and microscopic polyangiitis .In :Up to date, Oct 2010, Available from :< www.up to date.com>

Suzuki, Y .Takeda, Y .Sato, D .Kanaguchi, Y .Tanaka, Y .Kobayashi, S .Suzuki, K .Hashimoto, H.Ozaki, S .Horikoshi, S .& Tomino, Y.(2010).Clinico epidemiological manifestations of RPGN and ANCA-associated vasculitides :an 11-year retrospective hospital-based study in Japan .Mod Rheumatol, Vol.20, No.1, (Feb 2010), PP .54–62, 1439-7595

The Wegener's Granulomatosis Etanercept Trial [WGET]Research Group .(2005 .).Etanercept plus standard therapy for Wegener's granulomatosis .N Engl J Med, Vol. 352, No.4, (Jan 2005), PP.351-36

Tsujimoto, H .Takeshita, S .Nakatani, K.Kawamura, Y. Tokutomi, T .& Sekine, I .(2002) . Intravenous immunoglobulintherapy induces neutrophils apoptosis in Kawasaki disease .Clin Immunol, Vol.103, No.2, (May 2002), PP.161–8, 0271-9142

Vizjak, A.Rott, T .Koselj-kajtna, M.Rozman, B. Kaplan-Pavlovcic, SA .&Ferluga, DA. (2003 .) Histology and immunohistologic study and clinical presentationof anca-associated glomerulonephrits with correlationto ANCA antigen specificity.American Journal of Kidney Diseases, Vol. 41, No. 3, (November, 2002), pp. 539-549

Walters, GD .Willis, NS .& Craig, GC .(2010.)Interventions for renal vasculitis in adults .A systematic review .BMC Nephrology, Vol.11, (June 2010), PP.12, 1471-2369

Walton, EW.(1958) .Giant cell granuloma of the respiratory tract.Br J Med, Vol .2, No .5091, (August1958), PP.265-270

Wegener's granulomatosis etanercept trial [WGET]research group .(2005.) Etanercept plus standard therapy for Wegener's granulomatosis .N Engl J Med, Vol.352, No.4, (January 2005), PP.351-361

Yamagata, K .Hirayama, K. Mase, K. Yamaguchi, N. Kobayashi, M .Takahashi, H .& Koyama, A).(2004)(Apheresis for MPO-ANCA-AssociatedRPGN–Indications and Efficacy: Lessons Learned from Japan Nationwide Survey of RPGN .Journal of Clinical Apheresis, Vol .20, No.4, (December 2005), PP.244–251, 0733-2459

Zäuner, I. Bach, D.Braun, N. Krämer, BK. Fünfstück, R. Helmchen, U. Schollmeyer, P . & Böhler, J.(2002). Predictive value of initialhistology and effect of plasmapheresis on long-term prognosisof rapidly progressive glomerulonephritis .Am J Kidney Dis, Vol.39, No.1, (Jan 2002), PP .28–35

Part 2

Glomerular Disease in
Metabolic and Systemic Conditions

7

Diabetic Glomerulopathy

Mahmoud Barazi[1], Harneet Kaur[2] and Sharma Prabhakar[1]
[1]Department of Internal Medicine,
Texas Tech University Health Science Center, Lubbock, TX
[2]Department of Internal Medicine,
New York Medical College, Valhalla, NY
USA

1. Introduction

Diabetic nephropathy is the most common cause of end-stage renal disease (ESRD) in adults. In the United States, almost half of patients entering ESRD programs were diabetic, and most of them (≥80%) had type 2 diabetes. This is due to the facts that 1) diabetes, particularly type 2, is increasing in prevalence; 2) diabetes patients now live longer; and 3) patients with diabetic ESRD are now being accepted for treatment in ESRD programs where formerly they had been excluded. The annual cost of caring for these patients, in the United States alone, exceeds $10 billion. The mortality rate of patients with diabetic nephropathy is high, and a marked increase in cardiovascular risk accounts for more than half of the increased mortality among these patients.

The earliest clinical manifestation of renal involvement in diabetes is an increase in albumin excretion (microalbuminuria), a stage termed as incipient nephropathy at which renal histology may be relatively normal or may reveal glomerulosclerosis. Diabetes can cause a variety of pathological abnormalities: isolated glomerular basement membrane thickening, mesangial expansion, nodular intercapillary and/or diffuse glomeruloscelorsis or even advanced diabetic sclerosis. While glomerulopathy is quite the hallmark of diabetic nephropathy, the frequency and functional significance of interstitial lesions in diabetic kidney is now well recognized. Furthermore, the occurrence of non-diabetic glomerulopathy or vasculitis alone or superimposed on diabetic nephropathy is increasingly being documented in literature. The pathogenesis is incompletely understood and is very vigorously being investigated.

Once overt diabetic nephropathy (proteinuria) is present, ESRD can be postponed, but in most instances not prevented, by effective antihypertensive treatment and careful glycemic control. Treatment options currently are limited to obvious pathogenic factors while several innovative therapies are under evaluation. Therefore, in the last decades, there has been intensive research into pathophysiologic mechanisms of early diabetic renal injury, predictors of diabetic nephropathy risk, and early intervention strategies

2. Epidemiology

Type 1 diabetes – The epidemiology of diabetic nephropathy has been best studied in patients with type 1 disease, since the time of clinical onset is usually known. About 0.5% of the population in the United States and Central Europe has type 1 diabetes. The prevalence is higher in the northern Scandinavian countries and lower in southern Europe and Japan. Approximately 20 to 30 percent will have microalbuminuria after a mean duration of diabetes of 15 years (Orchard TJ 1990). Less than half of these patients will progress to overt nephropathy; microalbuminuria may regress or remain stable in a substantial proportion, probably related to glycemic and blood pressure control.

Prior to the current period of intensive monitoring and treatment, it was suggested that 25 to 45 percent of diabetic patients will develop clinically evident disease (the minimal criterion for which is a persistently positive urine dipstick for protein) (Parving HH, 1998). After so-called macroalbuminuria or clinical grade proteinuria (>300 mg albuminuria per day) develops, the majority of patients will progress to end-stage renal failure.

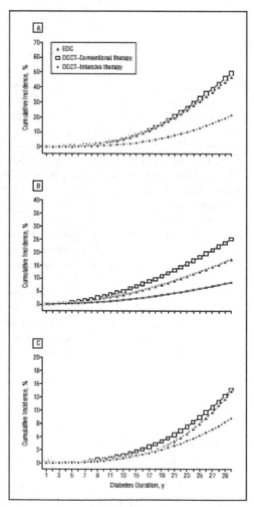

Fig. 1. Estimated cumulative incidences of proliferative retinopathy or worse (A), nephropathy (B) and cardiovascular disease over time.

The overall incidence of end-stage renal disease (ESRD) was also substantial, with reported rates of 4 to 17 percent at 20 years from time of initial diagnosis and approximately 16 percent at 30 years (Nathan DM 2009). A strong predictor of the development of ESRD was the level of glycemic control during the first two decades of IDDM. The risk of ESRD in the group with the poorest glycemic control was almost threefold higher than in the middle group, and fourfold higher than the group with the best glycemic control.

In comparison to these findings, subsequent studies have found that the renal prognosis of type 1 diabetes, including the rate of progression to ESRD, has dramatically improved over the last several decades. In addition to the importance of glycemic control, more aggressive blood pressure reduction and the use of angiotensin converting enzyme inhibitors have been shown to reduce the rate of progression of, though not prevent, diabetic nephropathy (Krolewski M 1996).

Type 2 diabetes is about nine times more prevalent than type 1 diabetes, accounting in part for the greater contribution of type 2 diabetic patients to ESRD incidence. In Caucasians, the prevalence of progressive renal disease has generally been lower in type 2 diabetes than in type 1 disease (Cowie CC, 1989). However, this observation may not apply to all groups with type 2 diabetes, some of whom have had a more ominous renal prognosis. Studies in type 2 diabetic patients from Western Europe and in Pima Indians from Arizona showed rates of progression to nephropathy similar to those of type 1 diabetic patients. The risk of developing ESRD is much higher in black than in white American patients with type 2 diabetes.

As previously described, however, the use of modern therapies lowers the incidence of ESRD, even in groups at extremely high risk such as the Pima Indians. In a subsequent study, for example, the incidence of diabetic ESRD was noted to have declined significantly from the period 1991-1994 to the period 1999-2002 (32 to 15 cases per 1000 patient-years, respectively).

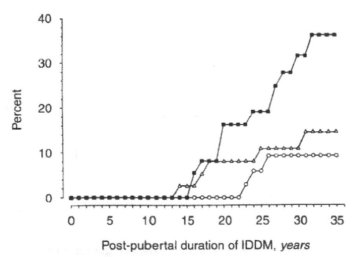

Fig. 2. Cumulative incidence of ESRD according to duration of IDDM and according to tertile of the index of hyperglycemia. Closed rectangles represent the tertile with the highest index of severe hyperglycemia; open triangles represent the middle tertile, and open circles represent the third with the lowest index of hyperglycemia. The differences among the curves are statistically significant, P = 0.017

Data suggest that the renal risk is currently equivalent in the two types of diabetes. Evidence in support of this hypothesis includes the observations in one report that the time to proteinuria from the onset of diabetes and the time to ESRD from the onset of proteinuria were similar in type 1 and type 2 disease (Ritz E, 1999).

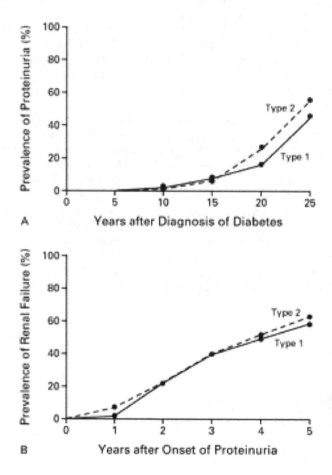

Fig. 3. Cumulative prevalence of persistent proteinuria among patients with type 1 or type 2 diabetes according to the duration of diabetes (Panel A), and cumulative prevalence of renal failure among patients with type 1 or type 2 diabetes according to the duration of proteinuria (Panel B).

Glycemic control, systemic blood pressure levels, and genetic factors seem to be very important in determining diabetic nephropathy risk. Other factors such as lipid levels, smoking habits, and vitamin D intake may also have a role in modulating this risk.

As with type 1 diabetes, some patients with microalbuminuria due to type 2 diabetes, particularly those with good glycemic control, experience regression of microalbuminuria (Araki S, 2005)

3. Natural history and clinical course

The course of renal involvement in type 1 diabetes can be divided in five stages. **Stage I,** present at diagnosis, is that of renal hypertrophy-hyperfunction. At this stage, patients at risk and not at risk of diabetic nephropathy cannot be clearly separated. A 25 to 50 percent elevation in the glomerular filtration rate (GFR) is seen early in the course in up to one-half of patients with type 1 diabetes mellitus, an abnormality that is exaggerated after ingestion of a protein load.

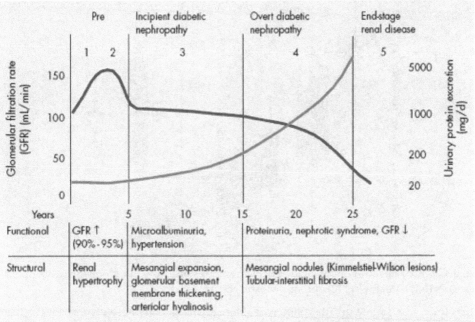

From Vora JP et al. Comprehensive Clinical Nephrology. 2000.[53] Used with permission.

Fig. 4. The five stages of renal involvement in type 1 diabetes

This increase in GFR could be explained by a relative increase in glomerular capillary pressure and/or ultrafiltration coefficient. Glomerular hypertrophy and increased renal size typically accompany the rise in GFR. In an inception cohort study of adult-onset type 1 diabetic subjects, a greater albumin excretion rate within the normal range, male gender, higher mean blood pressure and hemoglobin A1c, and shorter stature were independent predictors of development of microalbuminuria over 18 years of follow-up.

Hyperfiltration also occurs early in the course of type 2 diabetes (Vora JP, 1992). The degree of hyperfiltration and the course of the GFR in type 2 diabetes mellitus was evaluated in more detail in a study of 194 Pima Indians of the Gila River Indian Community in Arizona who have the world's highest incidence of Non-Insulin-Dependent Diabetes Mellitus (NIDDM) (Nelson RG, 1996). The following results were noted:

- In 31 patients with a normal glucose tolerance test, the mean GFR was 123 mL/min
- In 29 patients with impaired glucose tolerance, the mean GFR was 135 mL/min
- In 30 patients with newly diagnosed type 2 disease, the mean GFR was 143 mL/min

- In 70 patients with overt diabetes for more than five years and either normal albumin excretion or microalbuminuria, the mean GFR was 153 mL/min; in 34 similar patients with overt proteinuria, the mean GFR was 124 mL/min

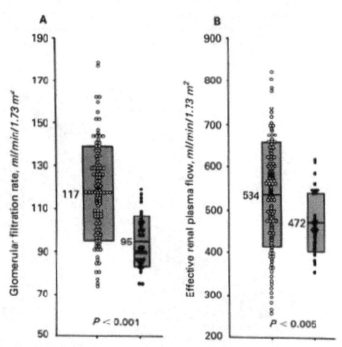

Fig. 5. Glomerular filtration rate and effective renal plasma flow in non-insulin dependent diabetics (NIDDMs) (N= 110) and normal subjects (N = 32).

After four year follow-up, the GFR rose 14 percent in patients with impaired glucose tolerance, 18 percent in newly diagnosed patients, was stable in those with microalbuminuria, and fell 35 percent in those with overt proteinuria. This pattern is consistent with the hypothesis that hyperfiltration causes progressive glomerular damage. However, the base-line glomerular filtration rate in the diabetic subjects predicted neither increasing urinary albumin excretion nor declining glomerular filtration during four years of follow-up, suggesting that hyperfiltration itself is not the principal factor in the development or progression of nephropathy. Higher urinary albumin excretion at base line, however, did predict increasing albuminuria and, in subjects with macroalbuminuria, declines in the GFR; these findings suggest that enhanced protein flux across the glomerular capillary wall contributes to progressive glomerular damage. Proteinuria also predicts the progression of renal disease in patients with nondiabetic renal disease.

Studies in experimental animals indicate that dilatation of the afferent (precapillary) glomerular arteriole plays an important role in the hyperfiltration response, by raising both the intraglomerular pressure and renal blood flow. (Bank N, 1991) A role for hormones is suggested by the ability of a chronic infusion of a somatostatin analogue octreotide to partially reverse both the early hyperfiltration and the increase in renal size in type 1 diabetic patients (Serri O, 1991). There was, however, a fall in the plasma concentration of insulin-like growth factor I (IGF-1), which is produced in part within the kidney. Although the pathogenetic role of IGF-1 is unproven, it is of interest that infusion of this hormone in normal subjects can replicate the findings seen in diabetics — renal vasodilatation and an elevation in GFR. Similar hemodynamic changes plus renal hypertrophy can be induced by IGF-I in experimental animals.

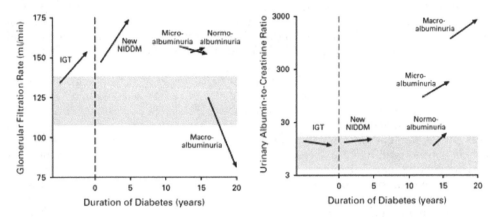

Fig. 6. Changes in the Mean Glomerular Filtration Rate and Median Urinary Albumin-to-Creatinine Ratio from Base Line to the End of Follow-up in Subjects with Impaired Glucose Tolerance (IGT), Newly Diagnosed Non-Insulin-Dependent Diabetes Mellitus (New NIDDM), NIDDM and Normal Urinary Albumin Excretion (Normoalbuminuria), NIDDM and Microalbuminuria, and NIDDM and Macroalbuminuria.

Each arrow connects the value at the base-line examination and the value at the end of follow-up. The dashed line indicates the time of diagnosis, and the shaded area the 25th through 75th percentiles of values in subjects with normal glucose tolerance. Albumin was measured in milligrams per liter and creatinine in grams per liter.

Several other factors directly related to hyperglycemia also may be important, including the intracellular accumulation of sorbitol and the formation of glycosylated proteins (Passariello N, 1993). The enzyme aldose reductase converts intracellular glucose to sorbitol, which then accumulates within the cells. Studies in hyperfiltering humans with type 1 diabetes have shown that the chronic administration of an aldose reductase inhibitor (tolrestat) lowers the GFR toward normal.

Stage II is defined by the presence of detectable glomerular lesions in patients with normal albumin excretion rates and normal blood pressure levels. Normoalbuminuric patients with more severe glomerular lesions might be at increased risk of progression. Patients can remain in stage 2 for the remainder of their lives. However, those in whom nephropathy is destined to progress further will at this stage exhibit a loss of the normal nocturnal blood pressure decline (i.e., night/day ratios >0.9 and non-dipping) as an early diabetic nephropathy indicator that often precedes the development of persistent microalbuminuria. Microalbuminuria, typically occurring in 2 to 5 percent of patients per year, defines **stage III**. Patients with microalbuminuria are referred to as having incipient nephropathy. Microalbuminuria (a sign of endothelial dysfunction that is not necessarily confined to the kidney) may be present earlier, particularly during adolescence and in patients with poor glycemic control and high-normal blood pressure levels. Compared with normoalbuminuric patients, patients with persistent microalbuminuria have threefold to fourfold greater risk of progression to proteinuria and ESRD. Current studies indicate that between 20% and 45% of microalbuminuric type 1 diabetic patients will progress to proteinuria after about 10 years of follow-up, whereas 20% to 25% will return to normoalbuminuric levels (Hovind P, 2004) and the rest will remain microalbuminuric. At this stage, glomerular lesions are generally more severe than in the previous stages, and blood pressure tends to be increasing, often into the hypertensive range. Other laboratory abnormalities, such as increased levels of cholesterol, triglycerides, fibrinogen, Von Willebrand's factor, and prorenin, can be detected in some patients. Diabetic retinopathy, lower extremity amputation, coronary heart disease, and stroke are also more frequent in this group.

The normal rate of albumin excretion is less than 20 mg/day (15 µg/min); persistent albumin excretion between 30 and 300 mg/day (20 to 200 µg/min) is called microalbuminuria and, in patients with type 1 diabetes, persistent microalbuminuria may be indicative of early diabetic nephropathy unless there is some coexistent renal disease.

It was initially thought that microalbuminuria precedes the loss of glomerular filtration rate (GFR) in patients with type 1 diabetes. However, some patients with normoalbuminuria or microalbuminuria have significant reductions in GFR prior to the development of macroalbuminuria. Loss of renal function, which was defined as an estimated decrease in GFR of more than 3.3 percent per year, occurred in 9 percent of patients with normoalbuminuria and 16 percent with regression of microalbuminuria. Loss of renal function occurred much more frequently (32 and 68 percent) in patients with stable or progressive microalbuminuria, respectively.

Patients with newly diagnosed type 2 diabetes in which 6.5 percent had microalbuminuria and 0.7 percent had macroalbuminuria at the time of diagnosis. The rate of microalbuminuria at the time of diagnosis of type 2 diabetes may be higher in older patients. There are at least two possible explanations for the presence of microalbuminuria at the time of diagnosis of type 2 diabetes: the patients had previously undiagnosed diabetes or some other disease was responsible for the microalbuminuria. Forty to 50 percent of patients with type 2 diabetes who have microalbuminuria eventually die of cardiovascular disease; this is three times as high a rate of death from cardiac causes as among patients who have diabetes but have no evidence of renal disease.

As with type 1 diabetes, some patients with microalbuminuria and type 2 diabetes regress to normoalbuminuria. At six years, regression occurred in 51 percent, while progression to macroalbuminuria occurred in 28 percent. Several factors (short duration of microalbuminuria, better glycemic and blood pressure control, and the use of ACE inhibitors or angiotensin II receptor blockers) were independently associated with remission.

Stage IV occurs after 10 to 20 years of diabetes and is characterized by the presence of dipstick-positive proteinuria: proteinuria of greater than 300 mg/d. Hypertension is present in about 75% of these patients, and reduced GFR and dyslipidemia are also common. Retinopathy and peripheral and autonomic neuropathy are present in most patients. In addition, the risk for cardiovascular events is extremely high, and asymptomatic myocardial ischemia is frequent. Without therapeutic interventions, GFR declines by about 1.2 mL/min/month in proteinuric type 1 diabetic patients. In type 2 diabetic patients, Once macroalbuminuria is present, creatinine clearance declines at a rate that varies widely from patient to patient; the average reduction is 10 to 12 ml per minute per year in untreated patients. Hypertension and proteinuria may accelerate the decline in the glomerular filtration rate and the progression to end-stage renal disease.

Progression to ESRD (**stage V**) occurs 5 to 15 years after the development of proteinuria. Renal replacement therapy — either dialysis or transplantation is required at this stage.

4. Pathogenesis

Diabetic nephropathy occurs as a result of a complex yet incompletely understood interaction between hemodynamic and metabolic factors (Cooper, M., 2001). Hemodynamic factors that contribute to the development of diabetic nephropathy include increased systemic and intraglomerular pressure, as well as activation of vasoactive humoral pathways including the renin angiotensin system and endothelin (G.M. Hargrove, 2000). These hemodynamic pathways activate intracellular second messengers such as protein kinase C (PKC), Mitogen-activated protein (MAP kinase) (M. Haneda, 1997), nuclear transcription factors such as NF-kB and various growth factors such as the prosclerotic cytokine, TGF-β and the permeability enhancing growth factor, vascular endothelial growth factor, VEGF.

Glucose dependent pathways are also activated within the diabetic kidney and result in enhanced oxidative stress, renal polyol formation (Dunlop ME, 2000) and the accumulation of advanced glycation end products (AGEs). In combination, these pathways ultimately lead to increased renal albumin permeability and extracellular matrix accumulation, resulting in increasing proteinuria, glomerulosclerosis and ultimately tubulointerstitial fibrosis.

5. Hemodynamic pathways

Glomerular hyperperfusion and hyperfiltration are the early signs resulting from decreased resistance in both the afferent and efferent arterioles of the glomerulus. Afferent arteriole seems to have a greater decrease in resistance than the efferent, which in fact may have increased resistance. Many factors have been reported to be involved in this faulty autoregulation, including nitric oxide, prostanoids, vascular endothelial growth factor (VEGF), TGF-β1, and the renin angiotensin system, specifically angiotensin II. These early hemodynamic changes predispose to albumin leakage from the glomerular capillaries and overproduction of mesangial cell matrix, as well as thickening of the glomerular basement membrane and injury to podocytes (Ziyadeh, F 2008). In addition, increased mechanical strain from these hemodynamic changes can induce localized release of certain cytokines and growth factors (Wolf, G.F.N, 2007)

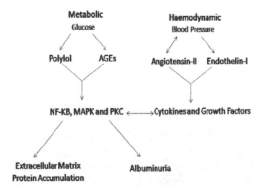

Fig. 7. Interaction of hemodynamic and metabolic pathway, cytokines and intracellular signaling molecules mediating diabetic nephropathy

The action of vasoactive hormones, such as angiotensin II and endothelin are mediator of renal hemodynamic changes. Glomerular hypertension and hyperfiltration contribute to the development of diabetic nephropathy because use of renin–angiotensin blockers preserves kidney function and morphology. Blockade of the renin-angiotensin–aldosterone system antagonizes the profibrotic effects of angiotensin II by reducing its stimulation of TGF-β1 (Hilker, KF, 2005). Support that such profibrotic effects underlie diabetic nephropathy has also been provided by study of an animal model of diabetic nephropathy (Nagai Y, 2005). Transient blockade of the renin–angiotensin system (for 7 weeks) in prediabetic rats reduced proteinuria and improved glomerular structure. Additionally, the administration of an angiotensin converting-enzyme inhibitor to patients with type 1 diabetes and nephropathy appears to reduce serum concentrations of TGF-β1. A correlation exists between decreased levels of TGF-β1 in serum and urine and renal protection, as determined by changes in the glomerular filtration rate.

5.1 Renin-angiotensin system in diabetic nephropathy

The renin-angiotensin system (RAS) has been extensively studied in diabetes. Earlier studies centered on the systemic RAS, and the data obtained have been conflicting, with stimulation, suppression, and no change in the system being reported (Wolf, G, 2007). The factors that influence the systemic RAS in addition to the different stages of disease and species studied may explain many of these divergent findings. However in various diabetic models, increased renal renin content relative to plasma renin levels has generally been found, thus suggesting impaired renal renin release into the circulation. In clinical diabetic nephropathy, there is decreased plasma rennin activity that may be due to nonenzymatic glycation of prorenin with decreased conversion to active renin. Thus, diabetic nephropathy has traditionally been considered a "low renin" state. However, plasma renin activity may not accurately reflect activity of the RAS in the kidney.

Another problem has been the difficulty of accurate measurement of plasma angiotensin-II (Ang II), which is an important issue because discordance can exist between plasma renin and Ang II levels. More recently, the intrarenal RAS has been the focus of extensive study. Abundant evidence indicates the existence of local tissue RASs that are regulated independent of plasma RAS (Ballerma, B.J., 1984). It was reported that glomerular Ang II receptors decrease in the diabetic rat 3 to 4 weeks after induction of the disease. Downregulation of glomerular Ang II receptors implies that intra- renal Ang II generation may be increased. The density of Ang II receptors in the proximal tubules was reported to be reduced in diabetic rats and was accompanied by decreased mRNA expression for the AT1 receptor (Cheng, H.F, 1994). Recently, AT1 receptor density has also been shown to be decreased in mesangial cells when incubated in high-glucose media (Amiri F, G, 1999). ACE activity in whole kidney is low in diabetes.

However, this is probably due primarily to mesangial RAS. Staining for ACE has been found to be enhanced in glomeruli and vasculature of diabetic rats and in patients with diabetic nephropathy (Mizuiri, S., 1998). These data suggest that the term "intrarenal" RAS is oversimplistic, in as much as the vascular RAS (vessels and glomeruli) appears to be regulated differently from the tubulointerstitial RAS. Angiotensin receptor blockers (ARBs) enhance the renal vasodilation in patients with diabetes (despite the presence of low plasma rennin activity), again supporting the concept that the renal vascular RAS is activated in several intrarenal compartments including the glomeruli by several orders of magnitude higher than those found systemically. This shows the existence of both local RAS acting is independently of the systemic RAS and also is consistent with the finding that in most renal cell culture studies, effects of Ang II are observed at substantially higher concentrations (about 0.01-1.0 mmol/L) than those found in the systemic circulation.

5.2 Vaso-active hormones

Endothelium is an interior covering of blood vessels. There are various biological functions of endothelium and it regulates vascular tone and maintains free flow of blood in vessels (Escandon, J.C, 2001). The luminal surface of every blood vessel, forms a physical and metabolic barrier to circulating elements. The endothelium is an important endocrine organ and releases a number of vasoactive hormones, including endothelin (ET-1) (Ulker, 2003), endothelium-derived hyperpolarizing factor (EDHF: nitric oxide and prostacyclin). Endothelin-1 is a potent vasoconstrictor, Endothelium-derived hyperpolarizing factor is still a controversial subject of vascular biology. Endothelial cells of every blood vessel release nitric oxide and prostacyclin and they form a particular partnership in the regulation of vascular and platelet function.

5.3 Nitric Oxide

Nitric Oxide (NO), originally identified as "endothelial derived relaxing factor," is a ubiquitously utilized signaling molecule that regulates a wide variety of organ and cellular functions, including renal hemodynamics and salt and water regulation. NO is generated enzymatically from the amino acid L-arginine by one of three specific nitric oxide synthases: "neuronal"(NOS1 or nNOS), "endothelial" (NOS3 or eNOS), or "inducible" (NOS2 or iNOS). Many, but not all, of the intracellular signaling pathways activated by NO are mediated by activation of guanylate cyclase, which increases intracellular levels of cyclic guanosine monophosphate.

All three NOS isoforms are present in the mammalian kidney, with both distinct and overlapping patterns of distribution. In normal kidney, NOS1 is highly expressed in the macula densa and glomerular parietal epithelium, as well as in the medulla in the collecting ducts and thin ascending limb. NOS2 is expressed in the endothelium of glomerular capillaries and afferent and efferent arterioles, renal arteries, and descending vasa recta, as well as in proximal tubule and medullary thick ascending limb. NOS3 is also expressed in tubules, including S3 segments of the proximal tubule, medullary thick ascending limb, and collecting duct, in addition to arcuate arteries and vasa recta bundles (Kone, BC, 1997). Both in vivo and in vitro studies have provided conflicting results regarding NOS expression and NO production in diabetes. Most but not all studies in cultured renal cells have determined decreased NO production in response to hyperglycemia (Komers R, 2003).

It has been established for a long time that the principal risk factors that affect the development and progression of diabetic nephropathy includes uncontrolled hyperglycemia, hypertension (systemic and glomerular) and activation of RAAS. All these three factors have been shown to modulate intra renal NO generation either directly or through signaling pathways. The role of NO in affecting the renal structure and function is very complicated and depends on several factors including the stage of diabetic renal disease, isoforms of NOS involved, structures in the kidney, and influence of other factors in diabetic milieu. The complex metabolic milieu in diabetes triggers several pathophysiological mechanisms that simultaneously stimulate and suppress intrarenal NO production. The net effect on renal NO levels depends on the mechanisms that prevail in a given stage of the disease process.

5.3.1 Dual role of Nitric Oxide in diabetic nephropathy

The currently available evidence enables us to reasonably conclude that early diabetic nephropathy is associated with increased renal NO production mediated primarily by constitutively released NO through eNOS or NOS III activation. There is some contribution to this augmented NO production through nNOS (NOS I) derived enhanced synthesis, particularly from macula densa region of the kidney. Together the increased intrarenal NO generation contributes to the development of glomerular hyperfiltration and microalbuminuria that characterize early diabetic nephropathy.

On the other hand, advanced diabetic nephropathy with severe proteinuria, hypertension and renal failure is associated with a state of progressive NO deficiency. As the duration of diabetic state increases, factors that suppress NO bioavailability prevail. Many factors including activation of protein kinase C, activation of TGF-beta, NO quenching by advanced glycosylation end products (AGE) contribute to the NO deficient state – either directly or by inhibiting and/or by post translational modification of activity of NOS isoforms. Other inhibitors of NOS enzyme such as asymmetric dimethylarginine (ADMA) accumulate in diabetic nephropathy and may contribute to progression of DN and such association has also been observed in other microvascular complications such as retinopathy. Most of these changes are mediated by endothelial and partly inducible NOS in the chronic advanced stage of DN. Progressive loss of renal parenchyma also contributes partially to the NO deficiency since kidney is a major source of L-arginine, the sole precursor of NO. These changes and the factors affecting them are discussed well in a review (Prabhakar 2005) and schematically represented in the figure below.

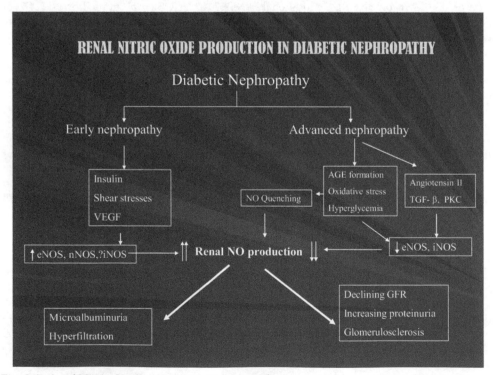

Fig. 8. Role of Nitric Oxide in Diabetic Nephropathy

In a recent study, the natural history of renal manifestations have been described in ZSF$_1$ rats, a recently developed rodent model of type 2 diabetes who developed obesity and hyperglycemia by 20 weeks of age on a high-carbohydrate diet. They also developed systolic and diastolic hypertension, hypercholesterolemia, profound hypertriglyceridemia, proteinuria, and renal failure. Renal histology demonstrated changes consistent with early diabetic nephropathy, including arteriolar thickening, tubular dilation and atrophy, glomerular basement membrane thickening, and mesangial expansion. Furthermore, renal nitric oxide production was decreased, and homogenates from renal cortices demonstrated reduced expression of renal endothelial and inducible nitric oxide synthases. These changes were associated with increased urinary levels and renal expression of 8-hydroxydeoxyguanosine, an indicator of mitochondrial oxidative stress, as well as with increased renal peroxynitrite formation. Administration of either insulin or the antioxidant alpha-lipoic acid decreased proteinuria and oxidative stress, but only the former slowed progression of renal failure (Prabhakar 2007).

5.4 Prostacyclin
The first step in prostacyclin synthesis is the liberation of arachidonic acid from membrane-bound lipids via the enzymatic actions of phospholipase A2 (PLA2). In endothelial cells, phospholipase A2 activation is a calcium-dependent step. Once liberated, arachidonic acid is available for metabolism by cyclooxygenase (COX). Cyclooxygenase is present in two isoforms: COX-1 and COX-2. Cyclo-oxygenase-1, like NOSI or NOSIII, is constitutively expressed, while COX-2, like NOSII, is induced at sites of inflammation and/or by PAMPs. In healthy endothelial cells, COX-1 is the predominate isoform. Cyclooxygenase has two enzymatic activities: firstly, an oxygenase step forms prostaglandin (PG) G2; and secondly, a peroxidase step, which forms PGH2 from PGG2. Prostaglandin H2 is the substrate for a range of downstream prostaglandin synthase enzymes, including prostacyclin synthetase (PGIS), the actions of which result in the formation of prostacyclin. Endothelial cells are enriched in cyclooxygenase-1(COX-1) and PGIS, which is why, when phospholipase A2 is activated, prostacyclin is the predominant metabolite made. It is important to note that in platelets, which also express predominantly COX-1, thromboxane is the principal product made. This is because platelets express mainly thromboxane synthase with negligible levels of PGIS.

5.5 Endothelin1
Endothelin-1 (ET-1) is a potent vasoconstrictor peptide produced by vascular endothelium from big ET-1 (Xu 1994) via specific cleavage by endothelium converting enzyme (ECE). ET-1 produces its actions by acting on endothelin ETA and ETB receptors (Haynes, 1993). ETA receptor predominates in vascular smooth muscle cells and mediates vasoconstriction in both large and small blood vessels where as ETB receptors on endothelial cells mediate vasodilation through the production of nitric oxide and prostacyclin (Verhaar, MC, 1998). ET-1 is involved in the pathogenesis of cardiovascular disorders such as hypertension and heart failure including diabetic nephropathy (Benigni 1998). Diabetes mellitus induces the renal overexpression of ET-1 in the glomeruli and tubular epithelial cells leading to progression of diabetic nephropathy. It was shown that diabetes-induced elevated level of renal ET-1 might induce glomerular hyperperfusion and damage tubulointerstitium in rats. The diabetes-induced elevated level of renal ET-1 was noted to accelerate the progression of diabetic nephropathy in rats31. It has been documented that ET-1 activates a variety of

signaling systems to induce contraction, hypertrophy, proliferation, and extracellular matrix accumulation in mesangial cells (Sorokin, 2003). The detrimental role of ET-1 in pathogenesis of diabetic nephropathy has been confirmed by the fact that diabetes induced elevated level of renal ET-1 is associated with an expansion of mesangial cells and collagen deposition in the glomeruli of diabetic mice. It has been recently demonstrated that ET-1 mediated activation of ETA receptor induced the renal TGF-β production and inflammation in diabetic rats (Sasser, 2007). Treatment with CPU0213, a dual ETA/ETB receptor antagonist has been found to improve the renal function in rats with diabetic nephropathy by suppressing Nicotinamide adenine dinucleotide phosphate (NADPH) oxidase, suggesting that ET-1 contributes to the pathogenesis of diabetic nephropathy via upregulation of NADPH oxidase mediated ROS production in renal cells (Xu, M., 2009). Thus under pathological conditions, prevention of endothelin-mediated various signaling pathways may provide an alternative approach to treat diabetic nephropathy.

5.6 Urotensin

Urotensin II (UII) is an 11-amino acid vasoactive peptide, recently identified as the ligand for a novel G protein-coupled receptor, GPR-14 (renamed urotensin receptor [UT]). In addition to its potentvasoconstrictive actions, UII also has trophic and profibrotic effects, leading to its implication in the pathogenesis of heart failure. However, it has been noted that elevated plasma levels of UII in association with renal impairment and diabetes and diabetic nephropathy. Urotensin-II, an endogenous vasoconstrictor, has been suggested to be involved in the pathogenesis of vascular endothelial dysfunction (VED) (Maguire, J.J., 2002). Urotensin-II increases the activity of NADPH oxidase and plasminogen activator inhibitor-1 (PAI-1) and cause decrease in endothelium dependent relaxation (Watanabe, T., 2006). The overexpression of urotensin-II in endothelial cells cause VED by increasing the expression of type 1 collagen and formation of ROS.

6. Metabolic pathway

Advanced glycosylation end products or AGEs are a chemically heterogeneous group of compounds formed as a result of the "Maillard reaction" when reducing sugars react non-enzymatically with amine residues, predominantly lysine and arginine, on proteins, lipids and nucleic acids. While the initial stage of the reaction leading to the formation of reversible glycosylation proteins termed Schiff bases is rapid and glucose dependent, a much slower reaction over a period of days results in the formation of the more stable Amadori product. These early glycosylation products accumulate predominantly on long lived proteins such as vessel wall collagen and crystallines (Brownlee, 2001), undergoing a series of in vivo rearrangements to form irreversible, complex compounds and cross-links, termed AGEs.

Once AGE related cross-links form on proteins, they become resistant to proteolytic degradation (Thomas, 2005). As well as their non-receptor mediated effects; AGES can exert their biological effects through receptor-mediated mechanisms, the most important of which is the receptor for advanced glycation end products (RAGE). RAGE is a signal transduction receptor that belongs to the immunoglobin superfamily and is expressed on a number of cell types including monocytes/macrophages, endothelial cells, renal mesangial cells and podocytes (Yan, S.F., 2004). Binding of AGEs to the RAGE receptor activates a number of pathways implicated in the development of diabetic complications, specifically diabetic renal disease. These include enhanced cytosolic reactive species formation, stimulation of intracellular molecules such as PKC and NF-kB and the activation and expression of a number of growth factors and cytokines such as TGF-β and VEGF (Wendt, T., 2003). Indeed, strategies to inhibit the formation of AGEs have been shown to ameliorate diabetic nephropathy.

In the initial study by Soulis-Liparota et al. aminoguanidine, an inhibitor of AGE formation, which acts by scavenging intermediates in the advanced glycation pathway attenuated the rise in albuminuria observed in diabetic rodents, while preventing increases in collagen related fluorescence in isolated glomeruli and renal tubules (Soulis-Liparota, T. 1991). Similar results have been obtained with alagebrium, a putative AGE cross-link breaker. In an experimental study, both aminoguanidine and alagebrium attenuated the albuminuria observed in diabetic rodents (Forbes, J.M., 2003). Furthermore, alagebrium was also beneficial when used as part of a delayed intervention protocol, suggesting that it may be useful in both preventing and retarding diabetic nephropathy (Ziayadeh, F.N., 1991).

A subsequent study confirmed and extended these findings. The early (weeks 16–32) and late (weeks 24–32) administration of alagebrium was again shown to reduce albuminuria in a type 1 diabetic rodent model. As a number of previous groups had demonstrated increases in collagen and other extracellular matrix components in experimental diabetic nephropathy, this study also sought to determine the mechanisms surrounding the improvements in microalbuminuria in diabetic rodent kidneys. The compound was shown to reduce diabetes induced increases in the gene expression of TGF-β1, connective tissue growth factor (CTGF) and collagen IV. Early treatment with alagebrium was also associated with significant structural improvement in the kidney including a reduction in the glomerulosclerotic index and tubulointerstitial area, in conjunction with a reduction in AGE peptide fluorescence in serum and the kidney. Furthermore, a reduction in renal accumulation of the specific AGE, carboxymethylysine (CML) and decreased RAGE immunostaining was also seen, providing further evidence that accumulation of AGEs is implicated in renal extracellular matrix accumulation in diabetes.

In the setting of diabetes mellitus and long-term hyperglycemia, nonenzymatic modification of proteins (or lipids) by glucose, or its metabolic products, results in their stable modification and altered function. This process is thought to underlie a major pathogenic pathway leading to tissue injury in diabetes. A major pathway for AGE formation involves triose phosphate intermediaries derived from metabolism of glucose. Triose phosphates build up as intracellular glucose increases and can nonenzymatically form the early glycosylation product methyglyoxal by spontaneous decomposition (Degenhardt 1998 and Frye 1998). Amine-catalyzed sugar fragmentation reactions then modify protein lysine residues directly, forming N- (epsilon) - (carboxymethyl) lysine (CML), a major product of oxidative modification of glycated proteins. Alternatively, reaction of terminal amino groups (e.g., on lysine) with glucose itself may form from early glycation products (i.e., Amadori products) that rearrange to produce stable moieties that possess distinctive chemical crosslinking and biologic properties, designated AGEs (Cohen 2003 and Vlassara 1981). Other glucosederived Amadori products and fructose are thought to be potential precursors of 3-deoxyglucosone (3-DG) in vivo. Fructose generated by the aldose reductase pathway is converted into fructose-3- phosphate by the action of 3-phosphokinase (3- PK). This leads to the generation of 3-deoxyglucosone, a central precursor in the generation of an array of AGEs, in particular, CML-adducts and others (3-Deoxyglucosone, 1999) 3-DG can further react with proteins to form pyrrolines or pentosidine.

AGEs have been suggested to represent a general marker of oxidative stress and long-term damage to proteins in aging, atherosclerosis, and diabetes (Wendt T.M., 2003). Renal CML-AGE is increased in diabetes. Immunolocalization of CML in skin, lung, heart, kidney, intestine, intervertebral discs, and particularly in arteries provide evidence for age-dependent increases in CML accumulation in distinct locations, and acceleration of this process in diabetes (Schleicher, E.D., 1997). Immunostaining and immunoblots of diabetic human kidneys show increased CML in diabetic glomeruli, especially in the mesangial matrix and capillary walls (Nathan, D.M., 2005).

6.1 Oxidative stress

Generally, large amount of reactive oxygen species are generated with in nephron by metabolic activity that is counter balanced by a large number of antioxidant enzymes and free radical scavenging systems. Peroxidation of cell membrane lipids, oxidation of proteins, renal vasoconstriction and damage to DNA are the negative biological effects of reactive oxygen species. Unfortunately, hyperglycemia tips the balance towards production of reactive oxygen species, most of which seem to be generated in the mitochondria (Nishikawa, T. 2007). The metabolism of glucose through destructive alternate pathways, such as via PKC activation and advanced glycation end-product formation, in the setting of hyperglycemia also seems partly dependent on reactive oxygen species. Oxidative stress specifically induced by hyperglycemia even before diabetes becomes clinically apparent. DNA damage marker induced by reactive oxygen species is higher in patients with severe nephropathy (i.e. proteinuria versus microalbuminuria). Diabetic nephropathy is linked with severe oxidative stress. This pathway may be responsible for the decreased bioavailability of nitric oxide in the kidney (Prabhakar 2007).

6.2 Reactive oxygen species

Diabetic nephropathy is characterized by excessive deposition of extracellular matrix (ECM) in the kidney, leading to glomerular mesangial expansion and tubulointerstitial fibrosis. Clinical studies have demonstrated that high blood glucose is the main cause of initiation and progression of diabetic vascular complications including nephropathy. High reactive oxygen species (ROS) induced by glucose upregulates TGF-β1 and extra cellular matrix protein (ECM) expression in the glomerular mesangial cells. Hyperglycemia induced ROS generation and ROS-activated signal transduction cascade and transcription factors and overexpression of genes and proteins in glomerular mesangial and tubular epithelial cells lead to ECM accumulation in diabetic kidney.

6.3 Nephrin

Podocytes (specialized visceral epithelial cells) are important for the maintenance of the dynamic functional barrier (Mundel 2002). Nephrin, a protein found in these cells, is crucial for maintaining the integrity of the intact filtration barrier. The renal expression of nephrin might be impaired in diabetic nephropathy. Patients with diabetic nephropathy have markedly reduced renal nephrin expression and fewer electron-dense slit diaphragms compared with patients without diabetes and minimal nephropathic changes or controls (Benigni. 2004). Furthermore, nephrin excretion is raised 17-30% in patients with diabetes (with and without albuminuria) compared with that in individuals without diabetes.

Thus, nephrin excretion could be an early finding of podocyte injury, even before the onset of albuminuria (Kobayashi, 2006). Treatment with blockers of the renin-angiotensin-aldosterone system might help protect nephrin expression. In a study of patients with type 2 diabetes, treatment with an angiotensin-converting-enzyme inhibitor for 2 years maintained nephrin expression at control levels compared with that in untreated patients with diabetes. By contrast, the expression of two other important podocyte and slit diaphragm proteins, podocin and CD2AP, was similar in the three groups. Comparable decreases in renal nephrin expression were reported in other studies of diabetic nephropathy.

6.4 Vitamin D

Vitamin D has a role beyond the regulation of calcium metabolism. There is evidence that the vitamin D system is also involved in regulation of the immune system, cell growth, and differentiation. Vitamin D binds to its nuclear receptor, and later to the vitamin D response element of target genes, to regulate gene transcription. It also interacts with pathways that are germane to the development and progression of diabetic complications, including the renin–angiotensin system (RAS), hypertension, inflammation, and albuminuria. Three recent randomized trials have shown that the vitamin D analogue−19-nor-1-α-dihydroxyvitamin D2 (paricalcitol) can reduce proteinuria in patients with chronic kidney disease, including those with diabetes.

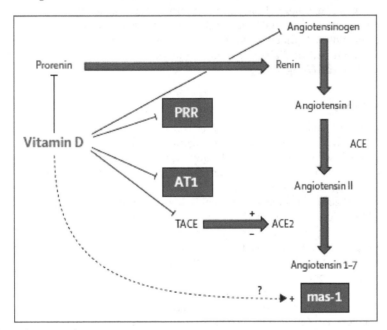

ACE=angiotensin-converting enzyme.
AT1=type 1 angiotensin receptor.
PRR=(pro)renin receptor.
ACE2=angiotensin-converting enzyme 2. TACE=tumor necrosis factor α converting enzyme. mas-1=receptor for angiotensin 1–7.

Fig. 9. Interactions between vitamin D and key elements of the renin–angiotensin system

Vitamin D is a negative regulator of RAS (Li YC, 2002). In experimental chronic kidney disease, paricalcitol reduces the renal expression of renin, the (pro)renin–receptor, angiotensinogen, and the type 1 angiotensin receptor (Freundlich M, 2008). Vitamin D also inhibits tumor necrosis factor α converting enzyme (TACE) (Dusso A, 2010), which regulates the shedding of angiotensin-converting enzyme 2 (ACE2), itself the major enzyme that metabolizes angiotensin II in the proximal tubule. Diabetes is associated with reduced ACE2 expression; therefore inhibition of TACE expression might improve the balance of RAS in the kidney, and might have additional renoprotective effects by inhibition of the TACE-dependent release of other pathogenic mediators.

Vitamin D has several anti-inflammatory actions, including effects on prostaglandin synthesis, inhibition of nuclear factor κB signaling, and innate immunity, all of which have been implicated in diabetic chronic kidney disease. Vitamin D deficiency is associated with raised concentrations of C-reactive protein. In previous studies, paricalcitol reduced C-reactive protein concentrations in patients with chronic kidney disease, which paralleled the decline in albuminuria

Patients with diabetes have increased rates of vitamin D deficiency (Tanaka H, 2009) especially in those with chronic kidney disease in whom the urinary loss of protein-associated vitamin D magnifies reduced activation of vitamin D by the proximal tubule, and reduced expression of the vitamin D receptor. For these patients, it seems rational to replace vitamin D. Selective analogues that restore vitamin D receptor signaling without risking hypercalcemia or hyperphosphatemia might have particular advantages, because of the aberrant calcification of diabetic vessels. Of note, vitamin D replacement reduced proteinuria in about half of diabetic patients with stage 3 or 4 chronic kidney disease in a placebo-controlled trial (Teng M 2003)

7. Histopathology

The pathogenesis of diabetic nephropathy is complex, and renal pathological lesions are diverse. Most likely, there are many pathogenic pathways, which through composite, interactive routes lead to the histological damage that we see in renal biopsies of patients with diabetic nephropathy (Elisabeth J.J, 2011). Though the number of patients with type 2 diabetes in a worldwide context is increasing and is predicted to be 438 million in 2030, paradoxically, diabetic nephropathy is probably becoming the renal disease per se for which the least renal biopsies are performed. In many centers, clinical parameters in the absence of a renal biopsy will diagnose the patient with diabetic nephropathy. Only if unusual signs or symptoms are present, such as sudden onset nephrotic syndrome, will a renal biopsy be performed, mostly with the aim to exclude other causes than diabetic nephropathy for the patient's clinical presentation. This means that in relation to diabetic nephropathy, co-morbidity is often seen by the pathologist in the renal biopsy, and cases in which diabetic nephropathy alone is present become less frequent. In many recent publications, the diagnosis of diabetic nephropathy was based on clinical symptoms, which, in many studies, also formed the gold standard on the evaluation of intervention therapies meant to prevent, slow down, or even reverse the processes causing diabetic nephropathy.

7.1 Histopathological classification system

Up to 2010, the terminology for histopathological lesions in diabetic nephropathy was variable. The new classification launched in 2010 (Thijs W, 2010) distinguishes four classes, essentially characterized by the absence of histological lesions (class I), mesangial changes (class II), nodular lesions (class III), or a predominance of global glomerulosclerosis (class IV).

Class	Description	Inclusion Criteria
I	Mild or nonspecific LM changes and EM-proven GBM thickening	Biopsy does not meet any of the criteria mentioned below for class II, III, or IV GBM > 395 nm in female and >430 nm in male individuals 9 years of age and older[a]
IIa	Mild mesangial expansion	Biopsy does not meet criteria for class III or IV Mild mesangial expansion in >25% of the observed mesangium
IIb	Severe mesangial expansion	Biopsy does not meet criteria for class III or IV Severe mesangial expansion in >25% of the observed mesangium
III	Nodular sclerosis (Kimmelstiel–Wilson lesion)	Biopsy does not meet criteria for class IV At least one convincing Kimmelstiel–Wilson lesion
IV	Advanced diabetic glomerulosclerosis	Global glomerular sclerosis in >50% of glomeruli Lesions from classes I through III

LM, light microscopy.
[a]On the basis of direct measurement of GBM width by EM, these individual cutoff levels may be considered indicative when other GBM measurements are used.

Table 1. Histological classification of Diabetic glomerulopathy

7.1.1 Class I: Glomerular basement membrane thickening

The biopsy specimen shows no or only mild, nonspecific changes by light microscopy that do not meet the criteria of classes II through IV. By direct measurements with EM the glomerular basement membrane (GBM) on average is thicker than 430 nm in males 9 years and older and thicker than 395 nm in females. These cutoff levels are based on a deviation from normal GBM thickness plus 2 standard deviations as recently determined. Light microscopic changes in the GBM and epithelial foot process effacement by EM have no influence on the classification.

Class I incorporates cases with certain degree of chronic and other reactive changes (e.g., changes of arterionephrosclerosis, ischemic type changes, or interstitial fibrosis). Diagnosing DN in cases without characteristic light microscopic glomerular lesions may be difficult, especially when a thicker GBM is also seen with aging or hypertension. The presence of arteriolar hyalinosis may be helpful in these cases, although it is not a prerequisite.

GBM thickening is a characteristic early change in type 1 and type 2 DN and increases with duration of disease. GBM thickening is a consequence of extracellular matrix accumulation, with increased deposition of normal extracellular matrix components such as collagen types IV and VI, laminin, and fibronectin. Such accumulations result from increased production of these proteins, their decreased degradation, or a combination of the two. GBM thickening may already be present in type 1 diabetes patients who are normoalbuminuric. GBM thickening has even been described as a "prediabetic" lesion: In patients with proteinuria and isolated GBM thickening but without overt diabetes, 20% were positive on a blood test for diabetes at the time of biopsy, whereas 44% were diagnosed with diabetes at 6 months, and 70% at 2 years after the biopsy was taken. Long-term glucose control and urinary albumin excretion (UAE) correlate strongly with basement membrane thickness.

7.1.2 Class II: Mesangial expansion, mild (IIa) or severe (IIb)

Class II encompasses those patients classified with mild or severe mesangial expansion but not meeting inclusion criteria for class III or IV and is analogous to the previously used term "diffuse diabetic glomerulosclerosis." Mesangial expansion is defined as an increase in extracellular material in the mesangium such that the width of the interspace exceeds two mesangial cell nuclei in at least two glomerular lobules. The difference between mild and severe mesangial expansion is based on whether the expanded mesangial area is smaller or larger than the mean area of a capillary lumen. If severe mesangial expansion is seen in more than 25% of the total mesangium observed throughout the biopsy, the biopsy is classified as IIb. If this is not the case, but at least mild mesangial expansion is seen in more than 25% of the total mesangium, the biopsy is classified as IIa.

Expansion of cellular and matrix components in the mesangium is a hallmark of type 1 and type 2 DN. It can be detected in some patients within a few years after the onset of type 1 diabetes. When the mesangium expands, it restricts and distorts glomerular capillaries and diminishes the capillary filtration surface.

Various indices have been proposed to describe the amount of mesangial expansion in DN. Mauer et al. define mesangial expansion by mesangial fractional volume or volume density (Vv), defined as the fraction or percentage of the cross-sectional area of the glomerular tuft made up by mesangium, expressed in the formula: Vv (mes/glom). Using this formula, many correlations have been made between mesangial expansion and clinical parameters of DN, particularly showing highly inverse correlations exist between Vv (mes/glom) and GFR. There is also a relationship between Vv (mes/glom) and UAE and blood pressure.

Another index to express mesangial expansion is the so-called "index of mesangial expansion" (IME) for DN. The IME is determined by a semiquantitative estimate of the width of mesangial zones in each glomerulus: grade 0 is normal, 1 is twice normal thickness, 2 is three times normal thickness, and so forth; half grades can also be assigned. The mean of the grades for each glomerulus for IME can thus be determined from a single biopsy. The IME closely correlates with the Vv (mes/glom).

In other classifications, mesangial expansion is defined in more practical ways, such as in the new classification for IgA nephropathy in which it is defined as an increase in the extracellular material in the mesangium such that the width of the interspace exceeds two mesangial cell nuclei in at least two glomerular lobules.

7.1.3 Class III: Nodular sclerosis (Kimmelstiel–Wilson lesions)

If at least one convincing Kimmelstiel–Wilson lesion is found and the biopsy specimen does not have more than 50% global glomerulosclerosis it is classified as class III. Kimmelstiel–Wilson lesions appear in type 1 and type 2 diabetes (only one-third of microalbuminuric type 2 diabetic patients had them) as focal, lobular, round to oval mesangial lesions with an acellular, hyaline/matrix core, rounded peripherally by sparse, crescent-shaped mesangial nuclei. Compared to type 1 diabetes, type 2 diabetes

Paul Kimmelstiel and Clifford Wilson first described nodular lesions in glomeruli from eight maturity-onset diabetes patients in 1936. According to Cameron, they barely noted the association with diabetes, and it was Arthur Allen who clarified the association in 105 patients with diabetes in 1941. Nodular sclerotic lesions may also occur in the absence of DN that are clinically related to hypertension, smoking, hypercholesterolemia, and extrarenal vascular disease.

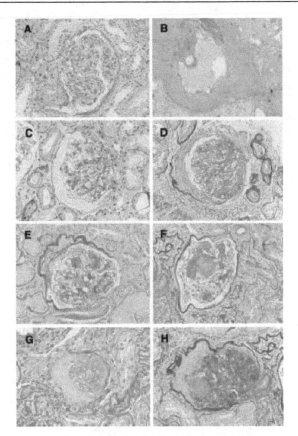

Fig. 10. Representative examples of the morphologic lesions in DN:

(A) Glomerulus showing only mild ischemic changes, with splitting of Bowman's capsule. No clear mesangial alteration.

(B) EM of this glomerulus: the mean width of the GBM was 671 nm (mean taken over 55 random measurements). EM provides the evidence for classifying the biopsy with only mild light microscopic changes into class I.

(C, D) Class II glomeruli with mild and moderate mesangial expansion, respectively. In panel C, the mesangial expansion does not exceed the mean area of a capillary lumen (IIa), whereas in panel D it does (IIb).

(E, F) In panel F is a class III Kimmelstiel–Wilson lesion. The lesion in panel E is not a convincing Kimmelstiel–Wilson lesion, therefore (on the basis of the findings in this glomerulus) the finding is consistent with class IIb. For the purpose of the classification, at least one convincing Kimmelstiel–Wilson (as in panel F) needs to be present.

In panel H, signs of class IV DN consist of hyalinosis of the glomerular vascular pole and a remnant of a Kimmelstiel–Wilson lesion on the opposite site of the pole.

Panel G is an example of glomerulosclerosis that does not reveal its cause (glomerulus from the same biopsy as panel H).

For the purpose of the classification, signs of DN should be histopathologically or clinically present to classify a biopsy with global glomerulosclerosis in > 50% of glomeruli as class IV

It is claimed that in the initial stage of developing nodular sclerotic lesions in DN, two important processes take place: lytic changes in the mesangial area called mesangiolysis and detachment of endothelial cells from the GBM. Exactly how these two processes relate remains uncertain. Paueksakon et al. detected fragmented red blood cells in Kimmelstiel–Wilson lesions, which supports the theory that microvascular injury contributes to the pathogenesis of these lesions. Dissociation of endothelial cells may disrupt the connections between the mesangial area and the GBM. This process precedes expansion of the Kimmelstiel–Wilson lesion. These lesions consist of an accumulation of mesangial matrix with collagen fibrils, small lipid particles, and cellular debris.

A completely developed Kimmelstiel–Wilson lesion destroys the normal structure of glomerular tuft with a decrease in mesangial cells, especially in the central area. In 1992, a graphic method of analysis of the position of Kimmelstiel–Wilson lesions demonstrated the nodules were distributed in a horseshoe-shaped area corresponding to the peripheral or intralobular mesangium, excluding the possibility of hyperfiltration as being their main cause of development.

The presence of at least one Kimmelstiel–Wilson lesion associates with longer duration of diabetes and less favorable clinical parameters. In a study of 36 patients with type 2 diabetes, patients with Kimmelstiel–Wilson lesions had more severe overall retinopathy and higher serum creatinine concentrations than those with mesangial lesions alone. In a study of 124 Chinese patients with type 2 diabetes, patients with at least one Kimmelstiel–Wilson lesion had relatively long duration of diabetes mellitus, a poor prognosis, and frequent evidence of diabetic retinopathy. Kimmelstiel–Wilson lesions are often found in combination with mesangial expansion. The occurrence of Kimmelstiel– Wilson lesions is widely considered transitional from an early or moderately advanced stage to a progressively more advanced stage of disease.

7.1.4 Class IV: Advanced diabetic glomerulosclerosis
Class IV implies advanced DN with more than 50% global glomerulosclerosis in which there is clinical or pathologic evidence that the sclerosis is attributable to DN. Glomerulosclerosis in DN is the end point of multifactorial mechanisms that lead to excessive accumulation of extracellular matrix proteins such as collagen types I, III, and IV and fibronectin in the mesangial space, which through stages of mesangial expansion and development of Kimmelstiel–Wilson lesions finally result in glomerulosclerosis. The clustering of sclerotic lesions in columns perpendicular to the kidney surface suggests that vascular factors relating to the interlobular arteries also contribute.

8. Tubulointerstitial lesions, vascular lesions and nondiabetic glomerular lesions

8.1 Tubular lesions
Concomitant tubular basement membrane thickening of nonatrophic tubules is apparent from the development of class II glomerular diabetic lesions and becomes more conspicuous in class III and IV, which is best seen in PAS or silver stains. Interstitial fibrosis and tubular atrophy (IFTA) follow glomerular changes in type 1 DN that ultimately lead to ESRD. A score of 0 is assigned when the biopsy specimen shows no IFTA, a score of 1 is assigned when less than 25% IFTA is present, a score of 2 is assigned when at least 25% but less than

50% of the biopsy has IFTA, and finally, a score of 3 is assigned when at least 50% IFTA is present, which is similar to the scoring in the recently published classification of IgA nephropathy.

Presence of mononuclear cells in the interstitium is a widely recognized finding in DN. Inflammatory interstitial infiltrates comprise T lymphocytes and macrophages. A score of 0 is assigned if interstitial infiltrates are absent, 1 if they only occur around atrophic tubules, and 2 if the inflammatory infiltrate is also in other areas than around atrophic tubules.

8.2 Vascular lesions

According to Stout et al., hyalinosis of the efferent arteriole is relatively specific for DN, but hyalinosis of the afferent arteriole occurs in numerous other settings. Chronic cyclosporine nephropathy is a typical example in which arteriolar hyalinosis occurs outside DN. Tracy et al. also report the presence of arteriolar hyalinosis in kidneys of young patients with coronary heart disease. Efferent arteriolar hyalinosis is an important lesion by which DN is distinguished from hypertensive nephropathy. However, most studies relate arteriolar hyalinosis to clinical parameters, not distinguishing between efferent and afferent arterioles, showing clear correlations with UAE and disease progression.

In addition to characteristic arteriolar hyalinosis, relatively nonspecific arteriosclerosis may be present in the biopsy specimen. Bohle and colleagues found increases in vascular disease associate with more severe glomerular disease. Osterby et al. use a so-called "matrix to media ratio" to investigate the role of arteriosclerosis and find this ratio is increased in patients with microalbuminuria, suggesting that arteriolar matrix accumulation occurs early in the course of DN. By assessing the most severely affected artery in the biopsy and assign a score of 0 if no intimal thickening is present, 1 if intimal thickening is less than the thickness of the media, and 2 if intimal thickening is more than the thickness of the media. Isolated or significant medial thickness may be associated with concurrent hypertension.

9. Other glomerular lesions

In 1994, Stout et al. defined "insudative lesions" as consisting of intramural accumulations of presumably imbibed plasma proteins and lipids within renal arterioles, glomerular capillaries, Bowman's capsule, or proximal convoluted tubules. Insudative lesions in Bowman's capsule are called capsular drop lesions, and in afferent and efferent arterioles they are called hyalinized afferent and efferent arterioles. In glomerular capillaries they are called fibrin cap lesions, although this term is considered obsolete and moreover is amisnomer because the lesion does not contain fibrin; we prefer the term hyalinosis for these lesions.

Capsular drops are mainly located between the parietal epithelium and Bowman's capsule of the glomerulus. Capsular drops are prevalent in advanced DN and associate with disease progression. The common belief, reviewed by Alsaad et al., is that capsular drops are specific but not entirely pathognomonic of DN. Stout et al. report a prevalence of capsular drops in 5.3% of biopsies without diabetes. However, finding a capsular drop in a biopsy can help distinguish DN from other causes of glomerulosclerosis.

By light microscopy, glomerular hyalinosis describes the same staining characteristics as the capsular drop lesion but it occupies the capillary lumen instead of being attached to Bowman's capsule. This lesion is not a specific finding in DN, because similar lesions are recognized in focal glomerulosclerosis, arterionephrosclerosis, and lupus nephritis.

Lesion	Criteria	Score
Interstitial lesions		
IFTA	No IFTA	0
	<25%	1
	25% to 50%	2
	>50%	3
interstitial	Absent	0
inflammation	Infiltration only in relation to IFTA	1
	Infiltration in areas without IFTA	2
Vascular lesions		
arteriolar hyalinosis	Absent	0
	At least one area of arteriolar hyalinosis	1
	More than one area of arteriolar hyalinosis	2
presence of large vessels	–	Yes/no
arteriosclerosis (score worst artery)	No intimal thickening	0
	Intimal thickening less than thickness of media	1
	Intimal thickening greater than thickness of media	2

Table 2. Interstitial and vascular lesions of DN

Finally, there is increasing recognition of abnormalities in the glomerulotubular junctions with focal adhesions called "tip lesions" and atrophic tubules with no observable glomerular opening (so-called "atubular glomeruli"). These lesions are typically found in more advanced stages of nephropathy associated with overt proteinuria.

One of the important questions that need to be validated is whether the new classification system, which makes no distinction between patients with type 1 and type 2 diabetes, is helpful for clinicians. Type 2 diabetes has more heterogenous clinical course with more heterogenous lesions. Type 2 diabetes also has different response towards treatments, and different relationship between diabetic nephropathy and retinopathy. In a study that published by Osterby R, Gall MA, Schmitz A, et al in 1993, virtually all patients with type 1 diabetes with overt nephropathy have retinopathy, whereas less than 50% of patients with type 2 diabetes and diabetic nephropathy have diabetic retinopathy. These figures may have been altered somewhat in the course of time. In 2010, Pedro et al. studied the prevalence and relationship between diabetic nephropathy and retinopathy in a population-based transversal study in northeastern Spain including 8187 type 2 and 488 type 1 diabetes patients. They distinguished between patients with microalbuminuria and those with overt nephropathy. The relationship between microalbuminuria and diabetic retinopathy was different between the types of diabetes, but the relationship between overt nephropathy and diabetic retinopathy was similar in both types. Overt nephropathy, in this study, was a risk factor for diabetic retinopathy in both types.

10. Biomarker studies

A number of studies reported on biomarkers in either plasma or urine for diabetic nephropathy, particularly in relation to type 2 diabetes. A group from Denmark reported on transthyretin, apolipoprotein A1, apolipoprotein C1, and cystatin C as promising biomarkers for diabetic nephropathy in the plasma of patients with type 1 diabetes (Overgaard AJ 2010). Proteomic analysis of plasma from a cross-sectional cohort of 123 type 1 diabetic patients previously diagnosed as normoalbuminuric microalbuminuric, or macroalbuminuric, gave rise to 290 peaks clusters. Independent component analysis identified 16 candidate peaks that contributed significantly in their respective components with high stability and ability to separate the groups. Four of the peaks were identified as transthyretin, apolipoprotein A1, apolipoprotein C1, and cystatin.

Soluble CD40 ligand derived from platelets and mediating atherothrombosis, was shown to be elevated in type 1 diabetes patients with diabetic nephropathy in comparison with controls. The study was a prospective, observational follow-up study of 443 type 1 diabetes patients with diabetic nephropathy and a control group of 421 patients with longstanding type 1 diabetes and persistent normoalbuminuria. High levels of sCD40L did not predict development of end-stage renal disease ($P = 0.85$) nor rate of decline in glomerular filtration rate (GFR) (Lajer M 2010).

There were several studies on biomarkers in type 2 diabetes giving rise to a number of new markers. A group from China reported an independent association between plasma levels of osteopontin and the presence and severity of diabetic nephropathy in type 2 diabetes (Yan X 2010). In another study on type 2 diabetes, plasma levels of methylglyoxal, a side-product of many metabolic pathways, was found to be higher in patients with diabetic nephropathy than in those without and, furthermore, were shown to correlate with the urinary albumin: creatinine ratio (Lu J 2011). Fibroblast growth factor 23 (FGF-23), previously reported as a marker for outcome in chronic kidney disease in general, was found to be predictive of renal outcome in type 2 diabetes patients with macroalbuminuric nephropathy (Alkhalaf A, 2010). At baseline, serum FGF- 23 showed a significant association with serum creatinine and proteinuria. FGF-23 was an independent predictor of the primary outcome in this study, defined as death, doubling of serum creatinine, and/or dialysis need. The moderate consistency observed between biomarkers reported in different studies is puzzling, which is probably due to different technologies used and the lack of statistical power in some studies resulting in the reporting of artifacts. Also the distinction between those patients with and without diabetic nephropathy in most of these studies is not proven by biopsy.

It is evident that a huge amount of effort is being put into how to identify diabetic nephropathy in patients with diabetes without being invasive, that is, without taking a renal biopsy, both in clinical practice and clinical research studies. A drawback in most of these biomarker studies pursuing this aim is that no renal biopsy was taken to determine the presence and severity of diabetic nephropathy in the diabetic patients in the first place. Virtually all studies rely on clinical parameters, mostly expressed as the amount of albuminuria, for the diagnosis of diabetic nephropathy. How reliable is this? Chronic renal insufficiency and/or proteinuria especially in type 2 diabetes may stem from chronic renal disease other than classic diabetic nephropathy. In a recent retrospective study of 69 patients with type 2 diabetes with renal biopsies, 52% had non diabetes-related nephropathy (Mou S, 2010). Selection bias most likely plays a role in these data, as renal biopsies are typically performed in these patients if co-morbidity is suspected. It remains, however, most likely that some of the patients included in the biomarker studies were unrightfully given the diagnosis of diabetic nephropathy, and it is uncertain how important this contamination of the data is for the study outcomes. Only one marker study in 2010 was found that did incorporate renal biopsy findings and interestingly, in this study, a classification model was able to reliably differentiate diabetic nephropathy from nondiabetic chronic kidney disease (Papale M 2010). Among the best predictors of this classification model were ubiquitin and b 2-microglobulin.

There are probably also a considerable proportion of patients without albuminuria who are at the beginning stages of diabetic nephropathy. These patients are unrightfully diagnosed as not having diabetic nephropathy. Interesting in this light was the 2010 study by Nielsen et al., which evaluated the new marker of tubulointerstitial damage kidney injury molecule 1 (KIM-1) in type 1 diabetes patients with either normoalbuminuria, microalbuminuria, or macroalbuminuria in comparison with normal controls. Urine KIM1 was elevated in all type 1 diabetes patients in comparison with the normal controls and irrespective of the presence of albuminuria. Thus, normoalbuminuric patients with type 1 diabetes also had elevated urine KIM1. It was therefore concluded that tubular damage may be present at an early stage in all patients, the so-called 'tubular phase' of diabetic nephropathy. Whether or not this means that in fact all patients with type 1 diabetes have a latent form of diabetic nephropathy remained undiscussed, but that would be an interesting hypothesis. Another study that investigated urinary changes in non-overt diabetic nephropathy in type 2 diabetes came from Japan (Araki S,2010). This study included 254 patients with type 2 diabetes of whom 185 were normoalbuminuric and 69 had microalbuminuria. At baseline, urinary type IV collagen levels. were higher in patients with microalbuminuria. During a follow-up study with a median duration of 8 years, the level of urinary type IV collagen inversely correlated with the annual decline in estimated GFR, whereas overt proteinuria did not appear in a majority of patients. Two studies from Malaysia gave similar results, with type IV collagen levels correlating with the amount of urinary albumin in 30 type 2 diabetes patients at baseline Sthaneshwar P, 2010), but also with subsequent GFR change (Katavetin P 2010). Also in New Zealand, urinary collagen IV was studied in diabetes: spot urine samples from 457 unselected patients attending a hospital diabetes clinic were analyzed for albumin, creatinine, and a number of biomarkers including collagen IV (Cawood TJ, 2010). The proportion of patients with abnormal collagen IV increased from 26, 58, and 65%, respectively, across the normoalbuminuria, microalbuminuria, and macroalbuminuria groups. The authors conclude that longitudinal studies are now required to assess whether these biomarkers can detect early renal disease with greater specificity and sensitivity than the albumin: creatinine ratio. Including histopathological findings in these types of studies would certainly make a great contribution to our better understanding of the mechanism leading to diabetic nephropathy.

11. Treatment

Interventions that have been found useful in preventing or retarding the progression of DN include
- Strict glycemic control
- Strict blood pressure control
- Cessation of smoking
- Control of hyperlipidemia and
- Restriction of protein intake.

12. Strict glycemic control

Hyperglycemia is an important risk factor for development of microalbuminuria, progression of established microalbuminuria to macroalbuminuria and impaired glomerular filtration rate (GFR). Additional risk factors for microalbuminuria include older age, male sex, long duration of diabetes, smoking, obesity, elevated blood pressure, and genetic predisposition. (de Boer IH 2011)

Studies have shown that strict glycemic control delays the development of microalbuminuria, stabilizes or reduces protein excretion in patients with microalbuminuria and overt proteinuria, and slows the rate of progression to chronic renal failure. The Diabetes Control and Complications Trial (DCCT) compared conventional with intensive glycemic management in 1,441 type-I diabetic patients. This study proved that intensive treatment reduced the risks of retinopathy, nephropathy, and neuropathy by 35% to 90% compared with conventional treatment. The absolute risks of retinopathy and nephropathy were proportional to the mean glycosylated hemoglobin (HbA1c) level over the follow-up period preceding each event. Intensive treatment was most effective when begun early, before complications were detectable. These risk reductions were achieved at a median HbA1c level difference of 9.1% for conventional treatment versus 7.3% for intensive treatment. ((The DCCT/EDIC Research Group 2000, The DCCT/EDIC Research Group 2002)) In the combined cohorts, intensive treatment reduced the development of microalbuminuria and clinical albuminuria by 39% and 56%, respectively. The benefits of intensive therapy were also long-lasting and persisted beyond the period of shortest intervention. (The DCCT/EDIC Research Group 2000, The DCCT/EDIC Research Group 2002) Thus, intensive treatment should be started as soon as possible safely after the onset of type 1 diabetes mellitus and maintained thereafter, aiming for a practicable target HbA1c level of 7.0% or less. (Writing Team for the Diabetes Control and Complications Trial/Epidemiology of Diabetes Interventions and Complications Research Group 2002). These findings suggest that hyperglycemia has long-term chronic effects on the underlying pathophysiology of microvascular complications. It takes time for improvements in control to negate the long lasting effects of prior prolonged hyperglycemia, and once the biological effects of prolonged improved control are manifest, the benefits are long lasting. However, using the current intensive treatment regimen led to a 3-fold increase in severe hypoglycemic events and to excess weight gain in the DCCT. (DCCT/EDIC research group 2002)

Efforts need to be made to eliminate preventable severe hypoglycemic episodes that result from unsafe patient behavior and decisions, and to avoid inordinate weight gain. Irregular food intake, failure to check blood glucose before planned or unplanned vigorous exercise or before operating a motor vehicle, and excess alcohol ingestion have been identified as risk factors for hypoglycemia and serious complications and must be scrupulously avoided. Mealtime bolus doses of rapid acting insulin must be based on the pre-injection blood glucose level, the anticipated amount of carbohydrate intake and upcoming exercise. Thorough diabetes education and its regular reinforcement should be provided by diabetes nurse and dietitian educators. These professionals can negotiate individualized care plans with patients, give them training in self-management, and provide stimulation, motivation, and positive reinforcement for good self-care behavior, such as frequent self blood glucose monitoring and regular eating habits. While these measures can interfere with patients' lifestyles, they are the current price that must be paid to delay or reduce the risk of microvascular complications. (DCCT/EDIC research group 2002)

13. Blood pressure control

Long term and aggressive antihypertensive treatment induces a progressive reduction in the rate of decline in kidney function. Thus, this modality of treatment can postpone renal insufficiency in patients with DN. Both systolic and diastolic hypertension markedly accelerate the progression of DN, and aggressive antihypertensive management has been shown to decrease the rate of fall of glomerular filtration rate, increase the median life expectancy, and reduce the need for dialysis and transplantation.

The primary goal of therapy for non-pregnant patients with DM older than 18 years is to achieve a blood pressure less than 130/80 mmHg for patients with proteinuria <1 g/day, and less than 125/75 mmHg for patients with >1 g/day of proteinuria. Angiotensin converting enzyme (ACE) inhibitors and ARBs are recommended as first-line antihypertensive therapy for patients with type-I and type-2 DM. Other agents that can be used include Beta blockers, calcium channel blockers, and diuretics. (American Diabetes Association 2003, Ayodele OE 2004).

Persistent clinical proteinuria is closely associated with the presence of hypertension in IDDM patients. In NIDDM patients the risk of developing clinical proteinuria is increased more than twofold in patients with blood pressure > 165/95 mm Hg compared to those with lower blood pressure after adjusting for age, sex and duration of diabetes. Moreover, in both insulin-dependent and non-insulin-dependent diabetes, the age adjusted total mortality rate is greatly increased in those patients with proteinuria or hypertension (Earle K 1994). Prospective studies have shown that normoalbuminuric patients who progress to microalbuminuria have higher blood pressures (albeit within the normal range) than those who persistently remain normoalbuminuric. Parents of insulin-dependent diabetic patients with nephropathy have a higher prevalence of hypertension and cardiovascular disease compared to patients without nephropathy (Earle K 1994).

ACE Inhibition versus Angiotensin II (Ang II) receptor type 1 blockade in the Renin-Angiotensin System (RAS). RAS is one of the most important physiological regulators of renal function. ACE inhibitors selectively dilate efferent arterioles. This decreases the arterial pressure and in turn reduces glomerular capillary pressure. In addition, Ang II causes mesangial cell growth and matrix production. Numerous animal studies and clinical trials have shown that ACE inhibitors significantly reduce the loss of kidney function in DN. They prevent progression of microalbuminuria to overt proteinuria and several studies evaluated the effect of ACE inhibitor on development and progression of DN.

The landmark study by Lewis et al. [1993], examined the effect of captopril on the progression of DN in patients with type 1 DM (Lewis, EJ 1993). This was measured as the rate of decline in creatinine clearance and the combined end points of dialysis, transplantation, and death. Treatment with captopril was associated with 48% risk reduction for doubling the serum creatinine as compared to placebo. The results of this study were subsequently confirmed by North American Microalbuminuria Study Group and EUCLID study group (EUCLID Study Group 1997, Laffel LM 1995). They extended the observation by showing a protective effect of ACE inhibitors in patients with a variety of renal diseases, including glomerulopathies, interstitial nephritis, nephrosclerosis, and DN. The exception was polycystic kidney disease. Importantly, the protective effect of ACE inhibition was independent of the severity of renal insufficiency. (Lewis, EJ 1993, Brown N 1998)

The MICRO-HOPE (Heart Outcomes Prevention Evaluation) studied the benefit of ramipril in type 2 diabetics. The diabetes sub-study of the Heart Outcomes Prevention Evaluation study showed ramipril reduced the risk of overt nephropathy by 24%. Moreover, ramipril reduced urinary albumin excretion at 1 year and at the end of the study. Thus, ACE inhibitors have also been shown to be renoprotective in patients with type 2 DM. (Heart Outcomes Prevention Evaluation Study Investigators 2000)

Two studies, Irbesartan in Patients with Diabetes and Microalbuminuria (IRMA-2) and Diabetics Exposed to Telmisartan and Enalapril (DETAIL) study examined the effect of ARB's in diabetic patients with microalbuminuria, but without overt DN (Parving HH 2001, Barnett A 2006). It is well known that, in patients with type 2 DM presence of microalbuminuria increases the risk of developing DN 10 to 20 times. IRMA-2 study showed that irbesartan significantly reduced the rate of progression of microalbuminuria to overt DN in patients with type 2 diabetes. Furthermore, the study discovered that irbesartan was associated with significantly more common restoration of normoalbuminuria as compared to standard therapy. All these effects were achieved independent of the systemic blood pressure. The more recent DETAIL study compared the renoprotective effects of ACE inhibitor enalapril and ARB telmisartan. In this head-to-head comparison the authors showed that both treatments were equally effective in preventing the progression of renal dysfunction, measured as decline in the GFR. Reduction of Endpoints in NIDDM with Angiotensin II Antagonist Losartan (RENAAL) study (Brenner BM 2001) showed that treatment with losartan was associated with a 25% decrease in the risk for doubling serum creatinine level. The risk of developing ESRD was also reduced by 28%.

Other individual factors may better define the impact of ACE inhibitors on the progression of renal insufficiency. In particular, Rigat et al described an insertion (I) and deletion (D) polymorphism in the ACE gene that correlates with ACE activity. ACE levels are highest in patients who are homozygous for the ACE D allele and lowest in patients homozygous for the ACE I allele (Rigat B 1990). They are intermediate in those who are heterozygous. Yoshida et al (Yoshida H 1995) later reported a greater reduction in proteinuria in response to ACE inhibition in patients with IgA nephropathy who were homozygous for the D allele. In contrast to this, other investigators have suggested a worse response to therapy in patients who carry the D allele (Parving HH 1996). Obviously, large-scale studies are needed to define the impact of genetic factors on the renal protective effects of ACE inhibition.

There are studies suggesting that dual blockade of renin-angiotensin system using a combination of ACE inhibitor and an ARB in patients with nephropathy is superior to the use of either drug alone. (Ayodele OE 2004, Mogensen CE 2000, Rosner MH 2003). The antiproteinuric effects of inhibitors of the renin angiotensin system are increased by sodium restriction and by concomitant administration of diuretics or non-dihydropyridine calcium channel blockers. (American Diabetes Association 2002, Ayodele OE 2004, Arauz-Pacheco C 2002).

In the United Kingdom Prospective Diabetes Study, atenolol showed beneficial effects comparable to captopril on diabetes-related mortality and microvascular complications in patients with type-2 diabetes. (United Kingdom Prospective Diabetes Group 1998) Beta-blockers have been shown to reduce mortality following myocardial infarction, and the absolute benefit of a given relative reduction is greater in diabetics compared to nondiabetics due to higher mortality from myocardial infarction in patients with diabetes. (Ayodele OE 2004) The nondihydropyridine calcium channel blockers have been shown to lower protein excretion in patients with diabetes. (Bakris GL 1990 and 1997) Their antiproteinuric effect may be due to reduction in intraglomerular pressure, reduction in glomerular hypertrophy, and improved glomerular size. The dihydropyridine calcium channel blockers have a variable effect on protein excretion ranging from increased protein excretion to no effect to a fall in protein excretion in various studies. (Melbourne Diabetic Nephropathy Study Group 1991, Vellussi M 1996, Salako BL 2002, Rosssing P, 1997)

14. Protein restriction

The role of dietary protein restriction in CKD is best described as controversial. However, restriction of protein (0.6 g/kg body weight per day) and phosphorus (0.5 to 1 g per day) were shown to reduce the decline in GFR, lower blood pressure, and stabilize renal function compared with higher intakes. This was suggested by a randomized trial involving patients with type-I DM and overt DN. In addition, another study showed that restriction of protein intake to 0.8 g/kg body weight per day reduced the rate of progression to ESRD in patients with type-I diabetes. The National Kidney Foundation recommends that patients with GFR <29 mL/min per m2 should have a daily protein intake of 0.6 g/kg body weight. More recently, a 4-year randomized controlled trial in 82 patients with type 1 diabetes with progressive DN showed that a moderately low–protein diet (0.9 g · kg−1 · day−1) reduced the risk of ESRD or death by 76%, although no effect on GFR decline was observed (Hansen HP, 2002)

A prospective, randomized controlled trial in patients with type 1 diabetes suffering from progressive diabetic nephropathy demonstrated beneficial effect of moderate restriction in dietary protein on the development of ESRD or death. The beneficial effect of protein restriction appeared within the first year, and persisted with continued treatment, as also has been demonstrated in non-diabetic nephropathies suggesting that type 1 diabetic patients with progressive diabetic nephropathy are highly sensitive to dietary protein restriction (Hansen HP, 2002).

The mechanisms by which a low-protein diet may reduce progression of DN are still unknown, but might be related to improved lipid profile and/or glomerular hemodynamics. (Jorge L, 2005) Since diabetic patients have other restrictions to the diet, this may reduce compliance to an additional low-protein diet, although better compliance can be obtained by applying much more intensive dietary counseling (Hansen HP, 2002)

15. Cessation of smoking

Smoking has been shown in many previous studies to effect diabetic complications. Cessation of smoking alone may reduce the risk of progression by 30% in patients with type-2 diabetes. (Ritz E, 2000) Recent studies demonstrated that smokers have increased systolic blood pressures and proteinuria amongst diabetics with nephropathy (Sawicki, PT 1996) More recent work by Chihuran et al has shown that renal function declines faster in smokers than nonsmokers with type 2 DN undergoing treatment to improve blood pressure including ACE inhibitors. Also, loss of renal function is slower in those who stopped smoking. Cigarette smoking remains a risk factor for renal function decline in type 2 DN despite currently recommended therapy (Chihuran T, 2002)

16. Hyperlipidemia

There is suggestion that elevation in lipid levels may contribute to the development of glomerulosclerosis in chronic renal failure. (Ravid M, 1995, Krolewski AS, 1994) Studies have shown that lipid lowering may have a beneficial effect on renal function. (Lam KSL, 1995) A meta-analysis of 13 controlled trials involving a total of 362 subjects, 253 of whom had diabetes, showed that statins decreased proteinuria and preserved GFR in patients with chronic renal disease. (Fried LF, 2001) Adequately powered randomized controlled trials will be needed to determine the role of lipid lowering therapy in retarding the rate of decline in kidney function in patients with chronic renal disease secondary to diabetes mellitus.

17. Renal replacement therapy

The renal replacement modalities available for patients with ESRD from diabetes include peritoneal dialysis, hemodialysis, and renal transplantation. Various studies have shown similar survival in hemodialysis and peritoneal dialysis, though patients are more likely to persist with hemodialysis than with peritoneal dialysis. Both hemo- and peritoneal dialysis limit social life, leisure, and sexual activity.(Hostetter TH, 1981) Patients with diabetes may manifest uremic symptoms at a relatively less-advanced degree of renal insufficiency than their nondiabetic counterparts. (Hostetter TH, 1982)

18. Emerging therapies

Extensive research is currently underway in this field and some new pathogenic mediators for DN have been discovered. These include
*   Renin
*   Advanced Glycosylation end-products [AGE]
*   Protein Kinase C [PKC]
*   Transforming growth factor – Beta 1 [TGF-1]
*   Nitric Oxide [NO]
*   Vascular endothelial growth factor [VEGF]
*   Oxidative stress

18.1 Direct renin inhibitor – Aliskiren
Blockade of RAS is a key therapeutic strategy in slowing progression of DN. Interruption of the RAS may also be accomplished by blocking the activity of renin. Aliskiren is a direct renin inhibitor and thus, decreases angiotensin II and aldosterone levels. Aliskiren is a potent antihypertensive and anti proteinuric.

18.2 Advanced Glycosylation end-products [AGEs]
The formation of AGEs and their cross-linked products is a phenomenon of normal aging; however, it is accelerated in the DM. AGE–cross-linked products accumulate in patients with DM and have been implicated in the pathologic process of diabetic complications. Several anti-AGE agents have been tested and shown to be renoprotective in experimental diabetic animal models. (Thomas MC, 2005)
Aminoguanidine is the prototype of an AGE formation inhibitor which acts by scavenging intermediates in the advanced glycation catalytic process.
ALT-946 is a more potent and selective AGE formation inhibitor than aminoguanidine. It has minimal effects on NO synthesis and appears to have fewer toxic effects, although it has not been studied in as much detail.
Pyridoxamine (PYR) - Pyridoxamine is one of the three natural forms of pyridoxine (vitamin B6). It scavenges pathogenic reactive carbonyl species and inhibits the formation of AGEs from Amadori compounds. (Voziyan PA, 2002, Chetyrkin SV, 2008)

18.3 Thiamine
Experimental studies have suggested that thiamine and benfothiamine (S-benzoylthiamine monophosphate), a vitamin B1 derivative, can also prevent or decrease kidney injury. These drugs decrease formation of AGE compounds and protein kinase C (PKC) activity in DN.

AGE Breakers - This group of compounds decreases AGE accumulation by breaking the glycation cross-links.

AGE Receptor Antagonists - AGEs mediate their effects both directly and indirectly through receptor-dependent mechanisms. They bind to the transmembrane receptor for AGE (RAGE) and prevent the development of diabetic microvascular complications. (Bierhaus A 2005, Wendt T, 2003) Thus, RAGE is a potential target to prevent AGE effects.

18.4 Pentoxifylline
Pentoxifylline (PTF) is a methylxanthine derivative with hemorheological properties that has favorable effects on microcirculatory blood flow. In vivo, it also functions as a phosphodiesterase inhibitor. (Navarro J.F., 1999)

18.5 Protein Kinase C inhibitors
Recent studies have identified that activation of PKC initiated by hyperglycemia is associated with many vascular abnormalities in retinal, renal, and cardiovascular tissues. The blocking of PKC-beta isoforms has been shown to decrease albuminuria, structural injury, and TGF-beta expression in animal models of DM. (Koya D, 2000) Ruboxistaurin is one such PKC beta inhibitor.

18.6 Glycosaminoglycans
Glycosaminoglycans are important determinants of GBM permeability. An emerging body of evidence supports the notion that glomerular capillary wall and mesangial alterations in DN involve pathobiochemical alterations of glycoproteins in these structures. Heparin and sulodexide are examples of this class of drugs.

18.7 Endothelin receptor antagonists
DN is associated with enhanced renal synthesis of endothelins. A number of preclinical reports suggested that endothelin might be an appropriate target to decrease DM-related albuminuria. (Turgut F, 2010) Avosentan (SPP301) is a new orally available endothelin 1 antagonist.

18.8 Antifibrotic agents and growth factor inhibitors
Characteristic morphologic lesions of DN include glomerular hypertrophy, thickening of the basement membrane, and mesangial expansion. This leads to glomerulosclerosis, tubulointerstitial fibrosis, and, eventually, loss of kidney parenchyma. Several growth factors which are normally expressed in the kidney have been implicated in the pathogenesis of DN.

TGF-β Inhibitors - Pirfenidone (PFD) is a low molecular weight synthetic molecule that exerts dramatic antifibrotic properties in cell culture and various animal models of fibrosis. SMP-534, another antifibrotic agent is also being studied. Several AGE inhibitors also decrease TGF-β levels. (Turgut F,2010, Sugaru E., 2006)

CTGF Inhibitors - Connective tissue growth factor (CTGF/CCN2) has been associated with fibrosis in various tissues including the kidney. It is up-regulated in most models of DN. Clinical trials evaluating anti-CTGF ab (FG3019) are underway.

18.9 Nitric Oxide (NO) modulation
Abnormalities of renal NO generation have been linked to pathogenesis of renal disease in diabetes. NO and / or NO Synthase are targets for drug development for treatment and/or prevention of DN.

18.10 Vascular endothelial growth factor (VEGF) inhibitors
VEGF is a main regulator of blood vessel growth and plays an important role in promoting endothelial survival and maintaining the microvasculature. Loss of capillaries is strongly associated with the progression of CKD to ESRD (Doi K, 2010).

19. Alternative and complementary therapies for diabetic nephropathy

19.1 Exercise and Yoga
The American Diabetes Association recommends a minimum of 30 minutes of moderate-intensity aerobic physical activity 5 days per week, or vigorous-intensity aerobic physical activity for 20 minutes 3 times per week is recommended for healthy adults aged 18 to 65. Currently, there is no clinical evidence to suggest that vigorous exercise increases the rate of progression of diabetic nephropathy. In fact, some studies have shown that aerobic exercise actually decreased urine protein excretion (Gordon LA, 2008). Additionally, it has been demonstrated that resistance training may have a beneficial effect on muscle mass, nutritional status, functional capacity, and glomerular filtration rate. Therefore, the American Diabetes Association feels that there is no need to restrict exercise in patients with diabetic nephropathy. A more recent study that examined the effects of Yoga and conventional exercise showed findings that suggest better glycemic and blood pressure control obtained in type 2 diabetic patients after Hatha yoga than conventional PT exercises (Gordon LA, 2008).

19.2 Life style modifications
Obesity is often associated with diabetes mellitus and also with nephropathy independent of diabetes (often focal sclerosis). However the impact of weight loss in diabetic subjects with nephropathy on renal function and proteinuria remains as a subject of intense investigation. Short term studies recently reported that weight reduction using dietary therapy for 4 weeks resulted in significant reduction in systolic pressure, proteinuria, and serum creatinine in obese patients with diabetic nephropathy. (A Saiki, 2005). Longer studies involving larger group of patients need to be evaluated to validate such conclusions.

19.3 Herbal and Food derivatives
19.3.1 Curcumin
Curcumin is the active component in Tumeric Rhizomes (Curcuma Long Linn). Curcumin has been shown to possess anti-inflammatory, anti-oxidant and antifibrotic properties in many tissues, in vivo and in vitro studies. Tikoo et al have shown that curcumin treatment prevented the development of DN by significantly lowering blood urea nitrogen and plasma creatinine/body weight ratio in diabetic animals. (Tikoo K, 2008) Various biological actions of curcumin are mediated by inhibiting cell proliferation (Sikora E, 1997), oxidative stress and inflammation (Sharma C, 2006). Several other investigators have also shown that the anti-inflammatory property of curcumin can significantly improve kidney function in animals with chronic renal failure.

19.3.2 Cinnamon
Cinnamon has been known for its antidiabetic effects for some time now. Mishra et al have investigated its effects on nephropathy in diabetes in rodent models of type I diabetes. Histological studies of the kidney proved the protective effect of cinnamon oil by reducing

the glomerular expansion, eradicating hyaline casts, and decreasing the tubular dilatations. (Mishra A, 2010). The authors concluded that the volatile oil from cinnamon contains more than 98 % cinnamaldehyde and that it confers dose-dependent, significant protection against alloxan-induced renal damage. While the mechanism of its action remains unclear, it is believed to be mostly due to its antidiabetic and antioxidant effects leading to reduced formation of AGEs.

20. Conclusions

During the last 3 decades, considerable progress has been made in delaying the progression of CKD even as the frequency of DN continues to increase. This is a truly a reflection of the advances made in understanding the pathogenesis. As reviewed in this chapter many pathogenic cytokines and growth factors have emerged in the recent years that either initiate or contribute to the progressive renal injury in diabetes. Current treatment options are still suboptimal. However with the rapid strides being made in the field, several new therapeutic targets are being recognized and effective treatment strategies being developed.

21. References

A Saiki, D Nagayama, M Ohhira, K Endoh, M Ohtsuka, N Koide, T Oyama, Y Miyashita and K Shirai . Effect of weight loss using formula diet on renal function in obese patients with diabetic nephropathy. International Journal of Obesity (2005) 29, 1115–1120.

Alkhalaf A, Zurbig P, Bakker SJ, et al. Multicentric validation of proteomic biomarkers in urine specific for diabetic nephropathy. PLoS One 2010; 5:e13421

American Diabetes Association. Treatment of hypertension in adults with diabetes. Diabetes Care. 2003;26 (Suppl 1):S80-S82.

Amiri F, G. R. Regulation of angiotensin II receptors and PKC isoforms by glucose in rat mesangial cells. Am J Physiol 1999; 276: F691–F699

Araki S, Haneda M, Koya D, et al. Association between urinary type IV collagen level and deterioration of renal function in type 2 diabetic patients without overt proteinuria. Diabetes Care 2010; 33:1805–1810.

Araki S, Haneda M, Sugimoto T, Isono M, Isshiki K, Kashiwagi A, Koya D, Factors associated with frequent remission of microalbuminuria in patients with type 2 diabetes. Diabetes. 2005;54(10):2983

Arauz-Pacheco C, Parrott MA, Raskin P. The treatment of hypertension in adult patients with diabetes. Diabetes Care. 2002;25:134-147.

Ayodele OE, Alebiosu CO, Salako BL Diabetic nephropathy: a review of the natural history, burden, risk factors and treatment. / Natl Med Assoc 2004;96: 1445-1454

Bakris GL, Coopley JB, Vicknar N, et al. Calcium channel blockers versus other antihypertensive drugs on progression of NIDDM-associated nephropathy. Kidney Int. 1996;50:1641-1650.

Bakris GL, Mangrum A, Copley JB, et al. Effect of calcium channel or beta blockade on the progression of diabetic nephropathy in African Americans. Hypertension. 1997;29:744-750.

Bakris GL. Effects of diltiazem or lisinopril on massive proteinura associated with diabetes mellitus. Ann Inter Med. 1990;1 12:707-708.

Ballerma, B.J., Skorecki,K.L., Brenner , B.M. Reduced glomerular angiotensin II receptor density in early untreated diabetes mellitus in the rats. Am J Physiol.1984; 247: F110-F116.

Bank N. Mechanisms of diabetic hyperfiltration. Kidney Int 1991; 40:792

Barnett A. Preventing renal complications in type 2 diabetes: results of the diabetics exposed to telmisartan and enalapril trial. J Am Soc Nephrol. 2006 Apr;17(4Suppl 2):S132-5.

Benigni ,A.,Colosio,V., Brena, C., et al. Unselective inhibition of endothelin receptors reduces renal dysfunction in experimental diabetes. Diabetes.1998;47:450-456.

Benigni A. A. Selective impairment of gene expression and assembly of nephrin in human diabetic nephropathy. Kidney Int 2004;65:2193-2200

Bierhaus A, Humpert PM, Morcos M, Wendt T, Chavakis T, Arnold B, Stern DM, Nawroth PP. Understanding RAGE, the receptor for advanced glycation end products. J Mol Med. 2005 Nov;83(11):876-86. Epub 2005 Aug 24.

Brenner BM, Cooper ME, de Zeeuw D et al. Effects of Losartan on Renal and Cardiovascular Outcomes in Patients with Type 2 Diabetes and Nephropathy. the RENAAL Study Investigators. N Engl J Med 2001 Sept; 345:861-869

Brown N and Vaughn D. Angiotensin converting enzyme inhibitors. . Circulation. 1998;97:1411-1420

Brownlee, M. Biochemistry and molecular cell biology of diabetic complications. Nature.2001;414 (6865): 813-820

Cawood TJ, Bashir M, Brady J, et al. Urinary collagen IV and piGST: potential biomarkers for detecting localized kidney injury in diabetes: a pilot study. Am J Nephrol 2010; 32:219-225

Cheng ,H.F.,Burns,K.V., Harris ,R.C. Reduced proximal tubule angiotensin II receptor expression in streptozotocin-induced diabetes mellitus. Kidney Int.1994;46:1603-1610

Chetyrkin SV, Zhang W, Hudson BG, Serianni AS, Voziyan PA. Pyridoxamine protects proteins from functional damage by 3-deoxyglucosone: mechanism of action of pyridoxamine. Biochemistry 47. (3): 997-1006.2008

Chihuran T and Wesson D E. Cigarette smoking predicts faster progression of type 2 established diabetic nephropathy despite ACE inhibition American Journal of Kidney Diseases. February 2002. Volume 39, Issue 2 , Pages 376-382.

Cohen ,M.P. Intervention strategies to prevent pathogenetic effects of glycated albumin. Arch Biochem Biophys.2003;419:25-30.

Cooper, M.Interaction of metabolic and hemodynamic factors in mediating experimental diabetic nephropathy. Diabetologia 2001;44 (11):1957-1972.

Cowie CC, Port FK, Wolfe RA, Savage PJ, Moll PP, Hawthorne VM, N Engl J Med. 1989;321(16):1074

de Boer IH, Rue TC, Cleary PA et al Long-term Renal Outcomes of Patients With Type 1 Diabetes Mellitus and Microalbuminuria: An Analysis of the Diabetes Control and Complications Trial/Epidemiology of Diabetes Interventions and Complications Cohort. Arch Intern Med. 2011 Mar 14;171(5):412-420.

Degenhardt T.P., Thorpe S.R. Baynes, J.W. Chemical modification of proteins by methylglyoxal. Cell, Mol Biol.1998;44:1139-1145.

Diabetes 1997; 46 (5): 847-853.

Doi K, Noiri E, Fujita T. Role of vascular endothelial growth factor in kidney disease. Curr Vasc Pharmacol. 2010 Jan;8(1):122-8.

Dunlop ME, M. E.Small heat shock protein alteration provide a mechanism to reduce mesangial cell contractility in diabetes and oxidative stress. Kidney Int 2000, 57, 464-475.

Dusso A, Arcidiacono MV, Yang J, Tokumoto M. Vitamin D inhibition of TACE and prevention of renal osteodystrophy and cardiovascular mortality. J Steroid Biochem Mol Biol 2010; 121: 193–98

Earle K, Viberti GC. Familial, hemodynamic, and metabolic factors in the predisposition to diabetic kidney disease. Kidney Int. 1994;45:434-437)

Escandon , J.C.,Cipolla ,M. Diabetes and endothelial dysfunction: a clinical perspective. Endocr Rev.2001;22:36-52

EUCLID Study Group. Randomised placebo-controlled trial of lisinopril in normotensive patients with insulin-dependent diabetes and normoalbuminuria or microalbuminuria. Lancet 1997;349:1787-92

Forbes,J.M. .,Thallas , V.,Thomas ,M.C. , et al. The breakdown of preexisting advanced glycation end products is associated with reduced renal fibrosis in experimental diabetes. FASEB J.2003;17(12):1762-1764

Freundlich M, Quiroz Y, Zhang Z, et al. Suppression of renin-angiotensin gene expression in the kidney by paricalcitol. Kidney Int 2008; 74: 1394–402.

Fried LF, Orchard TJ, Kasiske BL. The effect of lipid reduction on renal disease progression. A meta-analysis. Kidney Int. 2001;59:260-269.

Frye,E.B.,Degenhardt,T.P.,Thorpe,S.R.,et al . Role of the Maillard reaction in aging of tissue proteins. Advanced glycation end product–dependent increase in imidazolium cross-links in human lens proteins. J Biol Chem.1998;273:8714–8719.

G.M. Hargrove, J. D. Wong, Diabetes mellitus increases endothelin-1 gene transcription in rat kidney, Kidney Int.2000; 58 (4):1534-1545.

Gordon LA, Morrison EY, McGrowder DA, Young R, Fraser YT, Zamora EM, Alexander-Lindo RL, Irving RR. Effect of exercise therapy on lipid profile and oxidative stress indicators in patients with type 2 diabetes. BMC Complement Altern Med. 2008 May 13;8:21.

Hansen HP, Tauber-Lassen E, Jensen BR, Parving HH: Effect of dietary protein restriction on prognosis in patients with diabetic nephropathy. Kidney Int 62:220–228, 2002.

Haynes , W.G.,Webb, D.J. Venoconstriction to endothelin-1 in humans: role of calcium and potassium channels. Am J Physiol.1993;265:H1676-H1681.

Heart Outcomes Prevention Evaluation Study Investigators: Effects of ramipril on cardiovascular and microvascular outcomes in people with diabetes mellitus: results of the HOPE study and MICRO-HOPE substudy. Lancet 355:253–259, 2000

Hilker, KF ,R .,Veelken. Type 2 diabetic nephropathy : never too early to treat? J Am Soc Nephrol.2005;16:574-575.

Hostetter TH, Rennke GH, Brenner BM. The case for intrarenal hypertension in the initiation and progression of diabetic and other glomerulopathies. Am J Med. 1982;72:375-380.

Hostetter TH, Troy JL, Brenner BM. Glomerular hemodynamics in experimental diabetes. Kidney Int. 1981;19:410-415.

Hovind P, Tarnow L, Rossing P, et al. Predictors for the development of microalbuminuria and macroalbuminuria in patients with type 1 diabetes: inception cohort study. BMJ 2004; 328:1105

Jorge L. Gross Mirela J. De Azevedo, Sandra P. Silveiro, Luís Henrique Canani, Maria Luiza Caramori And Themis Zelmanovitz. Diabetic Nephropathy: Diagnosis, Prevention, And Treatment Diabetes Care, Volume 28, Number 1, January 2005.

Katavetin P, Katavetin P, Susantitaphong P, et al. Urinary type IV collagen excretion predicts subsequent declining renal function in type 2 diabetic patients with proteinuria. Diabetes Res Clin Pract 2010; 89:e33–e35.

Kimmestiel P, Wilson C. Intercapillary lesions in the glomeruli of the kidney. Am J Path. 1936;1 2:83-97.

Kobayashi N,Honda T,Yoshida K.et al. Critical role of bradykinineNOS and oxidative stress-LOX pathway in cardiovascular remodelling under chronic angiotensinconverting enzyme inhibition. Atherosclerosis,2006;87:92-100.

Komers R, A. S.Paradoxes of nitric oxide in the diabetic kidney. Am J Physiol Renal Physiol 2003;284:F1121–F1137.

Kone BC, B. C.Biosynthesis and homeostatic roles of nitric oxide in the normal kidney. Am J Physiol 1997;272:F561–F578

Koya D, Haneda M, Nakagawa H, Isshiki K, Sato H, Maeda S, Sugimoto T, Yasuda H, Kashiwagi A, Ways DK, King GL, Kikkawa R. Amelioration of accelerated diabetic mesangial expansion by treatment with a PKC beta inhibitor in diabetic db/db mice, a rodent model for type 2 diabetes. FASEB J. 2000 Mar;14(3):439-47.

Krolewski AS, Warram JH, Christlieb AR, Busick EJ, Kahn CR, Am J Med. 1985;78(5):785.

Krolewski AS, Warram JHG, Christlies AR. Hypercholesterolemia-A determinant of renal function loss and deaths in IDDM patients with nephropathy. KidneyInt. 1994;Suppl 45:S125-S131.

Laffel LM, McGill JB, Gans DJ. The beneficial effect of angiotensin-converting enzyme inhibition with captopril on diabetic nephropathy in normotensive IDDM patients with microalbuminuria. North American Microalbuminuria Study Group. Am J Med 1995;99:497-504

Lajer M, Tarnow I, Michelson AD, et al. Soluble CD40 ligand is elevated in type 1 diabetic nephropathy but not predictive of mortality, cardiovascular events or kidney function. Platelets 2010; 21:525–532

Lam KSL, Cheing IKP, Jamis ED, et al. Cholesterol-lowering therapy may retard the progression of diabetic nephropathy. Diabetologia. 1995;38:604-609.

Lewis, Ej, Junsinker, Lg, Bain, Rp, Rohde, Rd, The Collaborative Study Group: The effect of angiotensin converting enzyme inhibition on diabetic nephropathy. N Engl J Med 1993 329: 1456–1462

Li YC, Kong J, Wei M, Chen ZF, Liu SQ, Cao LP. 1,25-Dihydroxyvitamin D(3) is a negative endocrine regulator of the renin-angiotensin system. J Clin Invest 2002; 110: 229-38

Lorenzo Gordon, Errol Y. Morrison, Donovan A. McGrowder, Ronald Young, David Garwood, Eslaen Zamora, Ruby L. Alexander-Lindo, Rachael Irving, Elsa C. Perez Sanz. Changes in clinical and metabolic parameters after exercise therapy in patients with type 2 diabetes. Arch Med Sci 2008; 4, 4: 427–437.

Lu J, Randell E, Han Y, et al. Increased plasma methylglyoxal level, inflammation, and vascular endothelial dysfunction in diabetic nephropathy. Clin Biochem 2011; 44:307–311

M. Haneda, S. A.Mitogen-activated protein kinase cascade is activated in glomeruli of diabetic rats and glomerular mesangial cells cultured under high glucose conditions.

Maguire,J.J. Davenport, A.P. Is urotensin-II the new endothelin? Br J Pharmacol.2002;137:579-588.

Melbourne Diabetic Nephropathy Study Group. Comparson between perindopril and nifedipine in hypertensive and normotensive diabetic patients with microalbuminuria. BMJ. 1991;302:210-216.

Mishra A, Bhatti R, Singh A, Singh Ishar MP. Ameliorative effect of the cinnamon oil from Cinnamomum zeylanicum upon early stage diabetic nephropathy. Planta Med. 2010 Mar;76(5):412-7.

Mizuiri,S.,Yoshikawa ,H.,Tanagashima ,M.,et al. Renal ACE immunohistochemical localization in NIDDM patients with nephropathy. Am J Kidney Dis.1998;31:301-307

Mogensen CE, Neldam S, Tikkenen 1, et al. Randomized control trial of dual blockade of renin-angiotensin system in patients with hypertension, microalbuminuria, and noninsulin-dependent diabetes: the Candesartan and Lisinopril Microalbuminuria (CALM) study. BMJ. 2000;321:1440-1444.

Mou S, Wang Q, Liu J, et al. Prevalence of nondiabetic renal disease in patients with type 2 diabetes. Diabetes Res Clin Pract 2010; 87:354–359.

Mundel P and Shackland S. Podocyte biology and response to injury. J Am Soc Nephrol 2002;13: 3005–3015.

Nagai Y et al . Temporary angiotensin II blockade at the prediabetic stage attenuates the development of renal injury in type 2 diabetic rats . J Am Soc Nephrol.2005;16:703-711

Nathan DM, Zinman B, Cleary PA, Backlund JY, Genuth S, Miller R, Orchard TJ . Modern-day clinical course of type 1 diabetes mellitus after 30 years' duration: Diabetes Control and Complications Trial/Epidemiology of Diabetes Interventions and Complications(DCCT/EDIC) Research Group, Arch Intern Med. 2009;169(14):1307-16

Nathan, D.M.,Cleary, P.A .,Backlund, J.Y. Intensive diabetes treatment and cardiovascular disease in patients with type 1 diabetes. N Eng J Med.2005;353:2643–2653.

Navarro J.F., Mora C., Rivero A., et al: Urinary protein excretion and serum tumor necrosis factor in diabetic patients with advanced renal failure: effects of pentoxifylline administration. Am J Kidney Dis 33. (3): 458-463.1999

Nelson RG, Bennett PH, Beck GJ, Tan M, Knowler WC, Mitch WE, Hirschman GH, Myers BD, Development and progression of renal disease in Pima Indians with non-insulin-dependent diabetes mellitus. Diabetic Renal Disease Study Group, N Engl J Med. 1996;335(22):1636

Nielsen SE, Schjoedt KJ, Astrup AS, et al. Neutrophil Gelatinase-Associated Lipocalin (NGAL) and Kidney Injury Molecule 1 (KIM1) in patients with diabetic nephropathy: a cross-sectional study and the effects of lisinopril. Diabet Med 2010; 27:1144–1150.

Nishikawa ,T. et al. Impact of mitochondrial ROS production on diabetic vascular complications. Diabetes Res Clin Pract.2007;77 (Suppl 1):S41–S45.

Orchard TJ, Dorman JS, Maser RE, Becker DJ, Drash AL, Ellis D, LaPorte RE, Kuller LH, Diabetes. 1990;39(9):1116

Overgaard AJ, Hansen HG, Lajer M, et al. Plasma proteome analysis of patients with type 1 diabetes with diabetic nephropathy. Proteome Sci 2010; 8:4

P. T. Sawicki, I. Mühlhauser, R. Bender, W. Pethke, L. Heinemann, M. Berger. Effects of smoking on blood pressure and proteinuria in patients with diabetic nephropathy. J Internal Medicine 1996 239: 345-352.

Papale M, Di PS, Magistroni R, et al. Urine proteome analysis may allow noninvasive differential diagnosis of diabetic nephropathy. Diabetes Care 2010; 33:2409–2415.

Parving HH, Hommel E, Mathiesen E, Skøtt P, Edsberg B, Bahnsen M, Lauritzen M, Hougaard P, Lauritzen E, Br Med J (Clin Res Ed). 1988;296(6616):156

Parving HH, Jacobsen P, Tarnow L et al. Effect of deletion polymorphism of angiotensin converting enzyme gene on progression of diabetic nephropathy during inhibition of angiotensin converting enzyme: observational follow up study. BMJ. 1996;313:591–594.

Parving HH, Lehnert H, Bröchner-Mortensen J, Gomis R et al. The Effect of Irbesartan on the Development of Diabetic Nephropathy in Patients with Type 2 Diabetes N Engl J Med 2001 Sept; 345:870-878

Passariello N, Sepe J, Marrazzo G, et al. Effect of aldose reductase inhibitor (tolrestat) on urinary albumin excretion rate and glomerular filtration rate in IDDM subjects with nephropathy. Diabetes Care 1993; 16:789

Prabhakar S, Starnes J T, Shuping Shi, Lonis B and Tran R. Diabetic Nephropathy Is Associated with Oxidative Stress and Decreased Renal Nitric Oxide Production, J Am Soc Nephrol 18: 2945-2952, 2007

Prabhakar, SS. Pathogenic role of nitric oxide alterations in diabetic nephropathy. Curr Diab Rep, 2005 5(6), 449-54.

Ravid M, Neumann L, Lishner M. Plasma lipids and the progression of nephropathy in diabetes mellitus type-2: effect of ACE inhibitors. Kidney Int.1995;47:907-910.

Rigat B, Hubert C, Alhenc-Gelas F, Cambien F, Corvol P, Soubrier F. An insertion/deletion polymorphism in the angiotensin I converting enzyme gene accounting for half the variance of serum enzyme levels. J Clin Invest. 1990;86:1343–1346

Ritz E, Ogata H, Orth SR. Smoking: a factor promoting onset and progression of diabetic nephropathy. Diabetes Metab. 2000;26(Suppl 4):54-63.

Ritz E, Orth SR, Nephropathy in patients with type 2 diabetes mellitus, N Engl J Med. 1999;341(15):1127

Rosner MH, Okusa MD. Combination therapy with angiotensin-converting enzyme inhibitors and angiotensin receptor antagonist in the treatment of patients with type-2 diabetes mellitus. Arch Intern Med. 2003;163:1025-1029.

Rosssing P, Tarnow L, Boelskifte S, et al. Differences between nisoldipine and lisinopril on glomerular filtration rates and albuminura in hypertensive IDDM patients with diabetic nephropathy durng the first year of treatment. Diabetes. 1997;46:481-487.

Salako BL, Finomo FO, Kadiri S, et al. Comparative effect of lisinopril and lacidipine on urinary albumin excretion in patients with type-2 diabetic nephropathy. AfrJ Med Med Sci. 2002;31:53-57.

Sasser ,J.M., Sullivan,J.C., Hobbs, J.L., et al. Endothelin A receptor blockade reduces diabetic renal injury via an anti-inflammatory mechanism. J Am Soc Nephrol.2007;18:143-154

Schleicher,E.D.,Wagner, E.,Nerlich ,A.G. Increased accumulation of the glycoxidation product N(epsilon)-(carboxymethyl)lysine in human tissues in diabetes and aging. J Clin Invest.1997;99:457–468.

Serri O, Beauregard H, Brazeau P, et al. Somatostatin analogue, octreotide, reduces increased glomerular filtration rate and kidney size in insulin-dependent diabetes. JAMA 1991; 265:888

Sharma C, Kaur J, Shishodia S, Aggarwal BB, Ralhan R.Curcumin down regulates smokeless tobacco-induced NF-kappaB activation and COX-2 expression in human oral premalignant and cancer cells. Toxicology. 2006 Nov 10;228(1):1-15.

Sikora E, Bielak-Zmijewska A, Piwocka K, Skierski J, Radziszewska E.Inhibition of proliferation and apoptosis of human and rat T lymphocytes by curcumin, a curry pigment. Biochem Pharmacol. 1997 Oct 15;54(8):899-907.

Sorokin ,A., Kohan, D.E. Physiology and pathology of endothelin-1 in renal mesangium. Am J Physiol Renal Physiol.2003;285:F579–F589

Soulis-Liparota,T.,Cooper ,M.,Papazoglou , D., et al . Retardation by aminoguanidine of development of albuminuria, mesangial expansion, and tissue fluorescence in streptozocin-induced diabetic rat. Diabetes.1991;40(10):1328-1334.

Sthaneshwar P, Chan SP. Urinary type IV collagen levels in diabetes mellitus. Malays J Pathol 2010; 32:43–47.

Sugaru E., Nakagawa T., Ono-Kishino M., et al: SMP-534 ameliorates progression of glomerular fibrosis and urinary albumin in diabetic db/db mice. Am J Physiol Renal Physiol 290. (4): F813-F820.2006.

Tanaka H, Hamano T, Fujii N, et al. The impact of diabetes mellitus on vitamin D metabolism in predialysis patients. Bone 2009; 45: 949–55

Teng M, Wolf M, Lowrie E, Ofsthun N, Lazarus JM, Thadhani R. Survival of patients undergoing hemodialysis with paricalcitol or calcitriol therapy. N Engl J Med 2003; 349: 446–56

The DCCT/EDIC Research Group. Effect of Intensive therapy on the microvascular complications of type-I diabetes mellitus. JAMA. 2002;287: 2563-2569.

The DCCT/EDIC Research Group. Retinopathy and nephropathy in patients with type-1 diabetes four years after a trial of intensive therapy. NEJM. 2000;342:381-389.

Thijs W. Cohen Tervaert, Antien L. Mooyaart, Kerstin Amann, Arthur H. Cohen, H. Terence Cook, Cinthia B. Drachenberg,_ Franco Ferrario, Agnes B. Fogo, Mark Haas, Emile de Heer, Kensuke Joh, Laure H. Noe l, Jai Radhakrishnan, Surya V. Seshan, Ingeborg M. Bajema, and Jan A. Bruijn, on behalf of the Renal Pathology Society, Pathologic Classification of Diabetic Nephropathy, J Am Soc Nephrol 2010. 21: 556–563.

Thomas MC, Baynes JW, Thorpe SR, Cooper ME The role of AGEs and AGE inhibitors in diabetic cardiovascular disease. Curr Drug Targets 6. (4): 453-474.2005

Thomas,M.C.,Bayones,J.W.,Thorpe ,S.R . The role of AGEs and AGE inhibitors in diabetic cardiovascular disease.Curr. Drug Targets.2005;6 (4):453-474

Tikoo K, Meena RL, Kabra DG, Gaikwad AB. Change in post-translational modifications of histone H3, heat-shock protein-27 and MAP kinase p38 expression by curcumin in streptozotocin-induced type I diabetic nephropathy. Br J Pharmacol. 2008 Mar;153(6):1225-31.

Turgut F, Bolton WK. Potential New Therapeutic Agents for Diabetic Kidney Disease American Journal of Kidney Diseases, Vol 55, No 5 (May), 2010: pp 928-940

Ulker , S.,Mckeown ,P.,Bayraktutan,U. Vitamins reverse endothelial dysfunction through regulation of eNOS and NADPH oxidase activities. Hypertension.2003;41:534-541

United Kingdom Prospective Diabetes Group. Tight blood pressure control and rsk of macrovascular and microvascular complications in type-2 diabetes. UKPDS 38. BMJ. 1998;317.703-713.

United Kingdom Prospective Diabetes Group: efficacy of atenolol and captopril in reducing the rsk of macrovascular and microvascular complications in type-2 diabetes;UKPDS 39. BMJ. 1998;317:713-720.

Vellussi M, Brocco E, Frigato F, et al. Effects of cilazapril and amlodipine on kidney function in hypertensive NIDDM patients. Diabetes. 1996;45:216- 222.

Verhaar,MC., Strachan,F.E., Newby, D.E., et al. Endothelin-A receptor antagonist-mediated vasodilatation is attenuated by inhibition of nitric oxide synthesis and by endothelin-B receptor blockade. Circulation.1998;97:752-756.

Vlassara,H.,Brownlee, M.,Cerami,A. Nonenzymatic glycosylation of peripheral nerve protein in diabetes mellitus. Proc Natl Acad Sci U S A.1981;78:5190–5192.

Vora JP, Dolben J, Dean JD, Thomas D, Williams JD, Owens DR, Peters JR, Renal hemodynamics in newly presenting non-insulin dependent diabetes mellitus. Kidney International, 1992 Apr, 41 (4): 829-35.

Voziyan PA, Metz TO, Baynes JW, Hudson BG. A post-Amadori inhibitor pyridoxamine also inhibits chemical modification of proteins by scavenging carbonyl intermediates of carbohydrate and lipid degradation. J Biol Chem 277. (5): 3397-3403.2002

Watanabe,T., Kanome,T.,Miyazaki ,A. ,et al . Human urotensin II as a link between hypertension and coronary artery disease. Hypertens Res.2006;29:375-387

Wendt ,T.M.,Tanji ,N.,Guo.,et al. RAGE drives the development of glomerulosclerosis and implicates podocyte activation in the pathogenesis of diabetic nephropathy. Am J Pathol.2003;162:1123–1137.

Wendt T, Tanji N, Guo J, Hudson BI, Bierhaus A, Ramasamy R, Arnold B, Nawroth PP, Yan SF, D'Agati V, Schmidt AM. Glucose, glycation, and RAGE: implications for amplification of cellular dysfunction in diabetic nephropathy. J Am Soc Nephrol. 2003 May;14(5):1383-95.

Wendt,T.,Tanji ,N.Guo , et al. Glucose, glycation, and RAGE: implications for amplification of cellular dysfunction in diabetic nephropathy,. J. Am. Soc. Nephrol.2003;14 (5):1383-1395

Wolf,G.F.N.,Ziyadeh. Cellular and molecular mechanisms of proteinuria in diabetic nephropathy. Nephron Physiol.2007;106: 26-31.

Writing Team for the Diabetes Control and Complications Trial/Epidemiology of Diabetes Interventions and Complications Research Group. Effect of intensive therapy on the microvascular complications of type 1 diabetes mellitus. JAMA 2002; 287:2563–2569

Xu, D., Emoto , N., Giaid , A., et al. ECE-1: a membrane-bound metalloprotease that catalyzes the proteolytic activation of big endothelin-1. Cell.1994;78:473–485

Xu, M., Dai, D.Z.,Dai,Y. Normalizing NADPH oxidase contributes to attenuating diabetic nephropathy by the dual endothelin receptor antagonist CPU 0213 in rats. Am J Nephrol.2009;29: 252–256.

Yan X, Sano M, Lu L, et al. Plasma concentrations of osteopontin, but not thrombin-cleaved osteopontin, are associated with the presence and severity of nephropathy and coronary artery disease in patients with type 2 diabetes mellitus. Cardiovasc Diabetol 2010; 9:70-75

Yan,S.F.,Ramasamy ,R.,Bucciarelly ,L.G ., et al. RAGE and its ligands: a lasting memory in diabetic complications? Diab. Vasc. Dis. Res.2004;1 (1):10-20

Yoshida H, Mitarai T, Kawamura T et al. Role of the deletion polymorphism of the angiotensin converting enzyme gene in the progression and therapeutic responsiveness of IgA nephropathy. J Clin Invest. 1995;96:2162–2169

Ziyadeh ,G .,FN.,Wolf. Pathogenesis of the podocytopathy andproteinuria in diabetic glomerulopathy. Curr Diabetes Rev.2008;4:39-45.

Ziyadeh,F.N.,Goldfarb, S. The renal tubulointerstitium in diabetes mellitus. Kidney Int 1991;39 (3):464– 475

8

Glomerulonephritis and the Cystic Fibrosis Patient

Daniel Fischman,
Arvin Parvathaneni and Pramil Cheriyath
Pinnacle Health System-Harrisburg Hospital,
Harrisburg, Pennsylvania,
United States of America

1. Introduction

Cystic Fibrosis (CF) is a disease with an evolving definition. Through earlier diagnosis and newborn screening programs, as well as a robust world-wide research program, we are able to treat individuals afflicted with this life-threatening malady more aggressively and with earlier interventions. Despite our progress in extending the life expectancy of the typical CF patient, the disease is still viewed by the general medical community as one of childhood.

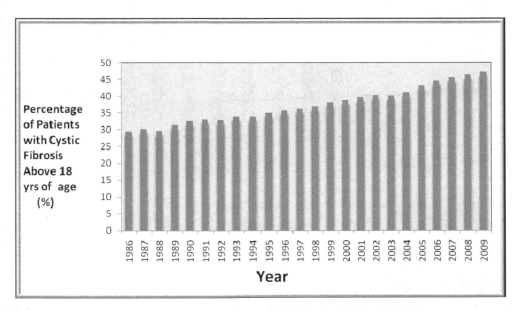

Source: Cystic Fibrosis Foundation Patient Registry Annual Data Reports, 1986-2009

Fig. 1. Prevalence of Cystic Fibrosis in North American Adults

This former "age constraint" on the natural history of CF is paralleled by other major developments, such as an expansion of the number of organ systems, which we now know are involved in this disease. We now know that this disease affects more than the pulmonary and gastrointestinal systems.

With the aging of the CF population, it has come to light that CF patients suffer from an increased risk of Diabetes Mellitus (Fischman & Nookala, 2008; Stecenko & Moran, 2010), Osteoporosis (Haworth, 2010), and malignancies (Hernandez-Jimenez et al., 2008). There is also a growing body of literature suggesting that as a result of treating other conditions associated with CF and as a result of the inflammatory and immunologic milieu associated with Cystic Fibrosis, these patients also suffer from renal disease (Stephens & Ridden, 2002; Katz et al., 1988) (Figure 2). In this chapter, we will discuss our current understanding of Cystic Fibrosis and review potential associations to renal disease with special attention to glomerulonephritis (GN).

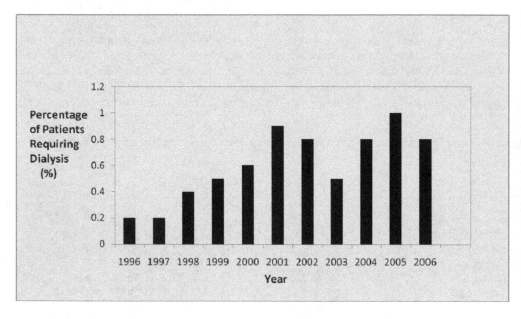

Source: Cystic Fibrosis Foundation Patient Registry Annual Data Reports, 1996-2006

Fig. 2. Prevalence of Cystic Fibrosis Patients Requiring Dialysis for Renal Failure

2. Background - Cystic Fibrosis

2.1 Genetics

Cystic Fibrosis is the most common, lethal, autosomal recessive disorder seen among the Caucasian population. For this reason, its disease prevalence throughout much of the world is 1 in 2,000 to 1 in 3200 individuals. Among non-Caucasian populations, and those not living in North America or Western Europe, the prevalence is approximately 1 in 4,000 to

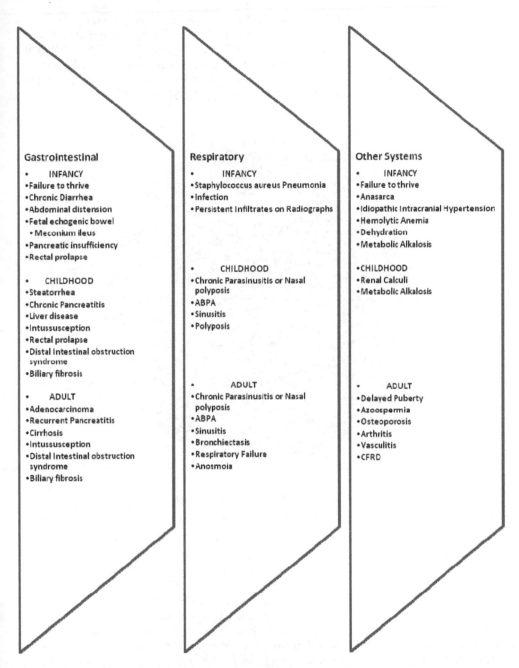

Gastrointestinal

- INFANCY
- Failure to thrive
- Chronic Diarrhea
- Abdominal distension
- Fetal echogenic bowel
  - Meconium ileus
- Pancreatic insufficiency
- Rectal prolapse

- CHILDHOOD
- Steatorrhea
- Chronic Pancreatitis
- Liver disease
- Intussusception
- Rectal prolapse
- Distal Intestinal obstruction syndrome
- Biliary fibrosis

- ADULT
- Adenocarcinoma
- Recurrent Pancreatitis
- Cirrhosis
- Intussusception
- Distal Intestinal obstruction syndrome
- Biliary fibrosis

Respiratory

- INFANCY
- Staphylococcus aureus Pneumonia
- Infection
- Persistent Infiltrates on Radiographs

- CHILDHOOD
- Chronic Parasinusitis or Nasal polyposis
- ABPA
- Sinusitis
- Polyposis

- ADULT
- Chronic Parasinusitis or Nasal polyposis
- ABPA
- Sinusitis
- Bronchiectasis
- Respiratory Failure
- Anosmoia

Other Systems

- INFANCY
- Failure to thrive
- Anasarca
- Idiopathic Intracranial Hypertension
- Hemolytic Anemia
- Dehydration
- Metabolic Alkalosis

- CHILDHOOD
- Renal Calculi
- Metabolic Alkalosis

- ADULT
- Delayed Puberty
- Azoospermia
- Osteoporosis
- Arthritis
- Vasculitis
- CFRD

Legend: ABPA = Allergic Bronchopulmonary Aspergillosis,
CFRD = Cystic Fibrosis-Related Diabetes Mellitus

Fig. 3. Common Signs and Symptoms of Cystic Fibrosis, by Stages of Life

1 in 20,000 (Figure 4) (Sullivan & Freedman, 2009). Although we have known for decades of the association between salty sweat, obstructive lung disease, and pancreatic insufficiency, which comprise the hallmark symptoms of CF, and it was postulated as early as 1949 that a gene defect was the cause of CF, it was not until 1989 that the gene defect was localized to chromosome 7 (Rowe et. al., 2005). Since that time, more than fifteen hundred mutations have been identified that can lead to the cystic fibrosis phenotype (Boyle, 2007).

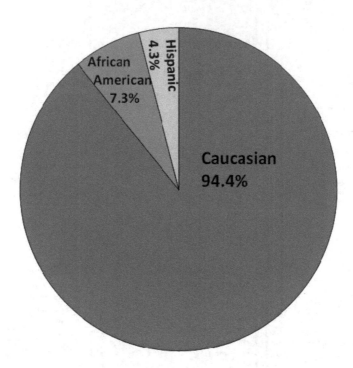

Source: Cystic Fibrosis Foundation Patient Registry Annual Data Report 2009

Fig. 4. Racial Demographics of Cystic Fibrosis Patients in North America

This specific gene encodes a protein called the Cystic Fibrosis Transmembrane Conductance Regulator (CFTR), which is found on many different types of cells. CFTR plays numerous regulatory roles throughout the body. The role most commonly associated with CFTR is that of chloride channel. However, the CFTR protein also plays a role in the inhibition of sodium transport, the regulation of ATP channels, and the inhibition of calcium-activated chloride channels. We now know that there are multiple types of CFTR gene mutations. They range in effect from complete lack of protein production (Class I Mutation), and defective protein processing and trafficking to the cell surface (Class II), to reduced production of normal-functioning CFTR protein (Class V) (Sullivan & Freedman, 2009) (Table 1). The F508del mutation, which accounts for two-thirds of Cystic Fibrosis in Northern Europe and North America, is a class II mutation, resulting in production of a defective CFTR protein.

Mutation Class	Effect on CFTR Protein	CFTR Ability to Function	Pancreatic Exocrine Dysfunction
I	Protein not produced	No	Severe
II	Protein trafficking defect with CFTR degraded in ER/GolB; CFTR does not reach cell membrane	No	Severe
III	Defective protein regulation; CFTR reaches cell membrane but not activated by ATP or cyclic AMP	No	Severe
IV	Reduced Cl transport through apical membrane CFTR	Yes	Mild
V	Splicing defect with reduced production of functioning CFTR	Yes	Mild
VI	CFTR reaches cell membrane, but more rapid CFTR turnover	Yes	Presumably Mild

Legend: CFTR = Cystic Fibrosis Transmembrane Regulator Protein, ER = Endoplasmic Reticulum, GolB = Golgi Body, ATP = Adenosine Triphosphate, AMP = Adenosine Monophosphate, Cl = Chloride ion

Table 1. CFTR Mutation Classes

Since Cystic Fibrosis is an autosomal recessive genetic trait, full expression of this disease requires that a defective gene be present on each chromosome. However, having one abnormal gene typically conveys a milder level of morbidity. As the level of CFTR metabolic regulatory function decreases below fifty percent, the chance of the individual developing sino-pulmonary conditions such as sinusitis, nasal polyps, or asthma increases. Men with the cystic fibrosis trait may experience infertility due to Congenital Bilateral Absence of the Vas Deferens (CBAVD). Despite the fact that it takes the presence of only one abnormal CFTR gene and fifty percent CFTR function for sino-pulmonary and genitourinary symptoms to occur; it typically takes CFTR function at levels less than five-percent of normal, usually seen with two mutations, before a patient's sweat chloride excretion rises to levels diagnostic of CF. Furthermore, it takes CFTR protein function to be decreased by ninety-nine percent for pancreatic insufficiency to occur (Strasbaugh & Davis, 2007). Moreover, despite our efforts to characterize the association between genetic defect and phenotypic disease, neither sweat chloride level nor pulmonary function test values correlate with number or type of CFTR mutation. In two studies looking at this association, a mutation known to lead to Cystic Fibrosis could be found in only three out of five patients (Groman et. al., 2005; Groman et al., 2002). However, it is interesting that a 2009 study of urinary protein excretion with regard to Cystic Fibrosis did find an apparent association between level of renal protein excretion and genotype, suggesting that although we cannot directly correlate gastrointestinal or pulmonary phenotype with a patient's genotype, we may be able to correlate renal phenotype with CF genotype (Cemlyn-Jones & Gamboa, 2009).

2.2 Pathophysiology
The pathophysiology of Cystic Fibrosis results from abnormalities localized to the CFTR gene site resulting in an abnormality in CFTR protein production or processing. Either

through this absence of CFTR protein, or through the production of abnormally functioning protein, an electrolyte imbalance occurs on luminal surfaces in multiple organ systems. The common result is the production of thick, tenacious secretions, which have impaired immunologic function and result in dysregulation of the patient's inflammatory response, leading to an imbalance between pro-inflammatory and anti-inflammatory chemokines. In addition, there has been some evidence to suggest that the abnormal CFTR protein may facilitate protein binding of bacteria, leading to CF-related lung disease involving such bacterial pathogens as Pseudomonas aeruginosa and Staphylococcus aureus (Sullivan & Freedman, 2009; Rowe, 2005).

2.3 Diagnosis

The diagnosis of Cystic Fibrosis is typically made based on a combination of clinical symptoms consistent with the disease along with confirmatory testing. Since 1959, the diagnostic standard for Cystic Fibrosis has been the measurement of sweat chloride levels, as stimulated through a process using Pilocarpine Iontophoresis. In children younger than six months of age, a normal concentration of sweat chloride is considered to be less than 30 mmol/liter. In patients older than six months, the normal range would be less than 41 mmol/liter. Regardless of age, any repeatable sweat chloride level greater than 59 mmol/liter is consistent with the diagnosis of Cystic Fibrosis, particularly if accompanied by symptoms of sino-pulmonary disease, a gastrointestinal malady such as fat-soluble vitamin deficiency, malnutrition, or intestinal obstruction, metabolic alkalosis, dehydration, or acute salt depletion (Figure 2) (Farrell et al., 2008).

Consistent with the phenotypic pancreatic insufficiency seen in 90-95% of Cystic Fibrosis patients, pancreatic enzyme levels may be measured to help confirm the diagnosis. As of 2010, fourteen European countries and all states in the United States have a process in place for screening newborns for this disease. Most of these testing programs, at least to some degree, rely on measuring levels of Immunoreactive Trypsinogen, a pancreatic enzyme found to be elevated in the first six weeks of life in infants with CF (Barto & Flume, 2010).

In the situation where the sweat chloride analysis is indeterminate or the symptomatic phenotype is subtle, genetic testing is often employed. If the patient is found to have two mutations known to be consistent with the cystic fibrosis phenotype, then the diagnosis can be made. If one mutation is found, and it is unclear if the patient has a second, less well-characterized mutation, then the patient is considered to have a possible diagnosis of Cystic Fibrosis. As noted previously, genetic testing may still be performed in the circumstance of confirmed disease, since the patient's specific mutations may have prognostic significance. Furthermore, as we attain a greater understanding of the myriad of ways that defective CFTR genes may lead to inadequate or defective protein production and function, we will be able to tailor our therapeutic regimens more effectively to the patient's genetic circumstance, in order to modulate or restore CFTR function (Ashlock et al., 2009).

2.4 Clinical manifestations

To date, it has been impossible to draw a direct link between the degree of genotypic abnormality and a particular patient's morbidity. However, there are some common clinical patterns and associations seen in cystic fibrosis patients. Based on these clinical findings, an all-encompassing definition of Cystic Fibrosis would be "a chronic and progressive, multi-system disease leading to sino-pulmonary disease, with probable exocrine pancreatic insufficiency, malnutrition, and gastrointestinal obstructive symptoms". Patients with

Cystic Fibrosis typically have some degree of obstructive lung disease and present with a distinguishing factor of early colonization and subsequent infection from organisms not typically seen except in immunosuppressed or severely bronchiectatic individuals, such as Pseudomonas aeruginosa, Burkholderia cepacia, or Stenotrophomonas maltophilia.

As a consequence of pancreatic insufficiency and associated malnutrition, many Cystic Fibrosis patients are deficient in fat soluble vitamins and suffer from a chronic, negative protein balance. Mouse studies have shown that the presence of CFTR gene defects leads to a heightened risk of Osteoporosis and subsequent bone fracture (Haworth, 2010). Along with this fracture risk, CF patients have an increased risk of kidney stones. One autopsy study of thirty-eight CF patients found that thirty-five had evidence of nephrocalcinosis, including one still-born and two neonatal infants (Katz et al., 1988). This predilection seems to be multifactorial and results from the interplay of 1) impaired vitamin D absorption leading to impaired calcium absorption, 2) chronic disease characterized by increased metabolic tempo, 3) immobility, 4) increased osteoclast activity, 5) inadequate caloric intake due to increase work-of-breathing, 6) an imbalance between protein anabolism and catabolism, and 7) loss of oxalate-degrading bacteria due to frequent, and often chronic antibiotic use (Stephens & Rigden, 2002). Furthermore, Andrieux et al., in their 2010 study, found that 75% of children in their study population had hypocitraturia and 70% had hyperoxaluria, both of which are risk factors for nephrolithiasis (Andrieux et al., 2010).

One interesting aspect of the renal expression of CFTR is that cystic fibrosis patients often have greater antibiotic excretion than their non-CF counterparts. This necessitates the use of higher-than-typical antibiotic doses. The classic example of this occurs with the use of aminoglycoside antibiotics for treatment of pseudomonal infections, where Tobramycin is dosed at 10 mg/kg, sometimes in conjunction with inhaled Tobramycin, instead of the usual 5-7 mg/kg (Barto & Flume, 2010, Bergman et al., 2007). Indeed, in one study of renal failure in children with Cystic Fibrosis, twenty of twenty-four cases of acute renal failure were associated with recent or concomitant aminoglycoside administration (Bertenshaw et al., 2007). As a result of this uncertain pharmacokinetic and pharmacodynamic profile encountered with cystic fibrosis patients, monitoring drug levels is critical to insure that therapeutic doses are being achieved for efficacy.

3. Renal disease and the CF patient

3.1 A broad picture of renal disease in Cystic Fibrosis

Since Dorothy Anderson first generated the term, "Cystic Fibrosis," in 1938, we have known that kidney disease may be part of this malady (Abramowsky & Swinehart, 1982). However, the natural history of CF-related renal disease has been elucidated in few studies. In Abromowksy and Swinehart's 1982 study, they found that all thirty-four of the patients studied had some form of glomerulopathy, with nineteen having glomerulosclerosis. Twenty-five had what was described as a "Mesangiopathy," and twenty-six had tubulointerstitial disease. In this study, the authors concluded that a number of factors had led to the myriad of renal lesions observed: 1) lung disease with resultant cyanosis, 2) liver disease, 3) Cystic Fibrosis-Related Diabetes Mellitus, 4) the effects of nephrotoxic medications, and 5) an altered immune response. Of note, the authors report that sixteen of thirty-four patients studied had complement-3 (C3) deposits in their kidneys while thirteen had evidence of immunoglobulin–M deposits (IgM) (Abramowsky & Swinehart, 1982).

A more contemporary, 2010 study investigating renal disease in Cystic Fibrosis followed 112 children, starting in the first year of life. This study revealed the presence of microalbuminuria in fifty-eight percent of patients. This finding was attributed to the presence of chronic inflammation as a result of the malfunctioning or absent CFTR protein, repeated infections, and the nephrotoxicity of many medications commonly used in the treatment of CF (Andrieux et al., 2010). Furthermore, a 2009 study following five hundred ten adults with CF, median age of thirty-one years, found that 13 developed renal disease severe enough to warrant renal biopsy, with eight different types of nephropathies found on histologic analysis. Twelve of these thirteen patients were found to have glomerular lesions. In this study, the main types of renal disease found were AA amyloidosis and diabetic nephropathy (Yahiaoui et al., 2009).

In literature reviewed for their 2002 article on renal disease in Cystic Fibrosis, Stephens and Rigden report that IgA Nephropathy appeared to be the most common form of glomerulonephritis described in CF patients, though the occurrence of this condition appeared rare (Stephens & Rigden, 2002). With respect to all renal disease in CF patients, the most common renal pathology found has been nephrocalcinosis. Drug-related nephrotoxicity also continues to be a common cause of renal morbidity among CF patients. Among the various agents responsible medication-induced renal disease, aminoglycosides continue to play a prominent role. As a result of the pharmacodynamic and pharmacokinetic eccentricities of the cystic fibrosis patient, Acute Tubular Necrosis (ATN) remains a constant concern when treating pulmonary exacerbations in this patient population. This risk of ATN is amplified by pulmonary biofilm formation and the need to use a combination of intravenous, oral, and inhaled antibiotics to effect a decrease in pathogen levels, and potentially facilitate bacterial eradication. It is for this reason that current Cystic Fibrosis Foundation guidelines recommend once-daily dosing of aminoglycosides to optimize treatment benefit, yet minimize risk of renal injury (Flume et al., 2009). Furthermore, a 2010 review of aminoglycoside toxicity in cystic fibrosis patients suggested that use of once-daily Tobramycin, particularly when dosed in the morning, may be superior to use of gentamicin in preventing aminoglycoside-induced renal injury (Prayle & Smyth, 2010).

3.2 Measurement of renal function in CF patients

Discussion of renal disease in CF patients is complicated by the fact that conventional methods of measuring renal function may not be accurate in this population (Prayle & Smyth, 2010). In Andrieux's 2008 study of renal disease in children with CF, his team observed that there was no correlation between a calculated Glomerular Filtration Rate (GFR), using the Schwartz Formula's manipulation of serum creatinine (SCr) values, and a urine creatinine-based (UCr) standard.

Schwartz Formula:

$$GFR(mL/min/1.73 \ m^2) = ((k)(Height \ in \ cm)/(SCr \ in \ mg/dL)) \ where$$

K = Constant as follows:
- 0.33 in premature infant
- 0.45 in term infants to 1 year-old
- 0.55 in children older than one, up to 13 years old
- 0.55 in adolescent females
- 0.65 in adolescent males

In one-third of children studied, the Schwartz Formula's serum-creatinine derived approach overestimated renal function (Andrieux et al., 2010). Furthermore, Yahiaoui's 2009 study investigating renal disease in thirteen adults with Cystic Fibrosis concluded that one of the reasons that renal disease is considered uncommon in CF patients is that measurements of SCr and calculations of GFR, using either the Cockcroft-Gault or MDRD equations, fail to adequately and reliably reflect a CF patient's true level of kidney function (Yahiaoui et al., 2009). To explain this apparent inadequacy in SCr-based evaluation of renal function observed in the CF population, it has been suggested that decreases in muscle mass seen among CF patients, and typically related to their underlying disease state, leads to decreased production of SCr. This would hinder the proportional rise in SCr levels in response to renal insufficiency, which has been observed in other studied populations. Recognizing this challenge of accurately measuring renal function in CF patients, methods that more directly measure kidney function have been proposed including methods using UCr collection, typically over twenty-four hours, or using plasma levels of an inert tracer which is only excreted via the kidneys (Prayle & Smyth, 2010).

In recognizing the fallacies of SCr-based formulae, the difficulties of collecting urine accurately over an extended period of time, and the invasiveness of nuclear tracer-based measurements of renal function, Beringer and colleagues studied levels of the biomarker Cystatin C (Cys C) as a potential method of estimating GFR. Their study showed that measurement of Cystatin C clearance was a suitable alternative to measurement of SCr or calculated GFR in following a CF patient's renal function. Furthermore, Cys C levels were not affected by age, gender, muscle mass, diet, or level of physical activity. Moreover, the authors make specific mention of using this method to follow CFRD patients for evidence of renal disease (Beringer et al., 2009). Unfortunately, at this time, Cys C levels have not become widely employed.

3.3 Cystic Fibrosis-Related Diabetes Mellitus and Renal Disease

Since Cystic Fibrosis-Related Diabetes Mellitus (CFRD) is becoming an increasingly common complication in the natural history of Cystic Fibrosis, and can lead to significant renal pathology, we discuss this type of renal disease as an independent section. By the time CF patients reach their thirtieth birthday, 45-50% will have developed CFRD, with an associated increase in morbidity and mortality. This complication of Cystic Fibrosis was formerly the most dreaded of sequelae, as it was associated with a six-fold increase in mortality, particularly among women (Fischman & Nookala, 2008). However, through aggressive efforts to increase screening for evidence of impaired glucose intolerance and overt diabetes, as well as through early use of oral diabetic medications and insulin, the mortality disparity associated with CFRD has all but disappeared (Stecenko & Moran, 2010) (Table 2).

As with other forms of Diabetes Mellitus, CFRD may lead to microvascular changes in such structures as the Eyes, Kidneys, Stomach, and Nerves. A 2007 study of the microvascular complications of CFRD suggested that CFRD-related nephropathy occurred less commonly than renal complications seen in association with other forms of Diabetes Mellitus (Schwarzenberg et al., 2007). The results found in Schwarzenberg's study appear to be consistent with our current understanding of CFRD, which suggests that the increased mortality risk that CFRD conveys is due to accelerated progression of the patient's underlying lung disease, not due to vascular complications (Stecenko & Moran, 2010). Moreover, the microalbuminuria that we typically associate with microvascular damage to the kidney was only seen among CF patients who had fasting hyperglycemia (Schwarzenberg et al., 2007) (Table 3).

Characteristic	CFRD	DM I	DM II
Age at Onset	18-21 years	< 20 years	>40 years
Prevalence	22% of CFFR population (2% of children, 19% of adolescents, 45-50% over age 30[a])	7% of US population	7% of US population (NB: > 15% of population > 50 years)
Body Habitus	Thin	Normal	Overweight/Obese
Insulin Secretion	Decreased, Release delayed	Absent	Decreased relative to need
Insulin Resistance	Increased or Unchanged	Increased Slightly	Increased Dramatically
Ketoacidosis	No	Yes	No
Microvascular Complications	Yes	Yes	Yes
Macrovascular Complications	Extremely Rare	Yes	Yes
Nutritional Support	**High calorie diet:** (120-150%) of RDA **Fat**: 40% of dietary intake (No restrictions on type) **Protein**: 10-20% of calories, not reduced for nephropathy **Sodium**: > 4 grams per day **Vitamins**: Routine supplementation	**Calories adjusted for goal:** growth, weight maintenance, or loss **Fat Restriction**: <30% of total calories, <10% from saturated fats **Protein**: 10-20% of total calories; reduced for nephropathy **Sodium**: <2.4 grams per day **Vitamin:** Supplementation for diagnosed deficiencies	**Calorie restriction for weight loss** **Fat Restriction**: <30% of total calories, <10% from saturated fats **Protein**: 10-20% of total calories; reduced for nephropathy **Sodium**: <2.4 grams per day **Vitamin:** Supplementation for diagnosed deficiencies
Pharmacologic Therapy	Insulin therapy(currently SOC); oral anti-diabetic agents(controversial)	Insulin replacement; SC synthetic Amylin analogues	Oral antidiabetic agents; Insulin therapy; SC Incretin Mimetic and synthetic Amylin analogues

Legend: CFFR = North American Cystic Fibrosis Foundation Registry; DM I = Diabetes Mellitus Type I; DM II = Diabetes Mellitus Type II ; RDA = recommended daily allowance; SOC = standard of care; SC = subcutaneously administered.

Table 2. A Comparison of Cystic Fibrosis-Related Diabetes Mellitus to Types 1 and 2 Diabetes Mellitus

Glucose Tolerance Catergory	Fasting Serum Glucose (mg/dl)	Two-Hour Oral Glucose Challenge: One-Hour Value (mg/dl)	Two-Hour Oral Glucose Challenge (mg/dl)
Normal Glucose Tolerance	<126		<140
Indeterminate	<126	>/= 200	<140
Impaired Glucose Tolerance	<126		140-199
Impaired Fasting Glucose	100-125		
CFRD *without* Fasting Hyperglcemia (CFRD FH-)	<126		>/= 200
CFRD *with* Fasting Hyperglycemia	>/= 126		>/= 200

Table 3. Cystic Fibrosis-Related Diabetes Mellitus Diagnostic Categories

It is interesting that a subsequent 2008 study comparing microvascular changes found in CF patients to a matched cohort of patients with Type I Diabetes Mellitus (DM1) found that while retinopathy occurred more frequently in DM1, renal disease as measured through microalbuminuria occurred with greater frequency in patients with CFRD. The authors of this study explained this discrepancy in microvascular findings by speculating that other factors, such as deficient CFTR function, chronic inflammation, repeated exposure to nephrotoxic agents, or genetic predispositions may be the cause (van den Berg et al., 2008). While the results of these two studies may appear to be conflicting, a closer analysis reveals that van den Berg's study methodology does not distinguish patients with fasting hyperglycemia from those without; thus, if van den Berg's CFRD population had a preponderance of patients with fasting hyperglycemia, then the results of these two studies may be consistent.

Within the last decade, case reports have emerged suggesting that Nodular Glomerulosclerosis (NGS) in cystic fibrosis patients may mimic the findings of Diabetic Nephropathy (DN) (Westall et al., 2004). Since the histopathology of these cases appears to be misleadingly reminiscent of that seen in Diabetic Nephropathy, we have chosen to discuss these cases in conjunction with our discussion of CFRD-related renal disease. In their case report, Westall's team reports that all three patients had pathologic findings thought consistent with DN, including Kimmelstiel-Wilson Nodules, without any evidence of impaired glucose tolerance. The authors speculate that the Focal and Nodular Glomerulosclerosis observed (e.g. the Kimmelstiel-Wilson nodules) may be an idiopathic occurrence, may be the result of CFTR deficiency or abnormal function, or may be the result of accumulation of toxic molecules. The authors explain that these toxic molecules are generated as the by-product of an inflammatory process or as a result of oxidative stress. Furthermore, they conjectured that these pathologic findings may be the consequence of undetected episodes of hyperglycemia, which would eventually become more persistent.

In an accompanying editorial to Westall's case series, Krous discusses the implications of Westall's work. In his commentary, Krous does raise the question of whether we should be routinely screening cystic fibrosis patients for proteinuria, since renal pathology similar to DN has been described, even without evidence of hyperglycemia. Krous also calls for further investigation of the specific pathologic process that leads to the NGS seen in both CF and Diabetes Mellitus. In the end, the only answer that Krous leaves us with is that it may be prudent to screen CF patients for proteinuria (Krous HF, 2004).

3.4 Glomeulonephritis
3.4.1 An introduction to glomerular disease in Cystic Fibrosis
Despite the fact that renal pathology among cystic fibrosis patients was described from the time that CF's constellation of symptoms was first delineated, there still remains relatively little written on renal involvement in CF. There are many explanations as to why this may be the case: lack of a clear CF renal disease phenotype, difficulty measuring renal impairment due to inadequacy of SCr-based renal function tests, and, possibly, reluctance of cystic fibrosis center care teams to pursue the presence of renal pathology with potentially intrusive, and possibly invasive testing (Yahiaoui et al., 2009). However, with the aging of this patient population, an increasing number of case reports have suggested that renal disease is part of the CF phenotype. In 1972, Openheimer described the presence of glomerular pathology in autopsied CF patients (Openheimer, 1972). Abramowsky's 1982 study showed that a majority of patients studied not only had evidence of glomerular involvement, but also immunoflourescence findings of immunoglobulin and complement deposition in glomeruli, with localization to the mesangial regions and capillary loops (Abramowsky & Swineheart, 1982). A more contemporary study of thirteen adults with CF and renal disease, who underwent a renal biopsy, revealed that twelve had glomerular lesions (Yahiaoui et al., 2009). Thus, it is clear that, beyond a CF patient's very real risk of experiencing a renal injury as a result of a medication adverse drug reaction or toxicity, Cystic Fibrosis, itself, may be associated with renal pathology. In this section we will discuss the types of glomerular lesions that have been observed and current theories on the development of glomerular pathology in Cystic Fibrosis.

3.4.2 IgA Nephropathy
In Stephens and Rigden's review of renal disease in Cystic Fibrosis, they report that among the glomerulonephritides, IgA Nephropathy is the most frequently reported (Stephens & Rigden, 2002). In a 1999 case series reported by Stirati and colleagues, four out of the five CF patients who underwent a renal biopsy for proteinuria had findings consistent with IgA Nephropathy. It should be noted that the authors do admit that since IgA Nephropathy is a common type of GN in young adults, and the patients in their study ranged in age from twenty-two to thirty years, their findings may be a chance occurrence.

However, another plausible explanation for this association, put forth by the authors is that recurrent bacterial infections result in a robust immune response leading to increased levels of circulating immunoglobulins and immune complexes. These immune-mediating molecules may deposit in the kidney and lead to the histopathology and morbidity observed (Stirati et al., 1999). Interestingly, in Abromowsky and Swinehart's 1982 study, the explanation of chronic bacterial infection leading to a high level of immune activity resulting in glomerular pathology was also raised. Abramowsky and Swinehart conjectured that the proximate cause was chronic pseudomonas aeruginosa infection. However, contemporary immunologic investigations using pseudomonas antiserum did not reveal any antigens in the studied glomeruli.

If chronic pseudomonal infection is not the nidus for this robust immune response, then what is? The answer may actually lie in staphylococcal infection. Staphylococcus epidermitis bacteremia and staphylococcus aureus-asssociated endocardititis have long been known to cause glomerulonephritis. Furthermore, histopathology of staphylococcal-associated GN typically reveals glomerular immune complex deposits containing complement, particularly C3, and immunoglobulins, typically IgG and IgM. These findings are consistent with those described in CF-related Glomerulonephritis, and have even greater significance in light of the fact that staphylococcus remains a common colonizing pathogen (Figure 5), and a major cause of lung infection early in a CF patient's life, typically causing pneumonia before pseudomonas aeruginosa infections become common. Moreover, idiopathic IgA Nephropathy is known to occur within a few days of the patient experiencing an upper respiratory infection. Thus, there appears to be a viable association between staphylococcal colonization and IgA Nephropathy in cystic fibrosis patients (Satoskar et al., 2006).

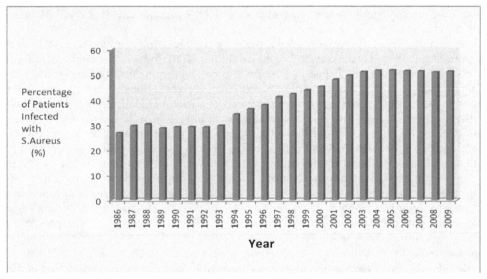

Source: Cystic Fibrosis Foundation Patient Registry Annual Data Reports, 1986-2009

Fig. 5. Prevalence of Staphylococcus Aureus Infection/Colonization Among Cystic Fibrosis Patients

In a 2006 case series by Satoskar and colleagues, they report eight cases of staphylococcus infection-associated mesangial and/or intracapillary proliferative glomerulonephritis (GN) associated with IgA-laden immune complex deposition. In this study, seven of the eight patients described had infections other than endocarditis, and the eighth suffered from an epidural abscess which resulted in endocarditis (Satoskar et al., 2006). The reason why staphylococcal infections may lead to GN remains unclear. One theory proposed by Satoskar suggests that staphylococcus enterotoxins may behave as superantigens that bind Major Histocompatibility Complex Class II (MHC II) molecules on Antigen-Presenting Cells (APC). This complex of MHC II and enterotoxin then binds to T-cell receptors, resulting in widespread T-cell activation and a surge of cytokine release. These cytokines, in turn, activate B-cells, which then produce IgA and IgG molecules. These immunoglobulins are then released, resulting in immune complex formation, and eventual deposition in the Kidney. Further elaborating on this mechanism of glomerular pathology, Koyoma's group described a specific staphylococcus aureus envelope antigen as a proximate cause for superantigen formation (Koyoma et al., 2004). Thus, research studying the association between staphylococcal skin and wound infections, as well as idiopathic IgA Nephropathy, may shed some light on the pathologic association between IgA Nephropathy and Cystic Fibrosis.

3.4.3 Membranoproliferative Glomerulonephritis

The occurrence of Membranoproliferative Glomerulonephritis (MPGN) in cystic fibrosis patients is not a new finding. Ambrowsky and Swinehart's 1982 autopsy study of thirty-four Cystic Fibrosis patients showed on eighteen patients who had evidence of immune complex deposition in the Kidney, and, of those, sixteen had evidence of mesangial proliferation with two also having evidence of membranoproliferative histopathology. Thus, this autopsy study would suggest that MPGN is a major cause of renal disease in the CF patient.

However, more contemporary reviews of the subject do not find nor discuss MPGN in the CF patient (Stephens & Rigden, 2002; Yahiaoui et al., 2009). Indeed, the only recent report of this association was published by Soriano and colleagues in 2008 (Soriano et al., 2008). In this paper, the authors discuss multiple, plausible explanations for the natural history of renal disease in CF. One mechanism proposed, the Factor H Deficiency Model, is based on the observation that genetic knockout mice who are deficient in alternate complement pathway Factor H not only develop MPGN, but also experience higher mortality with pseudomonas aeruginosa infections than factor H sufficient mice. Furthermore, factor H deficiency has been found to lead to aberrant activation of Complement Factor C3 and higher serum levels of various chemokines and cytokines (Soriano et al., 2008). This pathologic explanation is supported by the work of Wisnieski's group, who reported in 1985 that mortality among their cohort of one hundred thirty-nine patients was highly associated with decreased alternate complement pathway function and the presence of circulating immune complexes (Wisnieski et al., 1985).

Separate from the immunologic explanation proposed above, a plausible link between Cystic Fibrosis and Membranoproliferative Glomerulonephritis lies in the function of Toll-like Receptors (TLR), which are part of the Innate Immune System. This family of receptor proteins is responsible for recognizing recurring structures on pathogens, including single-stranded DNA, lipopolysaccharides, and RNA molecules. Upon recognition of a structure known to be associated with a pathogen, the TLR initiates inflammatory and immune responses whose end result is meant to be destruction of the pathogen. By modulating immune responses, including regulating helper T-cell immunologic responses, aberrant TLR function is conjectured to lead to kidney inflammation and glomerulonephritis (Smith & Alpers, 2005). A 2004 study by Muir and colleagues showed that TLR-2 expression was up-regulated in the lungs of CF patients (Muir et al., 2004). Moreover, in 2006, Shuto and colleagues suggested that this TLR-2 up-regulation and prolonged activation was critical to the pathogenesis of CF lung disease (Shuto et al., 2006). Separate from the Factor H Deficiency or the TLR models for the development of glomerulonephritis in cystic fibrosis patients, the presence of staphylococcal superantigens has been conjectured to lead to MPGN in CF patients (Soriano et al., 2008).

3.4.4 Treatment

To date, there has been very little written on the treatment of glomerulonephritis in CF patients. One available case series details the diagnosis and treatment of two adult patients. In this article, it is reported that one of the patients experienced an improvement in his renal disease to the point where he could safely forgo hemodialysis after undergoing a double-lung transplant and starting his anti-rejection regimen (Soriano et al., 2008). This would suggest that the conventional immunosuppressant therapy typically employed in the treatment of glomerulonephritis would be appropriate in this population as well. However, given the known pharmacokinetic and pharmacodynamic intricacies of the CF patient, further study is warranted.

4. Conclusion

Cystic Fibrosis is a disease in evolution. Through wide-spread newborn screening programs, patients are diagnosed earlier. Through an aggressive, world-wide therapy development network, new and revolutionary treatments for the manifestations of Cystic Fibrosis are shepherded from the lab bench to the patient's home. As we develop a better understanding of how genetic mutation translates into phenotypic dysfunction and symptoms, we will be able to regulate and modify protein function to ameliorate the symptoms of Cystic Fibrosis. However, with these revolutionary changes to how patients experience the morbidity of Cystic Fibrosis, and with the aging of the CF population, new manifestations of CF may emerge. Kidney disease, particularly glomerulonephritis, may be one of the more plausible morbidities to afflict CF patients with growing regularity in the future. Thus, we must stay ever vigilant, and not become complacent that we have a complete understanding of this disease process. Cystic Fibrosis is no longer a disease of children. We must, therefore, continue to broaden our understanding of what it means to be an adult with Cystic Fibrosis.

5. Acknowledgement

We thank Laurie Schwing, MLS, for editorial guidance in the preparation of this chapter.

6. References

Abramowsky, CR., & Swineheart, GL. (1982). The Nephropathy of Cystic Fibrosis. Vol. 13, No. 9, (October 1982), pp. (934-939)

Andrieux, A., Harambat J., Bui, S., Nacka, F., Iron A., Lianas B., & Fayon, M. (2010). Renal Impairment in Children with Cystic Fibrosis. *Journal of Cystic Fibrosis*, Vol. 9, No. 4, (July 2010), pp. (263-268), doi: 10.1016/j.jcf.2010.03.006

Ashlock, MA., Beall, RJ., Hamblett, NM., Konstan, MW., Penland, CM., Ramsey, BW., Van Dalfsen, JM., Wetmore, DR., & Campbell, PW 3rd.. (2009). A Pipeline of Therapies for Cystic Fibrosis. *Seminars in Respiratory and Critical Care Medicine*, Vol. 30, No. 5, (October 2009), pp. (611-626), ISSN: 1069-3424.

Barto, TL., & Flume, PA. (2010). Treatment of Pulmonary Exacerbations in Adult Cystic Fibrosis Patients. *Hospital Practice(Mineapolis),*Vol. 38, No. 1, (February 2010), pp. (26-34).

Bergman, JS., Speil, C., Short, M., & Koirala , J. (2007). Pharmacokinetic and Pharmacodynamic Aspects of Antibiotic use in High Risk Populations.

InfectiousDdisease Clinics of North America, Vol. 21, (2007), pp. (821-846), doi: 10.1016/j.idc.2007.07.004.

Beringer, PM., Hidayat, L., Heed, A., Zheng, L., Owens, H., Benitez, D., & Rao, AP. (2009). GFR Estimates Using Cystatin C are Superior to Serum Creatinine in Adult Patients with Cystic Fibrosis. *Journal of Cystic Fibrosis*, Vol. 8, No. 1, (January 2009), pp. (19-25), doi: 10.1016/j.jcf.2008.07.004.

Bertenshaw, C., Watson, AR., Lewis, S., & Smyth, A. (2007). Survey of Acute Renal Failure in Patients with Cystic Fibrosis in UK. *Thorax*, Vol. 62, No. 6, (January 2007), pp. (541-545), doi: 10.1136/thx.2006.067595.

Boyle, PM. (2007). Adult Cystic Fibrosis. *Journal of American Medical Association*, Vol. 298, No. 15, (October 2007), pp. (1787-1793), doi: 10.1001/jama.299.4.408-b.

Castellani, C., & Massie, J. (2010). Emerging Issues in Cystic Fibrosis Newborn Screening. *Current opinion in Pulmonary Medicine*. Vol. 16, No. 6, (2010), pp. (584-590), doi: 10.1097/MCP.0b013e32833e9e27.

Farrell, PM., Rosenstein, BJ., White, TB., Accurso, FJ., Castellani, C., Cutting, GR., Durie, PR., Legrys, VA., Massie, J., Parad, RB., Rock, MJ., & Campbell, P.W 3rd. (2008). Guidelines for Diagnosis of Cystic Fibrosis in Newborns through older adults. Cystic Fibrosis Foundation Consensus Report. *Journalof Pediatrics*, Vol. 153, No. 2, (August 2008), pp. (s4-s14), doi: 10.1016/j.jpeds.2008.05.005.

Fischman, D., & Nookala, V. (2008). Cystic Fibrosis Related Diabetes Mellitus: Etiology Evaluation and Management. *Journal of Endocrine Practice*, Vol. 14, No. 9, (December 2008), pp. (1169-1179).

Flume, PA., Robinson, KA., Mogayzel, PJ., Goss, CH., Rosenblatt, RL., Kuhn, RJ., & Marshall, B.C. (2009). Cystic Fibrosis Pulmonary Guidelines: Treatment of Pulmonary Exacerbations. *American Journal of Respiratory Critical Care Medicine*, Vol. 180, No. 4, (September 2009), pp. (802-808), doi: 10.1164/rccm.200812-1845pp.

Groman, JD., Karczeski, B., Sheridan, M., Robinson, TE., Fallin, MD., & Cutting, GR. (2005). Phenotypic and Genetic Characterization of Patients with Features of "Non-classic" Forms of Cystic Fibrosis. *Journal of Pediatrics*, Vol. 146, No. 5, (2005), pp. (675-680), doi: 10.1016/j.jpeds.2004.12.020.

Groman, JD., Meyer, ME., Wilmott, RW., Zeitlin, PL., & Cutting, GR. (2002). Variant Cystic Fibrosis Phenotypes in the Absence of CFTR Mutations. *New England Journal of Medicine*, Vol. 347, No. 6, (August 2002), pp. (401-407).

Haworth ,SC. (2010). Impact of Cystic Fibrosis on Bone Health. *Current Opinion in Pulmonary Medicine*, Vol. 16, No. 6, (November 2010), pp. (616-622), doi: 10.1097/MCP.0b013e32833e2e94.

Jimenez, HI., Fischman, D., & Cheriyath, P. (2008). Colon Cancer in Cystic Fibrosis Patients: Is This a Growing Problem? Vol. 7, (Feb 2008), pp. (343-346), doi: 10.1016/j.jcf.2008.02.006.

Jones, JC., & Gamboa, F. (2009). Protenuria in Cystic Fibrosis a Possible Correlation Between Genotype and Renal Phenotype. *Jornal Brasileiro de Pneumologia,*, Vol. 35, No. 7, (July 2009), doi: 10.1590/s1806-37132009000700008.

Katz, SM., Krueger, LJ., & Falkner, B. (1988). Microscopic Nephrocalcinosis in Cystic Fibrosis. *New England Journal of Medicine*, Vol. 319, (August 1988), pp. (263-266) In Stephens, SE., & Rigden, SP. (2002). Cystic fibrosis and Renal Disease. *Pediatric Respiratory Rreview*, Vol. 3, No. 2, (June 2002), pp. (135-138).

Krous, HF. (2004). Cystic Fibrosis Another Cause of Nodular Glomerulosclerosis. *Nephrology Clinical Practice*, Vol. 96, No. 3,(2004), pp .(70-75), doi: 10.1159/000076742.

Koyama, A., Sharmin, S., Sakurai, H., Shimizu, Y., Hirayama K., Usi, J., Nagata, M., Yoh, K., Yamagata, K., Muro, K., Kobayashi, M., Ohtani, K., Shimizu, Ta., & Shimizu, To. (2004). Staphylococcus Aureus Cell Envelope Antigen is a new Candidate for the Induction of IgA Nephropathy. *Kid Int*, Vol. 66, No. 1, (July 2004). PP. (121-132). In Satoskar, AA., Nadasdy, G., Plaza, JA., Sedmak, D., Shidham, G., Hebert, L., & Nadasdy, T. (2006). Staphylococcus Infection Associated Glomerulonephritis Mimicking IgA Nephropathy. *Clinical Journal of American Society of Nephrology*, Vol. 1, 1555-9041/106-1179.

Muir, A., Soong, G., Sokol, S., Reddy, B., Gomez, MI., Van Heeckeren, A., & Prince, A. (2004). Toll like Receptors in Normal and Cystic Fibrosis Airway Epithelial Cells. *American Journal of Respiratory, Cellular and Molecular Biology*, Vol. 30, No. 6, (June, 2004), pp. (777-783), doi: 10.1165/rcmb.2003-03290c.

Muller, OS., Drovin, MS., & Wetsel, AR. (2004). The Alternative Activation Pathway and Complement C3 are Critical for a Protective Immune Response Against Pseudomonas Aeruginosa in a Murine Model of Pneumonia. *Journal of Infection and Immunity*, Vol. 72, No. 5, (May 2004), pp. (2899-2906), doi: 10.1128/IAI.72.5.2899-2906.2004.

Nathan, BM., Laguna T., & Moran, A. (2010). Recent Trends in Cystic Fibrosis Related Diabetes Mellitus. *Current Opinion in Endocrinology, Diabetes and obesity*, Vol. 17, No. 4, (2010), pp. (335-341), doi: 10.1097/MED.0b013e32833a780d.

Opppenheimer, EH. (1972). Glomerular Leisons in Cystic Fibrosis: Possible Relation to Diabetes Mellitus, Acquired Cyanotic Heart Disease and Cirrhosis of the Liver. *Johns Hopkins Med J*, Vol. 131, No. 5, (November 1972), pp. (351-366). In Abramowsky, CR., & Swineheart, GL. (1982). The Nephropathy of Cystic Fibrosis. Vol. 13, No.9, (October 1982), pp. (934-939).

Prayle, A., & Smyth, RA. (2010). Aminoglycoside Use in Cystic Fibrosis: Therapeutic Strategies and Toxicity. *Current Opinion in Pulmonary Medicine*, Vol. 16, No. 6, (November, 2010), pp. (604-610) doi: 10.1097/MCP.0b013e32833eebfd.

Steven, MR., Stacey, M., & Eric, J.S. (2005). The Diagnosis of Cystic Fibrosis. *New England Journal OfMedicine*, Vol. 352, No. 19, (May 2005), pp. (1992-2001).

Satoskar, AA., Nadasdy, G., Plaza, JA., Sedmak, D., Shidham, G., Hebert, L., & Nadasdy, T. (2006). Staphylococcus Infection Associated Glomerulonephritis Mimicking IgA Nephropathy. *Clinical Journal of American Society of Nephrology*, Vol. 1, (September 2006), pp. (1179-1186), ISSN. 1555-9041/106-1179.

Schwarzenberg, SJ., Thomas, W., Olsen, TW., Grover, T., Walk, D., Milla, C., & Moran, A. (2007). Microvascular Complications in Cystic Fibrosis Related Diabetes. *Journal of Diabetes Care*, Vol. 30, No. 5, (May 2007), pp. (1056-1061), doi: 10.2337/dc06-1576.

Shuto, T., Furuta, T., Oba, M., Xu, H., Li, JD., Cheung, J., Gruenert, DC., Uehara, A., Suico, MA., Okiyoneda, T., & Kai, H. (2006). Promoter hypomethylation of Toll like Receptor 2 Gene is associated with Increased Proinflammatory Response Toward Bacterial Peptidoglycan in Cystic Fibrosis BronchialEpithelial Cells. *Faseb J*, Vol. 20, No. 6, (Feb 2006), pp. (728-734).

Stephens, SE., & Rigden, SP. (2002). Cystic fibrosis and Renal Disease. *Pediatric Respiratory Review*, Vol. 3, No. 2, (June 2002), pp. (135-138), doi: 10.1016/s1526-0550(02)00012-4.

Stecenko, AA., & Moran, A. (2010). Update on Cystic Fibrosis Related Diabetes. *Current Opinion in Pulmonary Medicine*, Vol.16, (2010), pp. (611-615), doi: 10.1097/MCP.0b013e32833e8700.

Stirati, G., Antonelli, M., Fofi. C., Fierimonte, S., & Pecci, G. (1999). IgA nephropathy in Cystic Fibrosis. *Journal of Nephrology*, Vol. 12, No. 1, (1999), pp. (30-32).

Strausbaugh, SD., & Davis, PB. (2007). Cystic Fibrosis a Review of Epidemiology and Pathobiology. *Clinical Chest Medicine*, Vol. 28, No. 2, (June 2007), pp. (279-288).

Smith, DK., & Alpers, EC. (2005). Pathogenic Mechanisms in Membranoproliferative Glomerulonephritis. *Current Opinion in Nephrology and Hypertension*, Vol. 14, No. 4, (July 2005), pp. (396-403).

Soriano, EP., Fischman, D., & Cheriyath, P. (2008). Membranoproliferative Glomerulonephritis in Patients with Cystic Fibrosis: Coincidence or Connected? A Case Series. *Southern Medical Journal*, Vol. 101, No. 6, (June, 2008).

Sullivan, BP., & Freedman, SD. (2009). Cystic Fibrosis. *Lancet*, Vol. 373, No. 9678, (May, 2009), pp. (1891-1904), doi: 10.1016/s0140-6736(09)60327-5.

Vanden Berg, JM., Morton, AM., Kok, SW., Pijl, H., Conway, SP., & Heijerman, H.G. (2008). Microvascular Complications in Patients with Cystic Fibrosis Renal Disease. *Journal of Cystic Fibrosis*, Vol. 7, May 2008), pp. (515-519), doi: 10.2337/dc06-1576.

Westall, GP., Binder, J., Kotsimbos, T., Topliss, D., Thomson, N., Dowling, J., & Wilson, JW. (2004). Nodular Glomerulosclerosis in Cystic Fibrosis Mimics Diabetic Nephropathy. *Clinical Nephrology*, Vol. 96, No. 3, (2004), pp. (70-75). ISSN: 0028-2766.

Wisnieski, JJ., Todd, EW., Fuller, RK., Jones, PK., Dearborn, DG., Boat, TF., & Naff, GB. (1985). Immune Complexes and Complement Abnormalities in Patients with Cystic Fibrosis. Increased Mortality Associated with Circulating Immune Complexes and Decreased Function of Alternative Complement Pathway. *American Review of Respiratory disorders*, Vol. 132, No. 4, (October, 1985), pp. (770-776).

Yahiaoui, Y., Jablonski, M., Hubert, D., Mosnier-Pudar, H., Noël, LH., Stern, M., Grenet, D., Grünfeld, JP., Chauveau, D., & Fakhouri, F. (2009). Renal Involvement in Cystic Fibrosis. Disease Spectrum and Clinical Relevance *Clinical Journal of American Society of Nephrologists*, Vol. 4, No. 5, (May, 2009), pp. (921-928), ISSN-1555-9041/405-0921.

9

Metabolic Syndrome Associated Kidney Damage

Hequn Zou[1], Yuxin Wang[2], Guimian Zou[3] and Jianxin Wan[4]
[1]Institute of Nephrology and Urology,
The 3rd Affiliated Hospital of Southern Medical University, Guangzhou,
[2]Department of Nephrology, The No. 2 Hospital of Xiamen,
Fu Jian Medical University, Xiamen,
[3]Nephrology Department of Guilin 181 Hospital &
Guangxi Provincial Key Laboratory of Metabolic Disease Research, Guilin,
[4]Department of Nephrology, The No. 1 Hospital of Fu Jian Medical University,Fuzhou
China

1. Introduction

We evaluated the incidences of metabolic syndrome (MS) and its components in the urban residents of southern China, analyzed their relationship to insulin resistance (IR), meanwhile compared the different of MS diagnostic criteria between Chinese Diabetes Society (CDS) and International Diabetes Federation (IDF) in clinic practice in the southern urban residents of China. The total incidence of MS was 8.7% according to the diagnostic criteria of CDS, but up to 19.8% according to the diagnostic criteria of IDF. The total incidences of hypertension, abdominal obesity and diabetes were 22.1%, 39.2% and 6.7%, respectively. The incidence of IR was 5.0% according the value of HOMA-IR. By means of binary logistic regression analysis, impaired fasting glucose, diabetes, obesity, abdominal obesity, elevated triglyceride and high sensitivity C reactive protein were independent risks of insulin resistance, but gender, hypertension, elevated low density lipoprotein and total cholesterol were not independent risks of insulin resistance. It is suggested by the data of our present screening in the residents of southern China that the incidence of MS according to the diagnostic criteria of CDS was lower than that according to the diagnostic criteria of IDF. Some residents with MS main presentation of abdominal obesity would be missed diagnosis by the criteria base on BMI. In the components of MS, hypertension, abdominal obesity and lower high density lipoprotein were more common than others. IR was associated to most of the components of MS and may be one of the main pathogenic factors.

By means of cross-section epidemiological analysis, we investigated the relationship of glycometabolic disorder and IR with chronic kidney diseases (CKD). The prevalence of CKD was 12.6% in the community population, with 11.2% in the youth group, 19.4% in the middle age group and 17.7% in the elder group. And there were a significantly difference between the three age groups (P<0.01). The awareness rates and treatment rates of CKD were very low in all of the three groups. In the whole screened population there was a higher CKD prevalence in IR residents when compared to non-IR residents, 36.9% versus 12.6% (P<0.01). Among population with only impair FBG but not diabetes, CKD prevalence in those residents with IR was higher than those without IR, 33.3% versus 16.0% (P<0.05).

Even among population with normal FBG, CKD prevalence in those residents with IR was higher than whose without IR, 39.1% versus 12.0% (P<0.01). It was observed in different age group that the prevalence of albuminuria and the mean albuminuria level were higher in the residents with IR when compared to the residents without IR. No difference existed between either the prevalence of decreasing eGFR or the mean level of eGFR in residents with IR and without IR in the middle age group and the old group, but not in the youth group in which. The mean level of eGFR was significantly higher in the residents with IR when compared to the residents without IR (P<0.01). It is indicated in our data that CKD is common and the awareness rate and treatment rate are very low in this investigated community population. IR might be associated with the increasing prevalence of CKD, especially with the increased prevalence of microalbuminuria, even in the population with normal FBG. Furthermore IR might also be associated with elevated eGFR in population at the early stage of diabetes but without CKD, while associated with decreased eGFR in those with CKD. It is suggested that IR might be a risk factor of CKD and also a prevention and treatment target of CKD in community residents.

We also explored the incidences of hyperuricemia (HUA) in the urban residents and the related risk factors. The total incidence of HUA was 23.5% in the cohort residents, and was 28.4% in the males and 19.7% in the females (P<0.01). The serum uric acid level was positively related to body weight (or BMI), waist circumference and the age (for females) when controling with serum creatinine (P<0.01). Alcohol consumption and smoke influences significantly on the serum uric acid level, and highest uric acid levels were in the residents frequently drunk and smoked in the past. More common prevalence of HUA was in the patients with chronic kidney disease and hypertension, and the serum uric acid levels were similar in these patients. There was no significant difference of the incidences of HUA between the patients with diabetes and non diabetes. It is suggested by our present investigation that the incidence of HUA is increasing in the residents of inland city of China, and that the change of their lifestyle with lose weight, prevention of obesity, avoid smoke and restriction of alcohol would be the most effective measures to change the high prevalence of HUA.

2. Pathogenesis of metabolic syndrome associated kidney damage

2.1 Insulin resistance and pathogenesis of metabolic syndrome-associated kidney damage
Insulin resistance and metabolic renal damage is closely related. So the metabolic syndrome were screened for kidney damage, assessment is very necessary. Regarding to the pathogenesis of insulin resistance and to improve the treatment based on will also be a metabolic control of renal damage in a new direction for the future.

2.1.1 Insulin resistance leads to kidney damage
The metabolic syndrome (MS) was defined as the presence of 3 or more of the following risk factors: elevated blood pressure, insulin resistance, low high-density lipoprotein cholesterol level, high triglyceride level, elevated glucose level, and abdominal obesity. MS disease risk factors in order to gather more focus is characterized by heart, kidney blood vessels and other target organs. The impact is clear. Now the increasing number of researches show that compared with simple hypertension, metabolic syndrome is more easily lead to kidney damage. Some studies further confirmed that the large vessels and kidney of metabolic syndrome patients damaged obvious. MS can cause kidney damage, and the kidney disease affects MS as well. This shows the relationship between MS and kidney disease is very close.

So people consensus that MS is started for obesity as the common factor. And insulin resistance is the central link of MS. This can be inferred that the relationship between insulin resistance and metabolic renal damage is close.

Insulin resistance refers to the uptake of insulin to promote peripheral tissue, the use of glucose output and inhibit the biological effects of glycogen decreased, with the changes in the compensatory ability of the body showed hyperinsulinemia and (or) high blood sugar status. The kidney damage mechanisms caused by high blood sugar is including that: ① polyol pathway activation; ② protein non-enzymatic glycation (advanced glycation end products formation); ③ activation of protein kinase C. The renal injury is caused by these lesions and GBM thickening. In addition, the recent study found, MS appears hypcrinsulinemia is also often high viremia of amylin, amylin is a high-fiber protein, mainly deposited in the glomerular mesangial area widened, K-W nodules, blood vessel walls and renal interstitial, which become one of the causes of injury about glomerular and interstitial. In vitro experiments showed that amylin may be higher in mesangial cells through induction of apoptosis and increased permeability in endothelial cells kidney damage, but the exact mechanism is still not very clear.[1, 2]

Now that insulin resistance occurs most often in patients with metabolic syndrome, is the central link in the pathogenesis and pathogenic basis. It not only prompts a new-onset diabetes mellitus, cardiovascular events and all-cause mortality in high-risk, but also the renal damage and failure are independent risk factors.[3-6] The primary kidney disease before there is often severely impaired renal function also showed insulin resistance.[4] Therefore, insulin resistance and renal damage can reinforce each other, so to clear the relationship between insulin resistance and metabolic renal damage is useful that in the prevention and treatment of kidney disease is especially prominent role in the process. This article is the review on the causes of pathogenesis why insulin resistance leads to metabolic kidney damage.

2.1.2 Insulin resistance and pathogenesis of metabolic syndrome-associated kidney damage

Insulin resistance is the central link of metabolic syndrome. The U.S. NHANES III data shows that the prevalence of metabolic syndrome has reached 23.7% for the adults who over 20 years 'old.[3] The study showed that In type 2 diabetes, more severe insulin resistance is independently associated with microalbuminuria.[5, 6] Animal experiments confirmed that clinical diabetes mellitus in the event of hyperinsulinemia stage before changes of structure and function in kidney have been.[7] Such early renal damage has its own characteristics and pathogenesis, which are different from diabetic nephropathy. Insulin resistance mechanisms lead to kidney damage mainly in the following areas.

Insulin-like growth factor (IGF) axis is involved in diabetic renal disease

Insulin-like growth factor I (IGF-I) is a potent mitogenic polypeptide under the regulation of growth hormone (GH). Evidence of significant involvement of the GH/IGF system in diabetic nephropathy and other nephropathies has been provided by several studies. Kidney tissue expresses receptors not only for IGF-I but also for GH, which suggests that although most of the biologic effects of GH are mediated by IGF-I, GH may also act independently of IGF-I. IGF-I may have pathogenic roles in diabetic nephropathy and other nephropathies. Serum IGF-I levels are reduced in hyperglycemic diabetic subjects, despite elevated GH levels. This phenomenon has been explained by inhibition of hepatic IGF-I synthesis, resulting from decreases in hepatic GHR expression and binding. The metabolic consequences of these alterations produce a "vicious cycle," wherein the hyperglycemia/insulinopenia induce decreases in serum IGF-I levels, which in turn induce GH hypersecretion, making optimal metabolic control more difficult to achieve.[8] People speculate that the mechanism underlying the renal effects of this GHR antagonist involves renal GHR inhibition of renal IGF-I (and IGFBP-1) protein accumulation. They also speculate that the mechanism underlying the renal effects of this GHR antagonist involves renal GHR inhibition of renal IGF-I (and IGFBP-1) protein accumulation. This study demonstrates that the GH/IGF axis plays a central role in the pathogenesis of early diabetic renal changes, and it suggests specific GHR blockade as a new concept in the treatment of diabetic kidney disease.[9]

Insulin resistance increase renal damage through the rennin-angiotensin system

Angiotensin II (Ang II) and insulin are implicated in the mesangial cell hypertrophy and excessive accumulation of mesangial matrix seen in glomerulosclerosis. Therefore, the effects of Ang II with and without insulin on mRNA levels of several important extracellular matrix genes and transforming growth factor beta-1 (TGF-beta 1) were examined. The results of the studies suggest that insulin, itself, significantly increases TGF-beta 1 and extracellular matrix gene expression in rat mesangial cells. Ang II alone has modest effects, while Ang II and insulin have additive effects. To explain the mechanism of these additive effects, we investigated the action of Ang II on insulin signaling and the effect of insulin on Ang II AT1 receptor mRNA expression. Ang II did not enhance insulin-induced insulin receptor substrate-1 (IRS-1) phosphorylation or phosphatidylinositol 3 (PI-3) kinase activity, but did enhance insulin-induced mitogen activated protein (MAP) kinase activity.[10] Insulin increased message levels of AT1 receptor by twofold. These results suggest that enhancement of MAP kinase activity and AT1 receptor regulation by insulin may contribute to the additive effects of insulin and Ang II in mesangial cells.

The direct impact of insulin resistance on kidney

Insulin major role in the tubules, but the specific sites of action are not yet entirely clear.It has a strong role in preserving sodium and dose dependent, while the presence of insulin to counter, this is still Paul sodium. Therefore, insulin resistance and hyperinsulinemia that occurs when the sodium sensitivity of blood pressure increase in glomerular pressure increased, resulting in microalbuminuria. A study was performed by Vedovato M to measure the effect of Na+ intake on blood pressure and albuminuria, in relation with insulin sensitivity and kidney haemodynamics, in Type 2 diabetic patients with and without microalbuminuria. They found that high salt intake increases blood pressure and albuminuria in Type 2 diabetic patients with microalbuminuria. These responses are associated with insulin resistance and increased glomerular pressure. Insulin resistance could contribute to greater salt sensitivity, increased glomerular pressure and albuminuria.[11]

Insulin resistance increase the renal damage by the plasminogen activator inhibitor 1

The insulin resistance syndrome typically features glucose intolerance and elevated fasting insulin and triglyceride levels. Elevated levels of PAI-1 and tPA antigens associated with glucose intolerance, hyperinsulinemia, and hypertriglyceridemia support inclusion of impaired fibrinolysis as an additional feature of the insulin resistance syndrome. Elevated fibrinolytic factors are also correlated with elevated markers of inflammation and endothelial dysfunction, which has been hypothesized to cause insulin resistance and thereby be the common pathogenic mechanism underlying atherosclerosis, insulin resistance, and glucose intolerance.[12] Hagiwara H's study proved that renal PAI-1 gene expression is up-regulated in both type 1 and type 2 diabetic rats, and changes in gene expressions of fibrinolytic factors may play important roles in the development and pathogenesis of diabetic nephropathy.[13] In addition, TGF-β, angiotensin Π and thrombin could stimulate the synthesis of PAI-1, the process by inhibiting fibrinolysis and plasmin-mediated matrix metalloproteinase activity, so that less matrix degradation, resulting in renal fibrosis.

Insulin resistance increases the rates of renal damage by endothelin (ET) -1

Endothelin-1, released from the vascular endothelium after cleavage from big endothelin-1, is a potent paracrine vasoconstrictor peptide. Small studies suggest that the circulating level of endothelin-1 is elevated in subjects with cardiovascular risk factors. High endothelin-1 level may better reflect endothelin-1 generation. It is indicated by studies that endothelin-1 level is not related to blood pressure, but higher in healthy young men with insulin resistance and obesity.[14] It was discovered in a diabetic mouse model treated with A-type ET receptor antagonist that glomerular TGF-β and collagen I, II, IV production were decreased.

Insulin resistance increase the renal damage through oxidative stress

Insulin-stimulated (or inhibited) pathways retain normal sensitivity to the hormone, hyperinsulinemia could, by its effects on antioxidative enzymes and on free radical generators, enhance oxidative stress. Other effects of insulin involve the inhibition of proteasome and the stimulation of polyunsaturated fatty acid (PUFA) synthesis and of nitric oxide (NO).[15] Prabhakar SS attempted to review the existing literature, discuss the controversies, and reach some general conclusions as to the role of NO production in the diabetic kidney. He found that genetic polymorphisms of the NOS enzyme also may play a role in the NO abnormalities that contribute to the development and progression of diabetic nephropathy.[16]

Insulin resistance increases renal damage through nitric oxide

The results of study performed by Steinberg HO argued that insulin effect on the endothelium is mediated by its own receptor and insulin signaling pathways, resulting in the increased release of nitric oxide. The vascular actions of insulin are impaired in insulin-resistant conditions such as obesity, Type II (non-insulin-dependent) diabetes mellitus and hypertension, which could contribute to the excessive rate of cardiovascular disease in these groups. Insulin-resistant state in obesity and Type II diabetes shows a multitude of metabolic abnormalities that could cause vascular dysfunction. Non-esterified fatty acid level increased long before hyperglycaemia becomes present.[17] Under the circumstance of insulin resistance, endothelial dysfunction leads to vascular complications in the central link, which results in microalbuminuria.

2.2 Hypertension and pathogenesis of metabolic syndrome-associated nephropathy

The abnormality of kidney structure and function caused by hypertension is called hypertensive renal damage. Arteriolar nephrosclerosis is the most characteristic pattern in hypertensive renal damage, including benign arteriolar nephrosclerosis and malignant arteriolar nephrosclerosis. The former caused by benign hypertension, the latter caused by malignant hypertension. Sustained hypertension can cause renal arteriolosclerosis for 5-10 years (tunica intimal thickening of arcuate artery and interlobular arteries, hyaline of afferent artery), wall thickening, lumens narrowing, and secondary ischemic renal parenchyma ischemic lesions, including glomerular ischemic shrinkage, sclerosis, tubular atrophy, interstitial infiltration of inflammatory cells and fibrosis, which lead to benign arteriolar nephrosclerosis. Malignant arteriolar nephrosclerosis is an accelerated hypertension or malignant hypertension-induced renal damage.

2.2.1 Pathogenesis of benign arteriolar nephrosclerosis

Factor of hemodynamics

Due to normal autoregulatory mechanism of renal vessels, renal blood flow (RBF) can be kept relatively stable, which can protect the kidney from blood pressure fluctuation. Renal arteriolar constrictive response occurs in the presence of hypertension, which increase renal vascular resistance and decrease renal blood flow (RBF). The degree of contraction of efferent arteries is more significant than afferent arteries in early stage. Glomerular filtration rate (GFR) can still be maintained within the normal range. With the progress of hypertension, there is renal arteriosclerosis, compliance decreasing, arterial wall thickening, lumens stenosis, and RBF further decline, GFR falling, which lead to ischemic renal lesions. Impairment of kidney tubules secondary to ischemia is more sensitive than glomeruli. Furthermore, renal tubular load does not reduce for maintaining normal GFR, thus more likely to increase renal tubular injury secondary to glomerular hyperperfusion.[18] However, benign arteriolar nephrosclerosis has obvious individual differences. There is not observed renal arteriolar sclerosis in some glomerulosclerosis secondary to hypertension. Hypertensive renal injury is not completely ischemic lesions. In addition to ischemic hypoperfusion nephron, the recent view is that most hypertensive renal damage is characterized by hypertransfusion compensatory nephron. The existence of glomerular hyperperfusion, high pressure and high filtration promote renal parenchyma lesions, especially is the major pathogenesis of glomerulosclerosis.[19].

Under hypertension state, renal vascular sensitivity to Ang II was significantly enhanced. Renal vascular resistance increased in the patients with hypertension who are injected low dose Ang II, and did not significantly change in normal people. The mechanism of proteinuria occurence is currently considered that increased RAS activity lead to podocyte fracture membrane damage and basilar membrane permeability increasing. High intra-glomerular pressure and high shear stress-induced endothelial cell injury and dysfunction, activated local lesions, increased Ang II and aldosterone, induced renal vascular remodeling and renal arteriosclerosis.[20]

Non-hemodynamic factors

In hypertension state, vascular endothelium bear high pressure and shear stress, cause endothelial cell injury, injured endothelial cell can lease cytokines, such as transforming growth factor β (TGF-β), plasminogen activator inhibitor (PAI).[21] Hypertension can directly cause renin-angiotensin-aldosterone system activation and oxidative stress. These factors can cause together kidney damage, matrixfibrosis and tissue hardening.[22, 23]

Clinically nephroangiosclcrosis may occur before significant elevation of blood pressure, such as unilateral nephrectomy or early type 1 diabetes mellitus (TIDM). Glomerular capillary blood flow is still significantly increased. Therefore, the renal capillary pressure overload, it can lead to nephrosclerosis. high pressure and high shear in glomerular cause endothelial cell dysfunction, which could lead to increase in some active factors such as angiotensin II (Ang II), endothelin-1(ET-1), thromboxane A2 (TXA2), TGF-β2 and platelet-derived growth factor (PDGF) factors, leading to vasoconstriction, mesangial cell proliferation and collagen deposition, promoting ECM synthesis and secretion. The high pressure in glomeruli can also lead to glomerular visceral epithelial cell injury, increasing permeability of the basement membrane, causing proteinuria, eventually leading to glomerulosclerosis, nephron loss. Therefore, the patients with essential hypertension have low perfusion of ischemic nephron and high perfusion nephron, the latter is more characteristic pattern.

In addition, reactive oxygen species, salt intake, lithium-sodium counter-transport abnormalities, racial and genetic backgrounds, metabolic disorders, age, gender, body mass index, smoking is also influencing factors.

In summary, hypertensive renal damage is secondary to vascular lesions caused by high arterial pressure. The main mechanism of hypertensive renal damage is hemodynamics abnormalities in glomerular, and cytokines, vasoactive substances and the ECM are involved in the disease process.

2.2.2 Pathogenesis of malignant arteriolar nephrosclerosis

The direct vascular injury of elevated blood pressure

When blood pressure is significant elevated, renal artery and glomerular capillary stress and shear stress can be changed, which induce endothelial cells to secrete varied adhesion molecules, promoting inflammatory cell adhesion to endothelial cells, leading to endothelial cell damage.[24] Vascular endothelial cell damage lead to increased permeability, plasma protein and fibrinogen deposition in the vessel wall, induce vascular fibrinoid necrosis and tunica intimal damage. Finally, it appears vascular lumen narrowed and renal ischemia. But some patients with severe and persistent hypertension, whose vascular injury can not become malignant state. It indicates that in addition to intravascular pressure, there are other factors involved in vascular damage.

Activation of renin-angiotensin-aldosterone system (RAAS) and endothelin

Malignant hypertension often accompanied with activation of RAAS, It should be noted that the activation of RAAS may be primary or secondary. Activation of RAAS can promote intermittent vasoconstriction, activate platelets, release thromboxane and platelet derived growth factor (PDGF), stimulate myointimal cell migration and proliferation, cause vascular lumen narrowed, increased level of blood pressure and renal ischemia. When the systolic pressure is over 180-190mmHg critical level, it can occur naturally natriuretic and diuretic phenomenon, the decline in blood volume can further activate the RAAS.[25] In addition, elevated angiotensin can promote inflammatory cells adhesion to endothelial cell, induce apoptosis of endothelial cells, damage the integrity of blood vessels, induce fibrinoid necrosis of arteriole by "vascular toxicity".[26] Endothelin is of powerful vasoconstrictor function, it can cause sustained elevation of blood pressure. Animal model of malignant hypertension has been confirmed to plasma endothelin and endothelin-mRNA expression in renal tissue increased.[27]

Microvascular coagulation and thrombosis

Hypertension damage vascular endothelial, which active directly coagulation system, lead to platelet aggregation and fibrin deposition in vascular lumen. When red blood cells pass through the damaged vascular lumen, it prone to result in damage and lead to microvascular coagulation. Meanwhile, both platelet aggregation and adhesion of leukocytes on vessel wall lead to turbulence, promoting to form platelet micro-thrombus.[28]

Genetic factors

It is reported that HLAB15, DR3, BW35 and CW4 are significantly associated with the incidence of malignant hypertension.[29, 30]

2.3 Lipid metabolic disorders and pathogenesis of metabolic syndrome-associated nephropathy

Lipid metabolism and kidney disease are closely related. As early as 1982, Moorhead[31] proposed that lipid accumulation can lead to chronic renal injury, it is not only a lot of primary or secondary renal diseases with common clinical manifestations, but also the progress of the diseases.[32] Hyperlipidemia, in addition to proteinuria and hypertension, promotes CKD progression outside the third most important factor. In polycystic kidney disease, obesity, diabetes and hypertension in animal models, hypercholesterolemia were found to accelerate the progress of kidney diseases, and high-fat diet can induce kidney macrophages and foam cell formation leaching, resulting in glomerular sclerosis.[33] In obese Zucker rats, lowering serum triglycerides improves glomerular sclerosis.[34] These results suggest that lipid metabolism is closely related with renal dysfunction, and a series of clinical studies have also been to the same conclusion. Samuelsson et al[35] found triglyceride-rich lipoproteins containing Apo-B in patients with CKD are closely related to the progress of the disease; Muntner et al[36] found in 12 728 subjects with normal renal function that low HDL cholesterol and hypertriglyceridemia in individuals with impaired renal function appeared more dangerous.

2.3.1 Mesangial cell function

Regulation of glomerular filtration of mesangial cells to produce matrix components, involved in the development of many glomerular diseases. Mesangial cell surface LDL, oxidized HDL and very low density lipoprotein act through receptor pathway and the corresponding lipoproteins. LDL can bind to mesangial cells and mesangial cell function can offset.[37] LDL stimulates mesangial cells and had a "phase effect", ie, low concentration of LDL stimulates cell proliferation, and high concentrations inhibits cell proliferation as toxic cells effect. The effect of LDL promoting mesangial cell proliferation may be related to arachidonic acid metabolism. Mesangial cells cytochrome P450 monooxygenase system produces epoxide metabolic pathways, it can promote cell proliferation, LDL oxidation and the formation of more toxic OX-LDL in a dose dependent manner, which can further increase mesangial cell injury. The mesangial cells and macrophages form foam cells and release cytokines and growth factors, such as transforming growth factor β, tumor necrosis factor, platelet derived growth factor and interleukin-1 and so on. These cytokines can stimulate the LDL receptor gene transcription and expression of epithelial cells, mesangial cells and macrophages, and promote the deposition of lipid in kidney cells and induced renal injury.[38] Mesangial cells themselves can be oxidized by LDL. OX-LDL can induce apoptosis of mesangial cells.

2.3.2 Mesangial matrix

Glomerular mesangial matrix includes type IV collagen, fibronectin and laminin. LDL and LDL oxidation in vitro can stimulate the increase of extracellular matrix components. LDL can be activated in mesangial cells by LDL protein kinase C, which promotes transforming growth factor-β synthesis in the cells, and TGF-β can stimulate the cells to produce tissue inhibitor of matrix metalloproteinases, inhibiting matrix degradation and leading to the increase of mesangial matrix.[39] It has been confirmed by in vitro experiments that lipids increased the expression of TGF-β mRNA in mesangial cells and epithelial cells.

2.3.3 Endothelial cells
Endothelial cells with LDL receptor, VLDL receptor and LDL receptor related protein. Lipoprotein receptors and related, or non-receptor pathway, causing cell proliferation, lipoprotein lipase and lipoprotein receptors can enhance and strengthen its effect in promoting cell proliferation. OX-LDL and Lp of endothelial dysfunction caused mainly by interfering with the vasodilators nitric oxide synthesis and direct inactivation; and increased thromboxane A2 and endothelin production, damage vascular endothelial NO dependent relaxation response, cause renal ball efferent arteries, increasing the pressure in the glomerular endothelial cells to further damage, the release of cytokines, to promote cell proliferation, glomerular sclerosis. In addition, the lipoprotein receptor pathway through the endothelial cells directly mediated endothelial cell injury, while activation of coagulation and fibrinolytic system activation and inhibition of platelet function, leading to fibrin deposition and thrombosis, increased glomerular injury.

2.3.4 Glomerular epithelial cells
Glomerular epithelial cell surface LDL, VLDL receptor and lipoprotein receptor related protein, which contains both apoB and apoE, respectively, with the lipoproteins, the annexation of the metabolism of cells. apoE with high affinity receptors, the degree of cellular cholesterol esterification increased, and inhibition of cholesterol synthesis, therefore, glomerular epithelial cellsith more and VLDL, thus not explain the clinical hypercholesterolemia, only lipoprotein formed an exception. Can also cause the deposition of lipids in the glomeruli, glomerulosclerosis occurring phenomenon.

2.3.5 Tubulo-interstitium
Tubular injury showed increased tubulointerstitial matrix proteins and fibrosis. Proximal tubular epithelial cells present LDL, very low density lipoprotein receptor, hyperlipidemia lipid deposition in the renal tubules, tubular epithelial cells by phagocytosis, the formation of foam cells, while LDL, OX-LDL for the expression and FN mRNA secretion, further stimulate tubulointerstitial synthesis, promoting fibrosis.

2.3.6 OX-LDL renal toxicity
OX-LDL can promote renal cell proliferation, apoptosis and phenotypic transformation, involved in the glomerulosclerosis process from cell to cell is too small too many states the state of the process of cell loss.[40] OX-LDL also has the monocyte chemotactic activity of macrophages can express clear the OX-LDL receptor, OX-LDL uptake by macrophages stimulated macrophages after the synthesis of growth factors, cytokines and other related matrix protein synthesis in the media. Extraordinary receptor exists in glomerular mesangial cells and epithelial cells. In the case of lipid metabolism, the oxidation of LDL can be modified first intake, OX-LDL accumulation in the kidney and stimulate the kidney cells to secrete TGF-β1 and other cytokines to promote renal fibrosis, leading to monocyte-

macrophage in the local infiltration. Moreover, the activation of macrophages and can promote LDL oxidation, secretion of TGF-β and PDGF-AD, caused by extracellular matrix and mesangial expansion, creating a vicious cycle.[41] Focal segmental glomerulosclerosis in animal models and human glomerular diseases, a number of chronic renal biopsy tissues were detected by OX-LDL deposition, and the extent of OX-LDL deposition and renal dysfunction and protein was positively correlated with urine.

2.4 Hyperuricemia and pathogenesis of metabolic syndrome-associated nephropathy

Hyperuricemia is highly prevalent in MS patients. A few studies showed that hyperuricemia was associated closely with progression of kidney disease.[42] About 20% to 60% of patients with gout have mild or moderate renal failure. The histological lesion named "gouty nephropathy" includes glomerulosclerosis, interstitial fibrosis, and renal arteriolosclerosis, often with focal interstitial urate crystal deposition.

The precipitation of uric acid in the renal medulla with formation of characteristic tophi was believed to activate an inflammatory response resulting in renal interstitial fibrosis, a loss of nephrons, and ultimately to irreversible chronic renal failure. When pH<5.5 in vivo or dehydration, urate can deposit in the renal tubules and interstitium which cause urate nephropathy. It also can form kidney stone in distal tubule and collecting duct and induce obstruction. Emmerson[43] found that some interstitial deposits of urate and uric acid in the kidney derived from intra-tubular deposits which react with the tubular epithelium and pass into the interstitium; loss of tubular integrity may not be a prerequisite for crystal migration. Toblli[44] confirmed that urate crystals deposit in renal tubular cells, evoke complement, platelet, inflammatory cell and macrophages by classical pathway or alternative pathway, induce the expression of cytokine and transforming growth factor beta increased; stimulate fibroblast to be fibrocyte, activate cross linkage of collagen and ultimately lead to renal fibrosis or renal failure.

However, it is difficult to ascribe the generalized renal damage in gout to the deposition of urate crystals, for they are often only focally present.

Recent studies have reported that mild hyperuricemia in normal rats induced by the uricase inhibitor, oxonic acid (OA), results in systemic hypertension, renal vasoconstriction, glomerular hypertension and hypertrophy, and tubulointerstitial injury independent of intra-renal crystal formation.[45-47] It has also been found that hyperuricemia can accelerate renal disease in the remnant kidney model and accelerate experimental cyclosporine nephropathy.[48,49] The main pathophysiological mechanism by which uric acid causes these conditions involves the inhibition of endothelial nitric oxide bioavailability and direct actions on endothelial cells and vascular smooth muscle cells.[50,51] The importance of these pathways is suggested by a recent prospective study in which lowering uric acid in individuals with hyperuricemia and renal dysfunction was associated with improved BP control and slower progression of renal disease.[52]

There are a lot of clinical evidences that hyperuricemia may induce endothelial dysfunction, as lowering uric acid with allopurinol can improve endothelial function as measured by brachial artery vasodilatation.[53] Interestingly, while both uric acid and nitric oxide (NO) exhibit circadian variation, serum uric acid peaks around 6 a.m. when the level of NO is lowest.[54] This relationship can be accounted for by the finding that uric acid also inhibits endothelial cell dependent vasodilatation of rat aortic rings[55] and NO production in endothelial cells.[56] Furthermore, uric acid blunts endothelial cell proliferation in response to serum. [56] The mechanism by which uric acid inhibits NO levels is complex. It may involve scavenging by

oxidants, which can be induced by NADPH oxidase under hyperuricemia.[57] A reduced NO bioavailability could also be due in part to inhibition secondary to CRP production.[56]
In addition, the activation of RAS plays an important role in the exacerbation of renal injury caused by uric acid, which has been shown to be an important mediator of progression of renal disease, not only by its hemodynamic effects to increase systemic and glomerular pressure, but also by its direct fibrogenic effect in kidney and vessels. The increase of renin expression is observed in hyperuricemic rats. The relationship between serum uric acid and plasma renin activity has been described in humans.[58] Blocking the renin angiotensin system can ameliorate hypertension and renal injury in hyperuricemic rats.[45] Furthermore, studies in humans suggest that uric acid acts on blood pressure and renal injury in part via the renin angiotensin system.[59] All of above discoveries suggest that the roles of uric acid may also be mediated by the activation of the renin angiotensin system.
Hyperuricemia also alters glomerular hemodynamics.[47] Hyperuricemia induces cortical renal vasoconstriction in rats as evidenced by a significant increase of afferent and efferent arteriolar resistances. A decrease in glomerular plasma flow and the ultrafiltration coefficient resulted in a 35% decrease in single nephron GFR whereas glomerular pressure was increased. These changes were restored by allopurinol treatment. Aberrant renal autoregulation appears to be responsible for the glomerular hypertension observed with experimental hyperuricemia. Under normal conditions, an increase in mean systemic arterial pressure causes a reflex vasoconstriction of the afferent arteriole, thus preventing the transmission of the increased pressure to the glomerular circulation. However, in the event that the afferent arteriolar vasoconstriction is insufficient, the transmission of increased pressure to the glomeruli results in glomerular hypertension.[47] While renal vasoconstriction occurs in experimental hyperuricemia, it may be insufficient for the degree of systemic hypertension, therefore glomerular pressures are increased. This may be due to the disease of the afferent arteriole that occurs in the hyperuricemic rats, as evidenced by an increase in the media to lumen ratio. Again, the observation that allopurinol was able to prevent arteriolar hypertrophy leading to a normal renal autoregulatory response indicates a potential role of uric acid on this process.[47]

2.5 Obesity and pathogenesis of metabolic syndrome-associated nephropathy
The metabolic syndrome is a cluster of the most dangerous heart attack risk factors: diabetes and prediabetes, abdominal obesity, high cholesterol and high blood pressure.[60] Abdominal obesity is the form of obesity most strongly associated with metabolic syndrome. Obesity and metabolic syndrome has been found to be independent risk factors for CKD.[3, 61, 62] Treating obesity might stabilize renal function or reverse early hemodynamic abnormalities and glomerular dysfunction.[63, 64] Since the first description of an association between massive obesity and nephrotic proteinuria in 1974, a specific histopathologic pattern characterized by glomerulomegaly, in many cases accompanied by focal segmental glomerulosclerosis, has been described repeatedly in obese patients without any other defined primary or secondary glomerular diseases (including diabetic nephropathy, hypertensive nephrosclerosis, and secondary focal segmental glomerulosclerosis) and now is referred to as "obesity-related glomerulopathy".[65, 66] Overweight, obesity, and the metabolic syndrome have recently emerged as strong independent risk factors for chronic kidney disease (CKD) and ESRD. The multivariate analysis made by Chen et al[3] showed that the risk for being affected by CKD was more than twice as high in patients with an increased waist circumference than in those without, suggesting that obesity may be an independent risk factor for CKD.

Obesity with the features of the metabolic syndrome causes renal dysfunction,[67] increase glomerular filtration rate (GFR), renal blood flow (RBF), and filtration fraction (FF) in experimental and clinical observations.[64, 68, 69] Obesity also increases the risk factor for diabetes and hypertension. Iseki[70] indicate that obesity, including metabolic syndrome, is a potential treatable cause of CKD and ESRD. In a large cohort of >320,000 patients who were followed at Kaiser Permanente, Hsu et al[62, 71] found that a higher BMI was a strong independent risk factor for ESRD even after adjustment for other major risk factors that are associated with ESRD, including smoking, baseline hypertension, and diabetes.

Hyperlipidemia, hyperinsulinemia, hyperleptinemia, hyperuricemia and hypercoagulability, together in obese patients may directly or indirectly affect renal structure and function, caused kidney damage.

The pathogenesis of ORG may be implicated:

1. Renal hemodynamic alterations: Studies in animals and in humans have shown that obesity is associated with elevated GFR and increased renal blood flow.[68, 71] This likely occurs because of afferent arteriolar dilation as a result of proximal salt reabsorption, coupled with efferent renal arteriolar vasoconstriction as a result of elevated Ang II. In addition, Ang II may have a role in the regulation of adipokine production in adipose tissue and may increase insulin resistance in the setting of obesity.[72, 73]

2. Sympathetic stimulation: Obesity-related there is widespread increased sympathetic nerve activity, its causes and obese patients with baroreceptor dysfunction and vasomotor centers less on the incoming inhibitory signals.[74]

3. Leptin: Wolf[75] studies have shown that Leptin levels in obese patients was significantly higher, it was upregulated in glomerular endothelial cells and mesangial cells. Increased TGF-β1 and its receptor mRNA expression promote glomerular endothelial cells and mesangial cell proliferation.

4. Inflammation: The results of several studies have suggested that adipose tissue, especially visceral adipose tissue, is a major source of cytokine secretion in the metabolic syndrome, and that inflammatory cells, especially mature bone marrow–derived macrophages, invade adipose tissue early in obesity.[76, 77] Inflammation was linked to obesity and the metabolic syndrome in patients with CKD. Ramkumar et al[78] found a strong association between inflammation as defined by a CRP level >3 mg/dl and a high BMI in patients with CKD.

5. Changes in fatty acid composition in kidney, causing kidney reduced the release of vasoactive substances, increased the pressure of glomerular capillary. Hall et al[79] show that the mechanisms responsible for increased sodium reabsorption and altered pressure natriuresis in obesity include activation of the renin-angiotension and sympathetic nervous systems, and physical compression of the kidneys due to accumulation of intra-renal fat and extracellular matrix.

2.6 Diabetes and pathogenesis of metabolic syndrome-associated nephropathy

Diabetic nephropathy is the most important long-term complication of diabetes mellitus and a major cause of end-stage renal disease. The condition is associated with excess cardiovascular morbidity and mortality, as well as other diabetic microvascular complications.[80] The etiopathogenesis of diabetic nephropathy appears to involve both genetic and environmental factors leading to disease in a subgroup of patients. Improved knowledge of the natural history and pathophysiology of the condition have enabled therapeutic strategies to be employed that have improved the outlook for patients with nephropathy.[81]

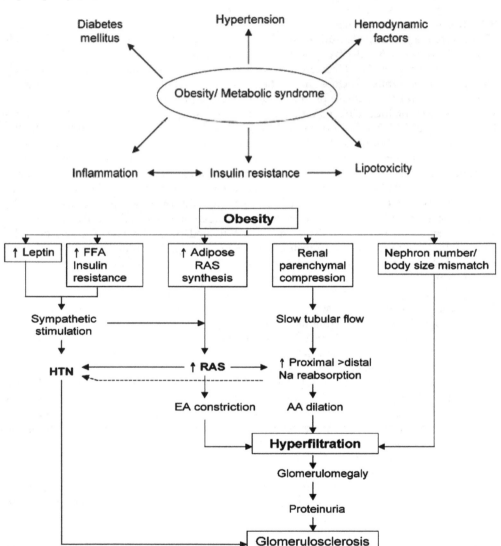

2.6.1 Historical background

DN has the characteristic of obvious family accumulation, but the incidence of the disease in different races is very different. Diabetic nephropathy is a serious problem resulted from microvascular complications of diabetes mellitus. Thus, genetic factors determining susceptibility plays an important role in DN, which was shown by studies about angiotensinogen (AGT) gene, angiotensin converting enzyme (ACE) gene, aloes reeducates (AR) gene, Glut21 gene, endothelial cells Nitric oxide synthase (eNOS) gene, cell receptor β-chain of fixed area (TCRβ) genes. Correlation between gene polymorphism and the occurrence and development of DN has also been discovered.[82]

2.6.2 Chronic hyperglycemia

Hyperglycemia can activate intracellular key catalytic glucose into sorbitol AR. With high glucose increased AR activity, polyol metabolism in kidney is active, so that excessive accumulation of sorbitol and fructose. Sorbitol polarity is strong, thus can not freely through the membrane, while fructose has little further metabolism. It results in fructose accumulation and the increase of intracellular osmotic pressure and therefore cell edema. While the level of intracellular inositol is decreased, glutathione, NADH / NAD + ratio increased, Na2K2ATP activity decreased, which results in tissue hypoxia and endothelial cell damage, contributing to the occurrence and development of DN.[83] Some studies suggest that AR gene polymorphism is related to AR mRNA levels in peripheral blood mononuclear cells and diabetic micro-vascular complications. High glucose can lead to non-enzymatic glycosylation reaction, formation of advanced glycation end products (AGEs) in many organs. AGEs bind the AGE receptor (RAGE) of vascular endothelial cells, macrophages, vascular smooth muscle cells, mesangial cells and other cells. RAGE, as a signal transduction receptor, activates mitogen-activated protein kinase pathway (MAPK) and nuclear factor (NF) -κB signaling pathway (cell proliferation and inflammatory response), Ras pathway (stress and apoptosis), Rac/Cdc-42 pathway (cell growth and movement), Jak / Stat pathway (regulation of gene expression), raising the expression of a variety of growth factors, such as platelet derived growth factor and transforming growth factor, basic fibroblast growth factor, and adhesion molecules, such as intercellular adhesion molecules-1 and vascular cell adhesion molecule.[84]

Reactive oxygen species (ROS), including superoxide radicals, hydrogen peroxide, hydroxyl radicals, and lipid peroxidation, are of in vivo biological activity of inducing aerobic metabolism. Studies demonstrated that increased oxidative stress existed in diabetes. High glucose increased the generation of ROS by inhibiting the activity of the three glycerol phosphate dehydrogenase, leading to the development of microvascular complications mediated by diabetes-related signaling pathways, such as PKC pathway, polyol pathway, hexosamine pathway and AGEs formation. High glucose can also increase the the gene transcription of adhesion molecules and inflammatory NF-κB. Increased levels of ROS can also increase peroxynitrite synthesis and nitrotyrosine formation, leading to DNA damage, prompting the development of diabetic microvascular complications.[85]

PKC activation in diabetes is a common pathway of vascular injury. PKC family, has more than ten isozymes and plays, mainly PKC-β, a role in vascular injury in diabetes. PKC can be activated through a variety of ways. Hyperglycemia within the tissue cells can increase PKC activation, increase NADH / NAD + ratio, increase oxidative stress.[86] PKC inhibited endothelial nitric oxide synthase (eNOS) activity, decreasing NO level and NO-mediated inhibition of cyclic guanosine monophosphate (cGMP) generation, leading to vasomotor dysfunction.[87] PKC stimulated platelet aggregation and increased the content and activity of PAI-1, promoting the hypercoagulability of patients with diabetes. PKC promoted vascular endothelial growth factor (VEGF) expression, promoting angiogenesis, increasing vascular permeability.[88] PKC regulated the expression of transforming growth factor (TGF)-β and increased the expression of fibronectin and collagen type IV, leading to extracellular matrix expansion. Researches had shown that TGF-β promoted local extracellular matrix deposition.

2.6.3 Microvascular disorders

Homodynamic changes in early diabetic micro-vascular disorders characterized by increased pressure, is generally reversible. High glucose increased the plasma osmolality, increasing blood volume and renal blood flow. Diabetes changed the ratio between the resistance of glomerular arterioles, resulting in glomerular capillary hyperperfusion and high pressure, the mesangial matrix expansion and basement membrane thickening, and therefore leading to focal glomerular sclerosis.[89] Meanwhile, the capillary endothelial cell was damaged, the normal filtration barrier was damaged, protein filtration was increased, which result in the loss of glomerular function.

Microvascular disorders in DN is the pathological basis of clinical manifestations, the most prominent is the basement membrane thickening and the damage of glomerular filtration barrier function. The pathogenesis includes continuing glomerular hyperperfusion and hyperfiltration, increased collagen synthesis. Sustained high glucose leads to the non-enzymatic glycation of basement membrane protein components. Another major pathological feature of DN is increased mesangial matrix. Mesangial expansion is mainly resulted from the following factors: glomerular hemodynamic abnormalities, increased capillary pressure. High filtration can stimulate the increase of mesangial matrix, the damage of glomerular filtration barrier. The leakage and accumulation of macromolecules in the membrane system stimulate mesangial cell proliferation and promote matrix production. High blood glucose activates protein kinase C in mesangial cell and the increase in mesangial matrix protein synthesis. Cellular growth factors are the important factors playing roles in increasing mesangial matrix. The most important of which is TGF-β. High blood glucose, glomerular capillary pressure and angiotensin (Ang) - II can promote the synthesis of extracellular matrix of mesangial and tubular epithelial cell. In addition endothelin (ET) also stimulate the proliferation of mesangial cells and the secretion of matrix. NO had inhibitory effect on mesangial cells. NO level is increased in early stage of diabetic nephropathy, which results in glomerular hyperperfusion and hyperfiltration. And it is reduced in the late stage due to endothelial cell damage, which leds to the increasing of mesangial matrix, playing a role in accelerating glomerular injury.[90]

In diabetes, blood flow slows down and micro-thrombosis is easy to form, mainly due to abnormal endothelial cell and platelet function. The increase in serum of von Willebrand factor (vWF) is considered a sign of vascular endothelial cell injury. vWF is synthesized by endothelial cells, mediates platelet adhesion to endothelium, promote thrombosis. Overseas studies suggest that vWF is an independent risk factor for microvascular disease in diabetes.[91] In addition endothelial dysfunction is also reflected by the decreased activity of tissue plasminogen activator (t-PA) or the incresed activity of plasminogen activator inhibitor (PAI) which result in decreased fibrinolytic activity. Decreased prostacyclin-2 (PGI-2) synthesis reduced platelet inhibition. Increased release of ET can promote platelet aggregation. Plasma β platelet globulin (β-TG) and platelet factor 4 (PF4) levels reflect platelet activation. Increased thromboxane (TXA) -2 synthesis promote platelet aggregation and thrombosis. Many studies shown that increased platelet aggregation plays a very important role in the development of microangiopathy in type-2 diabetes mellitus, in addition to long-term hyperglycaemia.

2.7 Metabolic syndrome in pathogenesis of allograft renal damage

The metabolic syndrome (MS) is a cluster of interrelated common clinical entities, which include obesity, insulin resistance, glucose intolerance, hypertension and dyslipidaemia. Insulin resistance is their common pathophysiological basis. Metabolic syndrome significantly increases the risk for cardiovascular disease and chronic kidney disease.[92] Recently it has been found that MS is also common in renal transplant recipients. How is kidney transplantation complicated with metabolic syndrome?

2.7.1 Immunosuppressive therapies

Immunosuppressive therapies induce post-transplantation diabetes

Post-transplantation diabetes is believed to be multi-factorial, probably involving β-cell toxicity and increased insulin resistance. In addition to other risk factors, studies suggest that immunosuppressive regimens may account for a large degree of the increased risk for the development of post-transplantation diabetes.

Corticosteroids and Calmodulin inhibitors (cyclosporine and tacrolimus) are widely used in kidney transplant recipients. They have long been recognized to potently affect glucose tolerance by a prevalent increase of peripheral insulin resistance.

Increasing daily prednisolone dose was independently associated with insulin resistance as glucocorticoids promote gluconeogenesis in the liver, inhibit glucose uptake, diminish glycogen synthesis in skeletal muscle cells and also may attenuate insulin secretion from pancreatic beta-cells. Several mechanisms displayed in vitro studies on murine β-cell or human cell lines incubated with dexamethasone, have been proposed: insulin secretion inhibition by increased expression of a2-adrenergic receptors, decreased cAMP levels, decreased Glut2 protein at the β-cell plasma membrane, down regulation of glucokinase mRNA, increased voltage-gated K+channel activity, β-cell apoptosis through the activation of the calcineurin phosphatase and the corticosteroid receptor.[93-96]

Calcineurin inhibitors, tacrolimus and cyclosporine cause reversible toxicity to islet cells and may directly affect the transcriptional regulation of insulin expression. Furthermore, both calcineurin inhibitors impair insulin gene transcription regulation through the inhibition of calcineurin signalisation. Other mechanisms have been proposed: closing of the ATP-sensitive potassium channel, interference with mitochondrial function of pancreatic β-cell, impairment of glucose-stimulated insulin secretion downstream of the rise in intracellular Ca2+ at insulin exocytosis, reduced ATP production and glycolysis derived from reduced glucokinase activity, decreased islet cell viability by a down regulation of anti-apoptotic factors and accumulation of pro-apoptotic mediators in cultures of freshly isolated human islets. Tacrolimus is more diabetogenic than cyclosporine.[97-99] At the first, it can be due to the steroid mimetic effect of tacrolimus. Tacrolimus binds to FK506-binding protein (FKBP), predominantly FKBP-12. Another immunophilin, FKBP-52 is associated with the cytoplasmic glucocorticoid (GC) receptor complex. When cells are exposed to glucocorticoids, the steroid binds to the GC receptor and liberates it from the complex. By binding to FKBP-52 in the GC receptor complex, tacrolimus may alter the affinity of interactions and either cause a release of the GC receptor at lower steroid concentrations, a steroid-sparing effect, or it may free the GC receptor I absence of steroids . Second, tacrolimus increases the bioavailability of steroids.

Immunosuppressive therapies induce obesity

Prednisone can induce overweight or obesity in transplant recipients, espically abdominal obesity, the abdominal fat which is sensitive to catecholamine can induce insulin resistance through elevating the level of low density lipoprotein and very low density lipoprotein, inhibiting the activity of phosphofructokinase, blocking glycolysis and glucose uptake.

2.7.2 Virus infection

Cytomegalovirus is one of the most important pathogenic microorganism after renal transplantation, Cytomegalovirus infection can infect insulin secretion, induce insulin resistance and impair the function of pancreatic β-cell, and it is independent infector of post-transplant diabetes mellitus (PTDM).[100] Cytomegalovirus infection increases the activity of tumor necrosis factor(TNF), TNF can affect the function of islet B cell and decrease the organism's sensitivity to insulin, that will promote insulin resistance in renal transplant recipients.

Patients with HCV infection were found to have a 8.3-fold higher risk of appearing PTDM compared with HCV(-) patient.[101] Patients with HCV disease have increased peripheral insulin resistance and are hyperinsulinemic, similar to those with type 2 DM. It also is postulated that patients with HCV have decreased β-cell responsiveness, possibly caused by direct viral effects. Other explanations include an autoimmune pathogenesis because HCV has been associated with several autoimmune diseases, including cryoglobulinemia, Hashimoto's thyroiditis, and Sjogren's syndrome. This would suggest antibody-mediated destruction of pancreatic β-cells. A potential role of viruses in the cause of type 1 DM has been suggested, as well as a role for enteroviruses. A greater prevalence of PTDM in patients with HCV therefore likely is caused by a combination of increased peripheral insulin resistance and either a direct viral- or immune-mediated effect of HCV on pancreatic β-cells that results in relative insulin deficiency.

2.7.3 Polycystic kidney disease

Insulin resistance with compensatory hyperinsulinaemia has been reported in adult polycystic kidney disease patients. It is reported that post-transplant diabetes mellitus (PTDM) occured in 10 adult polycystic kidney disease (APKD) patients and four controls (34.6% vs 15.3%; P<0.005).[102] It has been shown that increased membrane fluidity and abnormal erythrocyte Na/Li counter-transport, both abnormalities associated with insulin resistance, are present in APKD patient.[103, 104]

3. Diagnosis

Till now there is no formal denomination of metabolic syndrome associated kidney diseases which are often diagnosed as obesity-associated glomerulonephropathy, diabetic nephropathy, hypertension-associated kidney damage, lipid disorder associated kidney damage and hyperuricemia-associated kidney damage.

The diagnosis of metabolic syndrome associated renal disease is generally two levels criterion (Table 3-1). The first level is for large sample epidemiological screening, which is base on the diagnosis of MS and CKD, and often including MS complicated with CKD or CKD complicated with MS. The second is for clinical evaluation and treatment, which base on the diagnosis of MS and the clinical presentation and renal pathology of obesity-associated glomerulonephropathy, diabetic nephropathy, hypertension related renal damage lipid disorder associated kidney damage and hyperuricemia-associated kidney damage. Renal biopsy might be necessary for the investigation and clinical diagnosis of metabolic syndrome associated kidney diseases under some circumstances, and the pathological evaluation should be made with not only light microscope, but also immunofluorescence and electron microscope. The definite diagnosis of metabolic syndrome associated kidney diseases should exclude other primary or secondary kidney diseases. In clinical practice, metabolic syndrome associated kidney diseases are often accompanied with other primary or secondary kidney diseases. Post-transplant metabolic syndrome associated kidney diseases are often complicated with acute or chronic rejection in renal allograft.

Level 1 Metabolic syndrome complicated with chronic kidney disease
1. Consistent with the diagnosis criterion of metabolic syndrome (necessary).
2. Consistent with the chronic kidney disease (necessary).
Level 2 Metabolic syndrome associated kidney disease
1. Consistent with the diagnosis criterion of metabolic syndrome (necessary).
2. One of the following diagnosis criterions.
i. The obesity patient with the renal pathological character of obesity- associated glomerulonephropathy.
ii. The diabetes patient with the renal pathological character of diabetic nephropathy.
iii. The hypertension patient with the renal pathological character of hypertension related renal damage.
iv. The patients with hyperuricemian and the renal pathological character of uric acid nephropathy

Table 3.1. The diagnosis of metabolic syndrome associated renal disease: two levels of criterion

3.1 Diagnosis of MS

A diagnosis of metabolic syndrome associated kidney diseases must be based on the diagnosis of metabolic syndrome which is not only composed of central obesity, diabetes or prediabetes, hypertension, lipid metabolic disorder, etc., but also insulin resistance as its critical pathophysiological basis. the American Heart Association (AHA) along with the National Heart, Lung and Blood Institute issued an up-to-date version on the diagnosis of the metabolic syndrome.[105] The International Diabetes Federation (IDF) also provided a working definition for the syndrome (Table 3-2).[106]

Clinical diagnosis criteria	**Categorical cut points**
Insulin resistance	None
Body weight	Increased WC (population specific) plus any 2 of the following
Lipid	TG ≥150 mg/dL (1.7 mmol/L)or on TG Rx HDL-C <40 mg/dL (1.03 mmol/L)in men or <50 mg/dL (1.3 mmol/L) in women or on HDL-C Rx
Blood pressure	≥130 mm Hg systolic or ≥85 mm Hg diastolic or on hypertension Rx
Glucose	≥100 mg/dL(5.6 mmol/L), includes diabetes

Table 3.2. Criteria for Clinical Diagnosis of Metabolic Syndrome (IDF, 2005)

The present AHA/NHLBI statement, in contrast to IDF, maintains the ATP III criteria except for minor modifications (Table 3-3).

Measure (any 3 of 5 constitute diagnosis of metabolic syndrome)	Categorical cut points
Elevated waist circumference	≥102 cm (≥40 inches) in men, ≥88 cm (≥35 inches) in women
Elevated triglycerides	≥150 mg/dL (1.7 mmol/L) Or On drug treatment for elevated triglycerides
Reduced HDL-C	<40 mg/dL (1.03 mmol/L) in men<50 mg/dL (1.3 mmol/L) in women Or On drug treatment for reduced HDL-C
Elevated blood pressure	≥130 mm Hg systolic blood pressure, Or ≥85 mm Hg diastolic blood pressure Or On antihypertensive drug treatment in a patient with a history of hypertension
Elevated fasting glucose	≥100 mg/dL (5.6 mmol/L) or On drug treatment for elevated glucose

Table 3.3. Criteria for Clinical Diagnosis of Metabolic Syndrome (AHA/NHLBI)

It is suggested by the data of our recent community-based screening that the incidence of MS according to the diagnostic criteria of CDS was lower than that according to the diagnostic criteria of IDF. Some residents with MS mainly presentation of abdominal obesity would be missed diagnosis by the criteria base on BMI. In the components of MS, hypertension, abdominal obesity and lower high density lipoprotein were more common than others.

3.2 Diagnosis of CKD

The early evidences of metabolic syndrome associated kidney diseases might exist before the occurrence of clinical diabetes or hypertension, and it should include elevated or decreased GFR, microalbuminuria or even smaller proteins occurring in the urine before microalbuminuria, the presentation of renal pathological disorders existing before the clinical manifestation.

According the K/DOQI definition and classification, CKD is defined as kidney damage or glomerular filtration rate (GFR) <60 mL/min/1.73 m^2 for 3 months or more, irrespective of cause. Kidney damage in many kidney diseases can be ascertained by the presence of albuminuria, defined as albumin-to-creatinine ratio >30 mg/g in two of three spot urine specimens. GFR can be estimated from calibrated serum creatinine and estimating equations.[107]

There are many methods to determine GFR have been used, such as measuring GFR using exogenous markers, or endogenous markers, using exogenous marker is extremely inconvenience and is not used in clinical and epidemic practice. The often used endogenous markers are serum creatinine (SCr), usually calculated as creatinine clearance (CCr), and serum cystatin C. Most studies have shown that serum cystatin C levels correlate better with GFR than does serum creatinine alone, especially at higher levels of GFR. In practice, combining use of multiple indexes, such as SCr, age gender and race to evaluate GFR will be more accurate. So there many equations have been used to estimate GFR. The two most commonly used equations to estimate GFR are serum creatinine based: Cockcroft-Gault (CG) and the Modification of Diet in Renal Disease (MDRD) equations. A recent study involving a pooled analysis of individuals with chronic kidney disease proposed an

estimation equation that included serum cystatin C in addition to serum creatinine, age, sex, and race. Studies concluded this equation provided the most accurate estimates.
The CG equation is as follows:

$$CCr(ml/min) = \{[140 - Age(yr)] \times Weight(kg)\}/SCr(mg/dl) \times 72 \times (0.85, \text{ if female})$$

The six variable MDRD equation is as follows:

$$GFR = 170 \times (SCr)^{-0.999} \times (Age)^{-0.176} \times 0.762(\text{if female}) \times 1.18(\text{if black}) \times (BUN)^{-0.170} \times (Alb)^{0.318}$$

where BUN is blood urea nitrogen and Alb is albumin.
The abbreviated version or four variable version of the MDRD equation (ml/min per 1.73 m2) is as follows:

$$GFR = 186 \times (SCr)^{-1.154} \times (Age)^{-0.203} \times 0.742(\text{if female}) \times 1.212(\text{if black})$$

The equation base on SCr and serum CysC is as follow:

$$eGFR = 177.6 \times (SCr)^{-0.65} \times (CysC)^{-0.57} \times (Age)^{-0.20} \times 0.82(\text{if female}) \times 1.11 \text{ (if black)}$$

3.3 Renal pathological changes in metabolic syndrome

There is a small sample retrospective design.[108] The histopathologic presentation of patients with metabolic syndrome compared with controls had a greater prevalence of tubular atrophy, interstitial fibrosis, and arterial sclerosis, suggesting microvascular disease. Patients with metabolic syndrome had greater global and segmental glomerulosclerosis. Glomerular volume and cross-sectional surface area were not different. The combined end point of tubular atrophy greater than 5%, interstitial fibrosis greater than 5%, and presence of arterial sclerosis was more prevalent in patients with metabolic syndrome than controls.

4. Prevention and treatment

Aggressive multitargeted management of the metabolic syndrome can also improve cardio vascular and renal outcomes and is highly recommended by the American Heart Association. Although no study has evaluated whether multiple interventions can reduce the incidence or progression of CKD in patients with the metabolic syndrome.[109]

4.1 Lifestyle changes

Lifestyle interventions are the first line therapies recommended for treatment of the metabolic syndrome. The essential and important measurements include weight reduction, regular exercise, and a low-calorie, low-fat diet. Yet few data are available to indicate that such lifestyle interventions can prevent or reverse renal damage.[109]

4.2 Medication treatment

If lifestyle change is not sufficient, then drug therapies for abnormalities in the individual risk factors may be indicated. Such as medicine for treatment of diabetes, hypertension, lipid disorder and hyperuricemia.

4.2.1 Treatment of elevated blood glucose

In metabolic syndrome patients with IFG (or IGT if assessed), weight reduction, increased physical activity, or both will delay (or prevent) the onset of type 2 diabetes mellitus.

Intensive glucose control to lower the glycated hemoglobin value to 6.5% yielded a 10% relative reduction in the combined outcome of major macrovascular and microvascular events, primarily as a consequence of a 21% relative reduction in nephropathy.

Oral Antihyperglycemic Agents:[110] Metformin, thiazolidinediones and acarbose will lower risk for type 2 diabetes mellitus in people with IFG or IGT. The nonsulfonylurea insulin secretagogues repaglinide and nateglinide can be used in renal failure without dose adjustments. Metformin is contraindicated in renal failure because of the associated risk for lactic acidosis. It can be used at low dosages up to a creatinine clearance of 30 to 60 ml/min and should be avoided with clearances<30 ml/min. Although the metabolism of thiazolidinediones is unaffected by renal failure, they must be used with caution in this context because of their volume retaining effect with a risk for heart failure. The sulfonylureas (glyburide, gliclazide, glipizide, glibenclamide, tolbutamide, and chlorpropamide) have increased potency to prolong sulfonylurea induced hypoglycemia as the renal function decreases and are contraindicated in severe renal failure. α-Glucosidase inhibitors (acarbose and miglitol) are also contraindicated in renal failure.

Insulin therapy: Insulin therapy maybe benefits in glycaemic control, but not improves insulin resistance and metabolic syndrome. Insulin analogues, whose main objective is to stimulate physiologic insulin secretion, has opened new therapeutic possibilities in diabetic CRF patients.[111] Although only a few studies have evaluated the clinical efficacy and safety profile of insulin analogues in CRF patients, preliminary results appear hopeful. There is another concern of insulin injection for long term might be unfavourable, as ectogenous insulin may inhibit endogenous insulin secretion and results in the lack of the co-secretion of other beneficial substances such as C-peptide which is just now known to be potential in the treatment of diabetic nephropathy.[112]

4.2.2 Treatment of elevated blood pressure

In the presence of diabetes or chronic kidney disease, the blood pressure goal is <130/80 mm Hg. Mild elevations of blood pressure often can be effectively controlled with lifestyle therapies. Some investigators support angiotensin-converting enzyme (ACE) inhibitors as first-line therapy for hypertension in the metabolic syndrome, especially when either type 2 diabetes mellitus or chronic renal disease is present. ARBs may be used in those who cannot tolerate ACE inhibitors or as an alternative to ACE inhibitors.

4.2.3 Treatment of dyslipidemia

According to ATP III, as long as LDL-C remains above goal level, LDL-C is the primary target of therapy even in the metabolic syndrome. Other lipid risk factors are secondary. The LDL-C goals depend on estimates of absolute risk.

The main effects of Statin therapy are reduction of LDL-cholesterol, triglyceride and systemic inflammation, possible improvement of endothelial function and inhibition of renal endothelin 1-mediated proteinuria. The goal level of LDL-cholesterol: <1.80 mmol/l in very high-risk patients and <2.60 mmol/l in high-risk patients.[109]

Fibrates and nicotinic acid are the most commonly used drugs for elevated TG and reduced HDL-C. The main effects of fibrates therapy are decrease of triglycerides, increase of HDL, increase of insulin sensitivity, anti-inflammatory and antihypertensive action, and also reduction of mesangium-induced glomerular matrix deposition.[109]

4.3 New treatment

Islets transplantation or stem cell transplantation has shown very exciting future in more effectively controlling blood glucose and preventing and treating diabetes-associated organ damage. More early intervention and prevention targets have been found for metabolic syndrome associated kidney diseases.

4.3.1 Islets transplantation

Pancreas or Islets transplantation is indicated to treatment of type 1 diabetes which insulin is insufficient for normal glucose metabolism. After long term (more than five years) of normoglycemia, diabetic nephropathy will be reversed.[81] It is not clear that pancreas or Islets transplantation will be benefit to improve of type 2 diabetes. In fact, insulin resistance will be more serious after transplantation due to the use of immunosuppressive agent.[113] Our small sample of patients with type 2 diabetes and ESRD receive combined transplantation of islets and kidney shown reversion of the peripheral nerves and vascular diseases, and maybe a protection of renal graft from damage of hyperglycosemia.

Islet transplantation is an effective therapy for insulin-dependent diabetes mellitus, based on the research data which indicated that islet transplantation could not only retrieve the glycometabolism disorders but also prevent and reverse diabetes-associated microangiopathy. According to the registration data of the International Organ Transplantation Center, there had been up to 1300 patients received islet transplantation by the end of 2006. More than 40 institutes have developed islet transplantation for totally 550 cases of diabetic patients, since the Edmonton Islet Transplantation Protocol was available in 2000. The growth rate increased markedly compared to the era before 2000.

The islets isolated from donor's pancreatic tissue, by means of enzyme digestion and centrifugal purification, are injected into recipients' liver through portal vein. The transplanted islets locate in hepatic sinus, adjusting the synthesis of hepatic glycogen and reversing the disorders of glycometabolism through secreting insulin. Autogeneic islet transplantation is limited in patients received entire or partial resection of pancreas due to chronic pancreatitis and tumor. Allogeneic islet transplantation needs immunosuppressants and therefore is mainly suit for kidney transplant recipients with type I diabetes-associated renal failure. Along with the development of new immunosuppressants, the indications of islet transplantation are increasing. In recent years islet transplantation along has been applied in patients with "friable" type I diabetes with refractory severe hypoglycemia while without renal failure, and considered for patients with type II diabetes and complete lost of islets' function.

A four year cooperative study was carried out in 9 islet transplantation centers of USA, Canada and Europe and 36 cases of type I diabetes received islet transplantation according to coincident Edmondon Protocol. It was shown by the data that 16 cases were insulin-independent one year after transplantation (16/36, 44%) and, among them, 5 cases were still insulin-independent after 2 years follow-up (5/16, 31%). The study proved the efficacy of Edmondon Protocol in significantly increasing the success rate of islet transplantation. Besides, it is indicated by the success of Edmondon islet transplantation protocol that islet transplantation along is also fit to patients with type I diabetes while it is not always needed to be performed together with renal transplantation. In recent years some islet transplant recipients without renal failure were only administered short-term of immunosuppressive treatment (Daclizum administered on day 1 and day 3) and good efficacy achieved, which suggests that islet transplantation along may be do not need long-term immunosuppression therapy.

The surgical operation of islet transplantation is simple, but the isolation and the purification of islets belong to high-tech range. The skill and experience of operators are extremely important. Different operators have markedly different isolation results even they use the same pancreas from the same donor and apply the same isolation procedure. How to get enough functional islets from donor's pancreas is the key technique for islet transplantation. Islet transplantation is a program needs multi-department and multi-subject cooperation. A cooperation network should include endocrinologists, surgeons, transplantation center, net-serving staff, official administrators, transplant immunologists, transportation department. In addition, the qualities of a lot of procedures during transplantation can influence the result of islet transplantation, including patient selection, tissue matching, reservation and transportation, islet isolation and purification, islet implantation, blood glucose controlling during islet transplantation, immunosuppressant administration, and function evaluation after transplantation. The determination of islet cell auto-antibodies in recipients' blood after transplantation is important for the prognosis of long-term islet transplantation efficacy. We should further investigate the relationship between the production of islet cell auto-antibodies and the survival of transplanted islets, and make sure if the auto-antibodies is the main factor resulting in the damage of transplanted islets. Islet cell auto-antigens can be produced with gene recombination and immune absorption column can be prepare with the auto-antigens and used to in time eliminate the auto-antibodies in patients' blood, reducing islet damage induced by the antibodies and increase the long-term survival of transplanted islets.

4.3.2 Stem cell transplantation

Stem cell transplantation has shown effective in treatment of type 1 diabetes shown beta cell function increased,[114] and also in treatment of type 2 diabetes with significant increase of serum adiponectin and glucose tolerance.[115] Data from studies of NOD/SCID mice with diabetes shown that mesenchymal stem cells (MSCs) administration can prevent and treat diabetic nephropathy, prevent the pathological changes in the glomeruli and enhances their regeneration resulting in improved kidney function in diabetic animals.[116]

5. References

[1] Lim H. S., Patel J. V., Lip G. Y. Metabolic syndrome: a definition in progress. Circulation 2004, 110(4): e35; author reply e35.

[2] Lee H. B., Ha H., Kim S. I., et al. Diabetic kidney disease research: where do we stand at the turn of the century? Kidney Int Suppl 2000, 77S1-2.

[3] Chen J., Muntner P., Hamm L. L., et al. The metabolic syndrome and chronic kidney disease in U.S. adults. Ann Intern Med 2004, 140(3): 167-174.

[4] Fliser D., Kielstein J. T., Menne J. Insulin resistance and renal disease. Contrib Nephrol 2006, 151203-211.

[5] Parvanova A. I., Trevisan R., Iliev I. P., et al. Insulin resistance and microalbuminuria: a cross-sectional, case-control study of 158 patients with type 2 diabetes and different degrees of urinary albumin excretion. Diabetes 2006, 55(5): 1456-1462.

[6] Chen J., Muntner P., Hamm L. L., et al. Insulin resistance and risk of chronic kidney disease in nondiabetic US adults. J Am Soc Nephrol 2003, 14(2): 469-477.

[7] Cusumano A. M., Bodkin N. L., Hansen B. C., et al. Glomerular hypertrophy is associated with hyperinsulinemia and precedes overt diabetes in aging rhesus monkeys. Am J Kidney Dis 2002, 40(5): 1075-1085.

[8] Segev Y., Landau D., Rasch R., et al. Growth hormone receptor antagonism prevents early renal changes in nonobese diabetic mice. J Am Soc Nephrol 1999, 10(11): 2374-2381.

[9] Wang S., Denichilo M., Brubaker C., et al. Connective tissue growth factor in tubulointerstitial injury of diabetic nephropathy. Kidney Int 2001, 60(1): 96-105.

[10] Anderson P. W., Zhang X. Y., Tian J., et al. Insulin and angiotensin II are additive in stimulating TGF-beta 1 and matrix mRNAs in mesangial cells. Kidney Int 1996, 50(3): 745-753.

[11] Vedovato M., Lepore G., Coracina A., et al. Effect of sodium intake on blood pressure and albuminuria in Type 2 diabetic patients: the role of insulin resistance. Diabetologia 2004, 47(2): 300-303.

[12] Meigs J. B., Mittleman M. A., Nathan D. M., et al. Hyperinsulinemia, hyperglycemia, and impaired hemostasis: the Framingham Offspring Study. JAMA 2000, 283(2): 221-228.

[13] Hagiwara H., Kaizu K., Uriu K., et al. Expression of type-1 plasminogen activator inhibitor in the kidney of diabetic rat models. Thromb Res 2003, 111(4-5): 301-309.

[14] Irving R. J., Noon J. P., Watt G. C., et al. Activation of the endothelin system in insulin resistance. QJM 2001, 94(6): 321-326.

[15] Facchini F. S., Hua N. W., Reaven G. M., et al. Hyperinsulinemia: the missing link among oxidative stress and age-related diseases? Free Radic Biol Med 2000, 29(12): 1302-1306.

[16] Prabhakar S. S. Role of nitric oxide in diabetic nephropathy. Semin Nephrol 2004, 24(4): 333-344.

[17] Steinberg H. O., Baron A. D. Vascular function, insulin resistance and fatty acids. Diabetologia 2002, 45(5): 623-634.

[18] Cowley A. W., Jr., Mattson D. L., Lu S., et al. The renal medulla and hypertension. Hypertension 1995, 25(4 Pt 2): 663-673.

[19] Sealey J. E., Blumenfeld J. D., Bell G. M., et al. On the renal basis for essential hypertension: nephron heterogeneity with discordant renin secretion and sodium excretion causing a hypertensive vasoconstriction-volume relationship. J Hypertens 1988, 6(10): 763-777.

[20] Larochelle P. Glomerular capillary pressure and hypertension. Am Heart J 1991, 122(4 Pt 2): 1228-1231.

[21] Perticone F., Ceravolo R., Pujia A., et al. Prognostic significance of endothelial dysfunction in hypertensive patients. Circulation 2001, 104(2): 191-196.

[22] Koo J. R., Vaziri N. D. Effects of diabetes, insulin and antioxidants on NO synthase abundance and NO interaction with reactive oxygen species. Kidney Int 2003, 63(1): 195-201.

[23] Rodriguez-Iturbe B., Quiroz Y., Herrera-Acosta J., et al. The role of immune cells infiltrating the kidney in the pathogenesis of salt-sensitive hypertension. J Hypertens Suppl 2002, 20(3): S9-14.

[24] Piqueras L., Kubes P., Alvarez A., et al. Angiotensin II induces leukocyte-endothelial cell interactions in vivo via AT(1) and AT(2) receptor-mediated P-selectin upregulation. Circulation 2000, 102(17): 2118-2123.

[25] Mohring J., Mohring B., Petri M., et al. Studies on the pathogenesis of the malignant course of renal hypertension in rats. Kidney Int Suppl 1975, S174-180.

[26] Kumar D., Robertson S., Burns K. D. Evidence of apoptosis in human diabetic kidney. Mol Cell Biochem 2004, 259(1-2): 67-70.

[27] Jesmin S., Sakuma I., Togashi H., et al. Altered expression of endothelin and its receptors in the brain of SHR-SP at malignant hypertensive stage. J Cardiovasc Pharmacol 2004, 44 Suppl 1S11-15.

[28] Khanna A., McCullough P. A. Malignant hypertension presenting as hemolysis, thrombocytopenia, and renal failure. Rev Cardiovasc Med 2003, 4(4): 255-259.

[29] Gerbase-DeLima M., Paiva R. L., Bortolotto L. A., et al. Human leukocyte antigens and malignant essential hypertension. Am J Hypertens 1998, 11(6 Pt 1): 729-731.

[30] Forsberg B., Low B. Malignant hypertension and HLA antigens. Tissue Antigens 1983, 22(2): 155-159.

[31] Moorhead J. F., Chan M. K., El-Nahas M., et al. Lipid nephrotoxicity in chronic progressive glomerular and tubulo-interstitial disease. Lancet 1982, 2(8311): 1309-1311.

[32] Abrass C. K. Lipid metabolism and renal disease. Contrib Nephrol 2006, 151106-121.

[33] Hattori M., Nikolic-Paterson D. J., Miyazaki K., et al. Mechanisms of glomerular macrophage infiltration in lipid-induced renal injury. Kidney Int Suppl 1999, 71S47-50.

[34] Maddox D. A., Alavi F. K., Santella R. N., et al. Prevention of obesity-linked renal disease: age-dependent effects of dietary food restriction. Kidney Int 2002, 62(1): 208-219.

[35] Samuelsson O., Attman P. O., Knight-Gibson C., et al. Complex apolipoprotein B-containing lipoprotein particles are associated with a higher rate of progression of human chronic renal insufficiency. J Am Soc Nephrol 1998, 9(8): 1482-1488.

[36] Muntner P., Coresh J., Smith J. C., et al. Plasma lipids and risk of developing renal dysfunction: the atherosclerosis risk in communities study. Kidney Int 2000, 58(1): 293-301.

[37] Joles J. A., Kunter U., Janssen U., et al. Early mechanisms of renal injury in hypercholesterolemic or hypertriglyceridemic rats. J Am Soc Nephrol 2000, 11(4): 669-683.

[38] Sohn M., Tan Y., Klein R. L., et al. Evidence for low-density lipoprotein-induced expression of connective tissue growth factor in mesangial cells. Kidney Int 2005, 67(4): 1286-1296.

[39] Abrass C. K. Cellular lipid metabolism and the role of lipids in progressive renal disease. Am J Nephrol 2004, 24(1): 46-53.

[40] Bussolati B., Deregibus M. C., Fonsato V., et al. Statins prevent oxidized LDL-induced injury of glomerular podocytes by activating the phosphatidylinositol 3-kinase/AKT-signaling pathway. J Am Soc Nephrol 2005, 16(7): 1936-1947.

[41] Sugimoto K., Isobe K., Kawakami Y., et al. The relationship between non-HDL cholesterol and other lipid parameters in Japanese subjects. J Atheroscler Thromb 2005, 12(2): 107-110.

[42] Chonchol M., Shlipak M. G., Katz R., et al. Relationship of uric acid with progression of kidney disease. Am J Kidney Dis 2007, 50(2): 239-247.

[43] Emmerson B. T., Cross M., Osborne J. M., et al. Ultrastructural studies of the reaction of urate crystals with a cultured renal tubular cell line. Nephron 1991, 59(3): 403-408.

[44] Toblli J. E., DeRosa G., Lago N., et al. Potassium citrate administration ameliorates tubulointerstitial lesions in rats with uric acid nephropathy. Clin Nephrol 2001, 55(1): 59-68.

[45] Mazzali M., Hughes J., Kim Y. G., et al. Elevated uric acid increases blood pressure in the rat by a novel crystal-independent mechanism. Hypertension 2001, 38(5): 1101-1106.

[46] Nakagawa T., Mazzali M., Kang D. H., et al. Hyperuricemia causes glomerular hypertrophy in the rat. Am J Nephrol 2003, 23(1): 2-7.

[47] Sanchez-Lozada L. G., Tapia E., Santamaria J., et al. Mild hyperuricemia induces vasoconstriction and maintains glomerular hypertension in normal and remnant kidney rats. Kidney Int 2005, 67(1): 237-247.

[48] Kang D. H., Nakagawa T., Feng L., et al. A role for uric acid in the progression of renal disease. J Am Soc Nephrol 2002, 13(12): 2888-2897.

[49] Mazzali M., Kim Y. G., Suga S., et al. Hyperuricemia exacerbates chronic cyclosporine nephropathy. Transplantation 2001, 71(7): 900-905.

[50] Khosla U. M., Zharikov S., Finch J. L., et al. Hyperuricemia induces endothelial dysfunction. Kidney Int 2005, 67(5): 1739-1742.

[51] Kang D. H., Park S. K., Lee I. K., et al. Uric acid-induced C-reactive protein expression: implication on cell proliferation and nitric oxide production of human vascular cells. J Am Soc Nephrol 2005, 16(12): 3553-3562.

[52] Siu Y. P., Leung K. T., Tong M. K., et al. Use of allopurinol in slowing the progression of renal disease through its ability to lower serum uric acid level. Am J Kidney Dis 2006, 47(1): 51-59.

[53] Zoccali C., Maio R., Mallamaci F., et al. Uric acid and endothelial dysfunction in essential hypertension. J Am Soc Nephrol 2006, 17(5): 1466-1471.

[54] Kanabrocki E. L., Third J. L., Ryan M. D., et al. Circadian relationship of serum uric acid and nitric oxide. JAMA 2000, 283(17): 2240-2241.

[55] Nakagawa T., Tuttle K. R., Short R. A., et al. Hypothesis: fructose-induced hyperuricemia as a causal mechanism for the epidemic of the metabolic syndrome. Nat Clin Pract Nephrol 2005, 1(2): 80-86.

[56] Sautin Y. Y., Nakagawa T., Zharikov S., et al. Adverse effects of the classic antioxidant uric acid in adipocytes: NADPH oxidase-mediated oxidative/nitrosative stress. Am J Physiol Cell Physiol 2007, 293(2): C584-596.

[57] Feig D. I., Nakagawa T., Karumanchi S. A., et al. Hypothesis: Uric acid, nephron number, and the pathogenesis of essential hypertension. Kidney Int 2004, 66(1): 281-287.

[58] Saito I., Saruta T., Kondo K., et al. Serum uric acid and the renin-angiotensin system in hypertension. J Am Geriatr Soc 1978, 26(6): 241-247.

[59] Talaat K. M., el-Sheikh A. R. The effect of mild hyperuricemia on urinary transforming growth factor beta and the progression of chronic kidney disease. Am J Nephrol 2007, 27(5): 435-440.

[60] Sone H., Tanaka S., Ishibashi S., et al. The new worldwide definition of metabolic syndrome is not a better diagnostic predictor of cardiovascular disease in Japanese diabetic patients than the existing definitions: additional analysis from the Japan Diabetes Complications Study. Diabetes Care 2006, 29(1): 145-147.

[61] Kurella M., Lo J. C., Chertow G. M. Metabolic syndrome and the risk for chronic kidney disease among nondiabetic adults. J Am Soc Nephrol 2005, 16(7): 2134-2140.

[62] Hsu C. Y., McCulloch C. E., Iribarren C., et al. Body mass index and risk for end-stage renal disease. Ann Intern Med 2006, 144(1): 21-28.

[63] Agnani S., Vachharajani V. T., Gupta R., et al. Does treating obesity stabilize chronic kidney disease? BMC Nephrol 2005, 67.

[64] Chagnac A., Weinstein T., Herman M., et al. The effects of weight loss on renal function in patients with severe obesity. J Am Soc Nephrol 2003, 14(6): 1480-1486.

[65] Weisinger J. R., Kempson R. L., Eldridge F. L., et al. The nephrotic syndrome: a complication of massive obesity. Ann Intern Med 1974, 81(4): 440-447.

[66] Kambham N., Markowitz G. S., Valeri A. M., et al. Obesity-related glomerulopathy: an emerging epidemic. Kidney Int 2001, 59(4): 1498-1509.

[67] Hall J. E., Kuo J. J., da Silva A. A., et al. Obesity-associated hypertension and kidney disease. Curr Opin Nephrol Hypertens 2003, 12(2): 195-200.

[68] Henegar J. R., Bigler S. A., Henegar L. K., et al. Functional and structural changes in the kidney in the early stages of obesity. J Am Soc Nephrol 2001, 12(6): 1211-1217.

[69] Bosma R. J., van der Heide J. J., Oosterop E. J., et al. Body mass index is associated with altered renal hemodynamics in non-obese healthy subjects. Kidney Int 2004, 65(1): 259-265.

[70] Iseki K. Body mass index and the risk of chronic renal failure: the Asian experience. Contrib Nephrol 2006, 15142-56.

[71] Chagnac A., Weinstein T., Korzets A., et al. Glomerular hemodynamics in severe obesity. Am J Physiol Renal Physiol 2000, 278(5): F817-822.

[72] Engeli S., Schling P., Gorzelniak K., et al. The adipose-tissue renin-angiotensin-aldosterone system: role in the metabolic syndrome? Int J Biochem Cell Biol 2003, 35(6): 807-825.

[73] Goossens G. H., Blaak E. E., van Baak M. A. Possible involvement of the adipose tissue renin-angiotensin system in the pathophysiology of obesity and obesity-related disorders. Obes Rev 2003, 4(1): 43-55.

[74] Grisk O., Rettig R. Interactions between the sympathetic nervous system and the kidneys in arterial hypertension. Cardiovasc Res 2004, 61(2): 238-246.

[75] Wolf G., Ziyadeh F. N. Leptin and renal fibrosis. Contrib Nephrol 2006, 151175-183.

[76] Xu H., Barnes G. T., Yang Q., et al. Chronic inflammation in fat plays a crucial role in the development of obesity-related insulin resistance. J Clin Invest 2003, 112(12): 1821-1830.

[77] Weisberg S. P., McCann D., Desai M., et al. Obesity is associated with macrophage accumulation in adipose tissue. J Clin Invest 2003, 112(12): 1796-1808.

[78] Ramkumar N., Cheung A. K., Pappas L. M., et al. Association of obesity with inflammation in chronic kidney disease: a cross-sectional study. J Ren Nutr 2004, 14(4): 201-207.

[79] Hall J. E., Brands M. W., Henegar J. R. Mechanisms of hypertension and kidney disease in obesity. Ann N Y Acad Sci 1999, 89291-107.

[80] Kikkawa R., Koya D., Haneda M. Progression of diabetic nephropathy. Am J Kidney Dis 2003, 41(3 Suppl 1): S19-21.

[81] Fioretto P., Steffes M. W., Sutherland D. E., et al. Reversal of lesions of diabetic nephropathy after pancreas transplantation. N Engl J Med 1998, 339(2): 69-75.

[82] Abdel-Wahab N., Weston B. S., Roberts T., et al. Connective tissue growth factor and regulation of the mesangial cell cycle: role in cellular hypertrophy. J Am Soc Nephrol 2002, 13(10): 2437-2445.

[83] Hudson B. I., Schmidt A. M. RAGE: a novel target for drug intervention in diabetic vascular disease. Pharm Res 2004, 21(7): 1079-1086.

[84] Boyd-White J., Williams J. C., Jr. Effect of cross-linking on matrix permeability. A model for AGE-modified basement membranes. Diabetes 1996, 45(3): 348-353.

[85] Ceriello A. New insights on oxidative stress and diabetic complications may lead to a "causal" antioxidant therapy. Diabetes Care 2003, 26(5): 1589-1596.

[86] Inoguchi T., Yu H. Y., Imamura M., et al. Altered gap junction activity in cardiovascular tissues of diabetes. Med Electron Microsc 2001, 34(2): 86-91.

[87] Prabhakar S. S. Pathogenic role of nitric oxide alterations in diabetic nephropathy. Curr Diab Rep 2005, 5(6): 449-454.

[88] Scivittaro V., Ganz M. B., Weiss M. F. AGEs induce oxidative stress and activate protein kinase C-beta(II) in neonatal mesangial cells. Am J Physiol Renal Physiol 2000, 278(4): F676-683.

[89] Maxfield E. K., Cameron N. E., Cotter M. A. Effects of diabetes on reactivity of sciatic vasa nervorum in rats. J Diabetes Complications 1997, 11(1): 47-55.

[90] Michimata T., Murakami M., Iriuchijima T. Nitric oxide-dependent soluble guanylate cyclase activity is decreased in platelets from male NIDDM patients. Life Sci 1996, 59(17): 1463-1471.

[91] Karamanos B., Porta M., Songini M., et al. Different risk factors of microangiopathy in patients with type I diabetes mellitus of short versus long duration. The EURODIAB IDDM Complications Study. Diabetologia 2000, 43(3): 348-355.

[92] Vykoukal D., Davies M. G. Metabolic syndrome and outcomes after renal intervention. Cardiol Res Pract 2010, 2011781035.

[93] Davani B., Portwood N., Bryzgalova G., et al. Aged transgenic mice with increased glucocorticoid sensitivity in pancreatic beta-cells develop diabetes. Diabetes 2004, 53 Suppl 1S51-59.

[94] Hamamdzic D., Duzic E., Sherlock J. D., et al. Regulation of alpha 2-adrenergic receptor expression and signaling in pancreatic beta-cells. Am J Physiol 1995, 269(1 Pt 1): E162-171.

[95] Ullrich S., Berchtold S., Ranta F., et al. Serum- and glucocorticoid-inducible kinase 1 (SGK1) mediates glucocorticoid-induced inhibition of insulin secretion. Diabetes 2005, 54(4): 1090-1099.

[96] Ranta F., Avram D., Berchtold S., et al. Dexamethasone induces cell death in insulin-secreting cells, an effect reversed by exendin-4. Diabetes 2006, 55(5): 1380-1390.

[97] Vincenti F., Friman S., Scheuermann E., et al. Results of an international, randomized trial comparing glucose metabolism disorders and outcome with cyclosporine versus tacrolimus. Am J Transplant 2007, 7(6): 1506-1514.

[98] Duclos A., Flechner L. M., Faiman C., et al. Post-transplant diabetes mellitus: risk reduction strategies in the elderly. Drugs Aging 2006, 23(10): 781-793.

[99] Hoitsma A. J., Hilbrands L. B. Relative risk of new-onset diabetes during the first year after renal transplantation in patients receiving tacrolimus or cyclosporine immunosuppression. Clin Transplant 2006, 20(5): 659-664.

[100] Hjelmesaeth J., Asberg A., Muller F., et al. New-onset posttransplantation diabetes mellitus: insulin resistance or insulinopenia? Impact of immunosuppressive drugs, cytomegalovirus and hepatitis C virus infection. Curr Diabetes Rev 2005, 1(1): 1-10.

[101] Sun W, Zhang L, Tang Y W, et al. Role of C hepatitis on the morbidity of posttransplant diabetes mellitus in renal transplant recipients. Journal of Clinical Rehabilitative Tissue Engineering Research 2007, 11(38): 7529-7532.

[102] Ducloux D., Motte G., Vautrin P., et al. Polycystic kidney disease as a risk factor for post-transplant diabetes mellitus. Nephrol Dial Transplant 1999, 14(5): 1244-1246.

[103] Vareesangthip K., Thomas T. H., Tong P., et al. Erythrocyte membrane fluidity in adult polycystic kidney disease: difference between intact cells and ghost membranes. Eur J Clin Invest 1996, 26(2): 171-173.

[104] Vareesangthip K., Thomas T. H., Wilkinson R. Abnormal effect of thiol groups on erythrocyte Na/Li countertransport kinetics in adult polycystic kidney disease. Nephrol Dial Transplant 1995, 10(12): 2219-2223.

[105] Grundy S. M., Cleeman J. I., Daniels S. R., et al. Diagnosis and management of the metabolic syndrome: an American Heart Association/National Heart, Lung, and Blood Institute Scientific Statement. Circulation 2005, 112(17): 2735-2752.

[106] Alberti K. G., Zimmet P., Shaw J. Metabolic syndrome--a new world-wide definition. A Consensus Statement from the International Diabetes Federation. Diabet Med 2006, 23(5): 469-480.

[107] Levey A. S., Eckardt K. U., Tsukamoto Y., et al. Definition and classification of chronic kidney disease: a position statement from Kidney Disease: Improving Global Outcomes (KDIGO). Kidney Int 2005, 67(6): 2089-2100.

[108] Alexander M. P., Patel T. V., Farag Y. M., et al. Kidney pathological changes in metabolic syndrome: a cross-sectional study. Am J Kidney Dis 2009, 53(5): 751-759.

[109] Agrawal V., Shah A., Rice C., et al. Impact of treating the metabolic syndrome on chronic kidney disease. Nat Rev Nephrol 2009, 5(9): 520-528.

[110] Yale J. F. Oral antihyperglycemic agents and renal disease: new agents, new concepts. J Am Soc Nephrol 2005, 16 Suppl 1S7-10.

[111] Iglesias P., Diez J. J. Insulin therapy in renal disease. Diabetes Obes Metab 2008, 10(10): 811-823.

[112] Rebsomen L., Khammar A., Raccah D., et al. C-Peptide effects on renal physiology and diabetes. Exp Diabetes Res 2008, 2008281536.

[113] Sui W., Zou H., Zou G., et al. Clinical study of the risk factors of insulin resistance and metabolic syndrome after kidney transplantation. Transpl Immunol 2008, 20(1-2): 95-98.

[114] Voltarelli J. C., Couri C. E., Stracieri A. B., et al. Autologous nonmyeloablative hematopoietic stem cell transplantation in newly diagnosed type 1 diabetes mellitus. JAMA 2007, 297(14): 1568-1576.

[115] Abraham N. G., Li M., Vanella L., et al. Bone marrow stem cell transplant into intra-bone cavity prevents type 2 diabetes: role of heme oxygenase-adiponectin. J Autoimmun 2008, 30(3): 128-135.

[116] Volarevic V., Arsenijevic N., Lukic M. L., et al. Mesenchymal stem cell treatment of complications of diabetes mellitus. Stem Cells 2010.

10

Mild Forms of Alport Syndrome: Hereditary Nephropathy in the Absence of Extra-Renal Features

Han-Seung Yoon and Michael R. Eccles

Department of Pathology, Dunedin School of Medicine, University of Otago, Dunedin
New Zealand

1. Introduction

The type IV collagen nephropathies comprise a spectrum of abnormalities predominantly affecting the glomerular basement membrane (GBM) in the kidney, but also involving other organs such as the ear and eye. Type IV collagen nephropathies result from genetic mutations causing loss or deficiency of type IV collagen synthesis, and have been associated with Alport syndrome at one end of the spectrum, where individuals who are the most severely affected experience end-stage renal failure (ESRF) in their early teen-age years together with hearing loss and vision abnormalities. At the other end of the spectrum type IV collagen nephropathies are associated with mild defects, such as thin basement membrane nephropathy (TBMN) or benign familial hematuria where individuals may experience mild kidney abnormalities involving episodic hematuria but retain relatively normal renal function and show no extra-renal abnormalities. There are six different type IV collagen genes located on multiple chromosomes, and three of these genes (*COL4A3*, *COL4A4*, and *COL4A5*) are associated with X-linked, autosomal recessive or autosomal dominant inheritance patterns of Alport syndrome. In addition the type IV collagen genes are associated with the TBMN phenotype, involving heterozygous mutations of the *COL4A3* and *COL4A4* genes, with an autosomal dominant pattern of inheritance. The main focus of this chapter is the mild forms of Alport syndrome, and so in the following pages we review mild presentations of Alport syndrome, and illustrate this with a unique New Zealand family segregating mild X-linked Alport syndrome, some of whom display features of TBMN.

2. Synthesis and distribution of type IV collagen

The type IV collagen family is comprised of six homologous α-chains designated α1(IV)–α6(IV) encoded for by the *COL4A1-6* genes respectively, the corresponding genes of which are located pairwise on chromosomes 13q34, 2q36-37 and Xq22. Each α-chain has three domains composed of a short 7S domain at the amino terminus, a long collagenous domain of approximately 1400 residues of Gly-Xaa-Yaa repeats and a noncollagenous (NC1) domain of about 230 residues at the carboxyl terminus (Figure 1). Three α chains assemble into triple-helical molecules called protomers that then assemble into supramolecular networks by the association of four protomers at the N-terminus, forming a 7S tetramer, and the dimerization of two protomers at the C-terminus, forming an NC1 hexamer (Timpl et al., 1981). Interruptions in the Gly-Xaa-Yaa amino acid sequence at multiple sites along the collagenous domain give rise to flexibility, allowing for looping and supercoiling of protomers into networks (Hudson 2004, Miner 2003, Zhou & Reeders 1996).

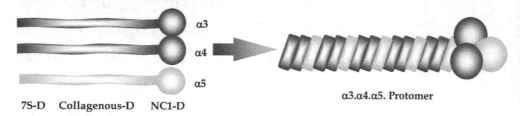

α3
α4
α5

α3.α4.α5. Protomer

7S-D   Collagenous-D   NC1-D

Fig. 1. A schematic drawing showing an example of α3-, α4-, and α5(IV)-chains and α3.α4.α5(IV) protomer formation. D: domain

To date, only three different types of collagen protomer have been identified; α1.α1.α2(IV), α3.α4.α5(IV) and α5.α5.α6(IV) (Hudson 2004). The protomer α1.α1.α2(IV) is ubiquitously present in most basement membranes (Hudson et al., 1993, Borza et al., 2001, Boutaud et al., 2000, Timpl et al., 1981). In contrast, α3.α4.α5(IV) and α5.α5.α6(IV) show restricted tissue distribution. In the kidney the α1.α1.α2(IV)-α1.α1.α2(IV) network predominates during early nephrogenesis in the GBM, the Bowman's capsular basement membrane, and tubular basement membrane. As the kidney becomes mature during the 2nd trimester of fetal development, the α3.α4.α5(IV)-α3.α4.α5(IV) network gradually becomes dominant and replaces the α1.α1.α2(IV)-α1.α1.α2(IV) network in the GBM and in tubular basement membranes while the α1.α1.α2(IV)-α5.α5.α6(IV) and the α1.α1.α2(IV)-α1.α1.α2(IV) networks are distributed in the Bowman's capsular basement membrane and in tubular basement membranes (Harvey et al., 1998, Milner 2003). The protomer α3.α4.α5(IV) is also expressed in the lung, testis, cochlea and eye while the α5.α5.α6(IV) network is present in skin, smooth muscle and esophagus (Cosgrove et al., 1998, Hudson et al., 2003, Kalluri et al., 1997). Alterations in any of the *COL4A3*, *COL4A4* and *COL4A5* genes may cause Alport syndrome.

3. Alport syndrome

Alport syndrome is a hereditary disorder with considerable genetic and clinical heterogeneity characterized by hematuria, proteinuria (1-2 gm of protein per day) and progressive renal failure and is frequently associated with diagnostic ocular abnormalities and high tone sensorineural deafness. Ocular abnormalities include lenticonus of the anterior lens capsule, retinopathy and cataracts. Other extra-renal manifestations include mental retardation or leiomyomatosis in rare cases (Alport 1927, Flinter et al., 1988, Hudson et al., 2003).

3.1 Genetics
In approximately 85% of patients with Alport syndrome there is X-linked inheritance of mutations in the *COL4A5* gene encoding the α5(IV) collagen chain on chromosome Xq22. *COL4A5* is a large gene comprising 51 exons. As many as 588 mutations have been described to date and are spread throughout the gene without any identified mutational hot spots. The types of mutations that involve *COL4A5* consist of missense, deletion, splice site, nonsense, insertion and duplication mutations (Hou et al., 2007, Mochizuki et al., 1994).

The remaining 15% of Alport syndrome patients show autosomal inheritance; of these 14% are recessive and 1% are dominant, which are caused by mutations either in the *COL4A3* or *COL4A4* genes on chromosome 2q36-37 encoding the α3(IV) or α4(IV) proteins. Heterozygous mutations of *COL4A3* or *COL4A4* could result in a less severe phenotype than that of homozygous or compound mutations in these genes (Jefferson et al., 1997). The authors also noted that heterogygous mutations of these genes could result in thin basement membrane nephropathy (TBMN) which typically does not result in renal failure. The authors postulated that mutations in the *COL4A3* or *COL4A4* gene can cause a spectrum of disease, ranging from TBMN/benign familial hematuria to autosomal dominant and recessive forms of Alport syndrome.

3.2 Pathogenesis

Ultrafiltration of plasma in the renal glomeruli is the major function of the kidney (Voskarides et al., 2008). The primary filtration barrier of the glomerular capillary consists of three layers: the fenestrated endothelial cells, the intervening GBM, and the epithelial podocyte foot processes. The foot processes are connected to each other by the slit diaphragm, and together these constitute an important component of the filtration barrier; the loss of podocyte foot processes results in massive proteinuria. The GBM is a special kind of acellular extracellular matrix, having properties of a viscous gel. The filtration barrier behaves as a selective sieve restricting the passage of macromolecules on the basis of their size, shape, and charge. Deterioration of the integrity of the GBM results in mild proteinuria. The major constituent of GBM is type IV collagen, which together with laminin, nidogen, and sulfated proteoglycans maintains the filtration barrier and provides the substrata and signals necessary for proper renal cell function (Hudson & Tryggvason 2003).

Mutations present in Alport syndrome that produce post-translational defects in α3(IV), α4(IV), or α5(IV) chains may result in incorrect folding or assembly of monomers. Such defective monomers are rapidly degraded. The mutations, therefore, arrest the normal developmental maturation during the fetal 2nd trimester period when the α1.α1.α2(IV) network is largely replaced by the α3.α4.α5(IV) network in the GBM. This maturation may be related to oxidative and physical stress in GBM (Kalluri et al., 2000) and perhaps also in the cochlea (Huang et al., 2000) and the lens capsule (Reddan et al., 1996). In the kidney, as plasma traverses glomerular capillaries, the protein content, including the levels of serum proteases, increases. The embryonic α1.α1.α2(IV) network is more susceptible to endoproteolysis than the more heavily cross-linked α3.α4.α5(IV) network (Kalluri et al 1997). It seems, then, that GBM that is more exposed to proteases or oxidants needs the protection of a resistant collagen IV network. Over time, patients with Alport syndrome probably become more sensitive to proteolysis, which may explain why their glomerular membranes thicken unevenly, split, and ultimately deteriorate (Kalluri et al., 1997, Kalluri et al., 2000). Immunohistochemical studies show that mutations in the *COL4A5* gene, which cause the X-linked form of Alport syndrome, frequently result in the loss of all three of the α3(IV), α4(IV) and α5(IV) chains in the GBM (Naito et al., 1996, Naito et al., 2003, Yoshioka et al., 1994). Thus, the absence of a functionally normal α5(IV) chain can disrupt assembly of the triple-helical protomer, and frequently leads to loss of the entire α3.α4.α5(IV) network in the GBM.

Mutations involving the NC1 domain of *COL4A5* result in no or severely reduced α3.α4.α5(IV) protomer formation within cells and/or in failure of secretion from cells

(Kobayashi T et al., 2008, Kobayashi & Uchiyama 2010). In the normal process of formation of the type IV collagen network, the NC1 domain plays an important role in forming protomers as three α chains specifically interact with each other. Additionally, in forming NC1 hexamers, two protomers dimerize at the C-terminus. Defective monomers or protomers of type IV collagen networks may be degraded rapidly.

4. Genotype-phenotype correlation in X-linked Alport syndrome

Approximately six hundred mutations in COL4A5 have been reported, 588 of which are causally linked with X-linked Alport syndrome (Arup Laboratories 2011). Considerable allelic heterogeneity is observed by the high number of mutations and the associated phenotypic variability. Clinically the natural history of the nephropathy and other extra-renal lesions are quite variable. A number of researchers have attempted to link genotypes in Alport syndrome to phenotypes (Bekheirnia et al., 2010, Gross et al., 2002, Jais et al., 2000). Gross and colleagues have proposed a classification linking phenotype and genotype into three categories (Gross et al., 2002).

- Type S (severe); genotypic alterations in COL4A5 include major gene rearrangements, premature stop codons, frameshift mutations, and donor splice site alterations. Also includes mutations involving the NC1 domain. The phenotype is characterised by early onset of ESRF at about 20 years of age and significant extra-renal manifestations including 80% with sensorineural deafness and 40% with ocular lesions.
- Type MS (moderately severe). The genotype in this group is characterised by non-glycine-XY missense alterations, in-frame deletions/insertions, acceptor splice site changes and glycine-XY substitutions involving exons 21-47. This type is associated with ESRF appearing in the mid-twenties with about 65% of individuals having hearing loss and 30% ocular defects.
- Type M (moderate). The genotype is glycine-XY substitutions involving exons 1-20. The phenotype appears to be milder with a later onset of ESRF at about 30 years of age, including a significant number of individuals with sensorineural deafness (70%) and ocular lesions (30%).

Bekheirnia and colleagues have confirmed previous reports (Gross et al., 2002, Jais et al., 2000) in that there is a strong genotype-phenotype correlation in X-linked Alport syndrome (Bekheirnia et al., 2010). The authors conclude that missense mutations are associated with the best prognosis with an average age at onset of ESRF of 37 yr, followed by splice site mutations at 28 yr, truncating mutations at 25 yr and small deletions at 22 yr. The authors also point out a strong relationship between mutation position and age onset of ESRF, with younger ages at onset of ESRF associated with the 5' end of the gene. Affected males with splice mutations or truncating mutations showed two-fold greater odds of developing eye problems and hearing loss than those with missense mutations. Mutations associated with hearing loss and ocular changes are located closer to the 5' end of the gene.

5. Mild forms of Alport syndrome

While many affected males of X-linked Alport syndrome show moderate to severe forms of nephropathy and extra-renal abnormalities between the second and third decades, it is also well known that there are occasional milder cases where ESRF may be delayed until the fifth or sixth decade along with variable age occurrence of deafness (Bekheirnia et al., 2010, Kobayashi et al., 2008, Smeets et al., 1992). Of the six hundred or so *COL4A5* mutations that have been reported to date (Arup Laboratories 2011), 588 mutations were pathogenic for X-linked Alport syndrome, whereas 12/600 mutations were benign (silent). A total of 81/588 mutations (13.8%) were associated with a mild form of Alport syndrome where the age of onset of ESRF was over 30 yr old. These 81 mutations of a mild form are shown in Figure 2 and consist of 66 mutations within exons (red column) and 15 mutations within introns (blue column), widely distributed over the *COL4A5* gene. It appears that mutations involved in a mild form of Alport syndrome are widely distributed within 51 exons of the *COL4A5* gene with a tendency for more mutations between Exon 25 to 51.

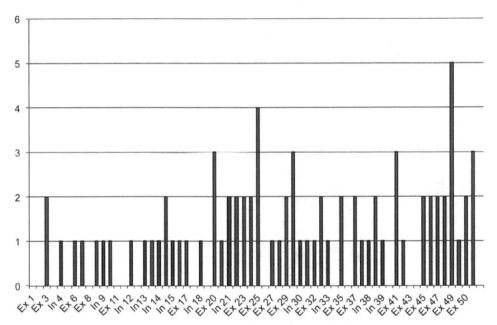

Fig. 2. Distribution and frequency of mutations in exons (red column) and introns (blue column) within the *COL4A5* gene causally relating to X-linked Alport syndrome (Arup Laboratories 2011).

6. A unique mild form of Alport syndrome in New Zealand families

We previously described a novel Cys1638Tyr alteration in the NC1 domain of *COL4A5* identified in a large New Zealand family (Fig 3) with a hereditary nephropathy (Wilson et al., 2007). This family was identified when two sisters (IV26 and IV28) presented to the clinic to be considered as potential live kidney donors for their sons (V29 and V35, respectively) who had ESRF (see Tables 1 and 2). Both women were found to have significant proteinuria and hypertension and so it was decided to carry out renal biopsies. Following the results of the biopsies each family member was then evaluated for the presence of renal disease as indicated in Table 1, and only three male members of the extensive pedigree were found to exhibit ESRF. Extra-renal manifestations such as sensorineural deafness or ocular changes were not observed in any family member. Further renal biopsies were carried out on additional family members, so that renal biopsies now totalled eight members of the family. The biopsies from a 39 year-old male with proteinuria of 1.1 g/24h and normal auditory and eye examination (V42) showed mild increase of mesangial matrix and mild periglomerular Bowman capsular fibrosis (Fig 4A). There were occasional areas showing focal interstitial accumulation of foam cells (Fig 4B), interstitial fibrosis (Fig 4C) and thick-wall hyalinized vessels surrounded by scattered aggregates of lymphocytes (Fig 4D).

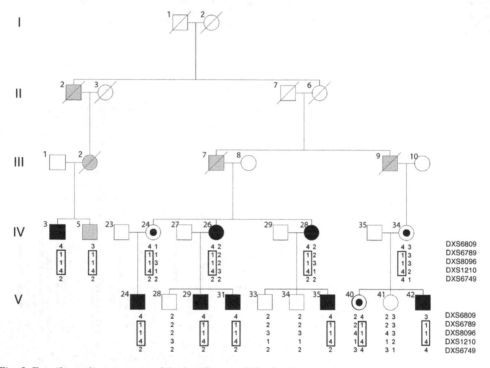

Fig. 3. Family pedigree. A simplified pedigree of the family showing males (squares) and females (circles) depicted by generation (I-V) is shown. While the disease appears severe in this pedigree, the extended pedigree was published previously (Wilson et al., 2007), and only 32/155 members of the extended pedigree are shown in this diagram. Some of the individuals indicated in Tables 1 and 2 are represented in this pedigree and are identified in each case by their corresponding number. Black symbols indicate individuals with biopsy-confirmed GN. Black dots inside the symbols indicate obligate carriers. Grey symbols indicate individuals who were not biopsied, with clinical manifestations of renal disease and therefore presumed GN. Open symbols indicate individuals without clinical signs of renal disease. X chromosome region markers (Xq21.33-Xq23) informative for linkage analysis are indicated on the right, and shown below the symbols are the genotypes for each individual that are associated with the relevant marker. The boxed region indicates a common haplotype inherited from the father or the mother, corresponding to genotypes of the 3 markers that segregate with the disease. The genomic region of chromosome X corresponding to this haplotype contained the COL4A5 gene locus.

Identification number	Age Gender	Presentation	Renal Function and Blood Pressure	Biopsy *	Inheritance
III2	Female		Died on dialysis	Not done	Affected/ Carrier
IV3	57 yrs old male		ESRF at 40 yrs old. Dialysis. Renal transplant.	Not done.	Affected
IV5	46 yrs old male	Proteinuria 4.7g/24h Hypertension	Chronic kidney disease BP 200/120	Not done	Affected
V24	39 yrs old male	Proteinuria. Hematuria	BP 148/90	Mild mesangial matrix expansion	Affected
V29	41 yrs old male	Acute nephritic syndrome. Hypertension	ESRF at 28 yrs old. Dialysis. 2nd renal transplant	Chronic glomerulo-nephritis	Affected
V31	36 yrs old male	Proteinuria. Hypertension	Chronic kidney disease BP 136/86	Mesangial cell proliferation.	Affected
V35	32 yrs old male	Proteinuria. Hematuria	Chronic kidney disease. Progressed to ESRF, at 26 yrs old and renal transplant	Chronic glomerulo-nephritis	Affected
V42	39 yrs old male	Proteinuria 1.1g/24 hr	BP 126/80	Mesangial cell proliferation.	Affected

* Ig immunofluorescence negative

Table 1. Renal disease identified prior to mutation screening in the New Zealand family

Electron microscopy of a renal biopsy from (V42), of which histology is shown in Fig 4, demonstrated a classical basket weave pattern or splitting of the basement membrane characteristic of Alport syndrome (Fig 5A and 5B). However, a diagnosis of Alport syndrome was not necessarily an obvious diagnosis in this family, since the disease in all three males was relatively mild and there was a lack of extra-renal manifestations in any of the family members, raising some doubts as to whether this was Alport syndrome prior to carrying out genetic analysis.

To determine the genetic cause of the disease in this family, genomic DNA was isolated from whole blood of each of the family members, and used in linkage analysis with genetic markers spanning chromosome X carried out as described in Wilson et al (2007). Strong evidence for linkage to markers DXS6789, DXS8096, DXS1210, adjacent to the COL4A5 (and COL4A6) genes located on chromosome X was obtained, indicating that this corresponded to a collagen nephropathy in the family, and that it was most likely due to a mutation in COL4A5.

Identification number	Age Gender	Presentation	Renal Function and Blood Pressure	Biopsy *	Inheritance
IV24	69 yrs old female	Trace microscopic hematuria	Normal renal function. BP 168/86	Not done	Carrier
IV26	64 yrs old female	Proteinuria 1.8g/24 hr Hypertension.	Normal renal function BP 152/76	Mesangial cell proliferation. Hypertensive arteriosclerosis	Affected/ Carrier
IV28	60 yrs old female	Proteinuria 1.4g/24 hr Hypertension	BP 160/98	Mesangial cell proliferation. Hypertensive arteriosclerosis	Affected/ Carrier
IV31	69 yrs old female	Hypertension Negative urine	Normal renal function	Not done	Carrier
IV34	65 yrs old female	Hypertension Negative urine	Normal renal function	Not done	Carrier
IV36	61 yrs old female	Microscopic hematuria	Normal renal function	Not done	Carrier
IV39	72 yrs old male	Proteinuria 1.6g/24 hr No hematuria Hypertension	Mild chronic kidney disease BP 144/76	Not done	Affected
IV47	54 yrs old female	Hematuria Hypertension	Normal renal function BP 148/70	Not done	Carrier
V44	36 yrs old female	Intermittent microscopic hematuria	Normal renal function BP 120/76	Not done	Carrier
V49	43 yrs old female	Negative urine	Normal renal function BP 120/70	Not done	Carrier
V37	39 yrs old female	Negative urine	Normal renal function	Not done	Carrier
V40	42 yrs old female	Hematuria	Normal renal function. BP 118/70.	Mild mesangial cell proliferation	Carrier

* Ig immunofluorescence negative

Table 2. Renal disease or carrier status identified after mutation screening in the NZ family

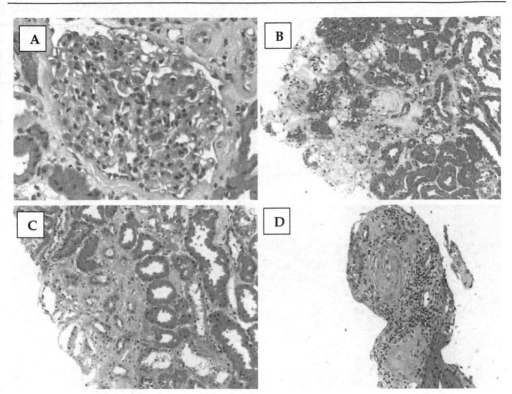

Fig. 4. Histological findings of the kidney of a patient, 39 yr old male with hematuria, proteinuria 1.1 g/24h and normal auditory and eye examination. (A) Glomerulus from kidney biopsy of this patient showing mild periglomerular fibrosis and mild mesangial matrix increase. Tubular atrophy is seen at the right upper corner. (B) Focal accumulations of foam cells in the interstitium. (C) Multiple focal areas of interstitial fibrosis associated with atrophic tubules. (D) Sclerosed vessels surrounded by lymphocytes.

Eventually the mutation, comprising a c.4913G>A nucleotide substitution in exon 50 of *COL4A5*, was identified by PCR amplification and sequenced following analysis using a series of primer pairs corresponding to each of the 51 exons making up the *COL4A5* transcript (Genbank accession number NM_000495) as well as the entire promoter region between *COL4A5* and *COL4A6*. Therefore, this analysis conclusively showed that the disease in this family was a mild form of Alport syndrome.

Since it is known that most cases of Alport syndrome result in loss of the synthesis or secretion of the collagen protein and/or protomer, which can be detected by the absence of the collagen staining by immunohistochemistry, in order to further understand whether the pathogenesis of this disease in the New Zealand family was due to the loss of synthesis of COL4A5, immunohistochemical studies of the α1 to α5 type IV collagens in kidney biopsies from affected and carrier individuals were carried out. This analysis showed that in affected men (V31, V35 and V42) and carriers (IV26 and IV28) the GBMs were positive for α1 to α5 type IV collagens, as exemplified in Fig 6 (α3, α4 and α5). These findings were considerably different from the previous reports of Alport syndrome, where the X-linked form of Alport syndrome was generally found to result in the loss of all three of the $\alpha3$(IV), $\alpha4$(IV) and $\alpha5$(IV) chains in the GBM.

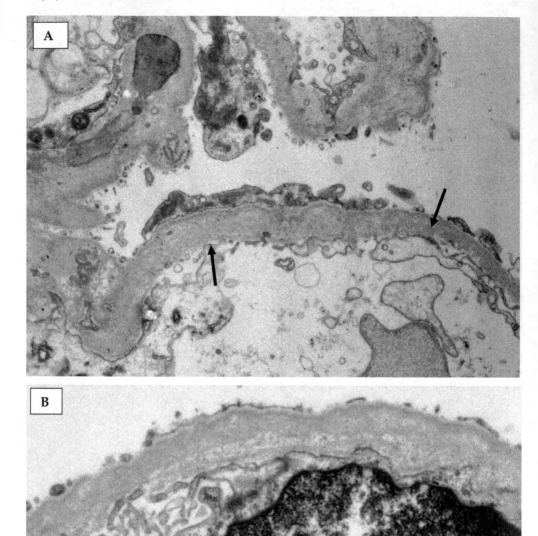

Fig. 5. Electron microscopy of glomerular basement membranes of the same patient (V42) of Figure 4. (A) Characteristic splitting or basket weave appearance of GBM (arrows) and abnormal podocyte foot processes. (original magnification x9,700). (B) Higher magnification of a basket weave appearance. (original magnification x13,500). Note, the ultra-structural changes in the glomerular basement membrane of patients with Alport syndrome were variably associated with areas of thick and thin basement membrane, and/or presence of a basket-weave pattern.

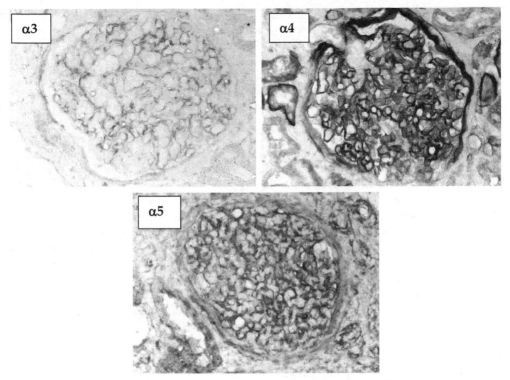

Fig. 6. Immunohistochemistry using monoclonal antibodies against αIV collagen in a kidney biopsy shows α3, α4 and α5 positivity in the GBM.

Unlike most other reports of Alport syndrome, and inconsistent with the disease severity and multi-organ involvement that is generally associated with NC1 mutations, the major manifestation of the renal abnormality in the New Zealand family was proteinuria, which occurred in six of the nine male members who carried the *COL4A5* mutation. Only three of the nine males in the family who inherited the mutation presented with glomerulonephritis and ESRF.

The NC1 domain plays an important role in the selection of α chains for assembly into heterotrimers. In general, substitution and missense mutations in the NC1 domain, as in other regions of *COL4A5*, lead to hematuria, proteinuria, ESRF and sensorineural hearing loss with an overwhelming predominance in males (Barker et al., 1996, Barker et al., 1997, Gross et al., 2002, Hertz et al., 2001, Inoue et al., 1999, Knebelmann et al., 1996, Nakanishi et al., 1994, Netzer et al., 1996, Zhou et al., 1991). A previous study classified X-linked Alport syndrome patients caused by mutations involving the NC1 domain into Type S (severe) phenotype (Gross et al., 2002). Mutations involving other cysteine residues in the NC1 domain have also been reported and include C1486S (Zhou et al., 1991), C1567R (Knebelmann et al., 1996) and C1586R (Hertz et al., 2001) and others (see Figure 7).

Using the proposed classification suggested by Gross and colleagues, the New Zealand family would be placed in 'type S' on the basis of the mutant genotype involving the NC1 domain. However, none of the family members had a phenotype as severe as reported previously in association with NC1 domain mutations. In all cases the presentation of renal disease in the affected male members of the New Zealand family was relatively late. The lack of extra-renal manifestations in the males is also contrary to previous reports correlating NC1 mutations with 'type S' Alport syndrome.

Therefore, while NC1 domain mutations in *COL4A5* are thought to be associated with severe forms of Alport syndrome, the pattern of disease in this family was comparatively mild, and only 27% of the affected or presumed obligate mutant males in the family developed end-stage renal disease. Indeed, considerable variability and phenotypic heterogeneity in the extent of renal disease was observed in the affected males and carrier females. For example, one family member, a 72 year-old male (IV39) shown in Table 2, was later found to carry the sequence alteration, and was initially apparently phenotypically unaffected, but then further investigation revealed proteinuria (1.6g/24h) and hypertension. This man was not biopsied. Furthermore, the presentation of ESRF in one female carrier in this study (III2) leads to the conclusion that female carriers were also affected. Skewed inactivation of the X chromosome could account for this, although other genetic or environmental factors, such as hypertension, could also be contributing factors to the variability in disease progression. This amount of phenotypic variation between males and females is unusual in Alport syndrome, and even more unusual is the fact that none of the family members exhibited the full spectrum of renal, auditory and ocular abnormalities typifying Alport syndrome. The inheritance pattern was clearly consistent with an X-linked dominant mode, albeit with reduced penetrance, as the linkage analysis, together with the scan of the entire *COL4A5* gene for the mutation, clearly identified that the NC1 domain mutation identified in *COL4A5* was the causative mutation in this family.

The Cys1638Tyr alteration in the New Zealand family is predicted to affect the 10th conserved cysteine residue among 12 cysteine residues in the NC1 domain, thus disrupting the disulfide bond linking the C-terminal β3'-β4' hairpin (Fig 7). In the kidney GBM the β3' to β4' disulfide-bridge could be involved in inter-molecular rather than intra-molecular interactions. For example, inter-protomer disulfide cross-links, or interactions with other molecules, such as integrins could involve formation of disulfide linkages to the cysteine residues at positions 66, 72, 177 or 183 in the N-terminal or C-terminal β3-β4 sheets in the type IV collagen NC1 domain.

During protomer assembly the NC1 domains of the α3(IV), α4(IV) and α5(IV) chains specifically interact to select chains for triple-helix formation. In Alport syndrome, NC1 domain cysteine substitutions (see Figure 7) are thought to affect the folding of the monomeric NC1 domain, preventing its participation in trimer assembly. The NC1 domain is also important for network assembly, whereby the NC1 trimers of two protomers specifically interact forming a NC1 hexamer. Variants that result in a loss of, or a defect in any of the α3(IV), α4(IV), or α5(IV) chains result in incorrect folding or assembly of the entire protomer leading to a complete absence of the α3.α4.α5(IV) network from the GBM. However in kidney biopsies from affected patients in this family the α3(IV), α4(IV) and α5(IV) collagens were still present in the GBM, implying that the p.Cys1638Tyr alteration must still allow for the correct assembly of the triple helical protomer. It is possible, however, that an organ-specific defect in protomer function rather than assembly could explain the lack of sensorineural hearing loss or ocular defects in this family, although it remains to be determined whether the p.Cys1638Tyr variant could indeed disrupt the dimerization of two protomers at the C-terminus, thus affecting network assembly.

Further to the New Zealand family, there have been 7 other mutations involving cysteine residues in the NC1 domain (Bekheirnia et al., 2010, Gross et al., 2002, Hertz et al., 2001, Inoue et al., 1999, Knebelman et al., 1996, Wang et al., 2005., Wilson et al., 1997, Zhou et al., 1991) affecting males and females (Figure 7). These mutations are shown together with information of age at the time of diagnosis. From refs 2, 3, 6, 7 and 8 patients were detected during the ages of 6–16 yrs while one was at 31 yrs old. From refs 3 and 2 two males showed ESRF at 14 and 16 yr old, respectively. When clinical information was available, all of the affected individuals appeared to show hearing loss, except for three individuals who had mutations involving C226 (Wang et al, 2005), C177 (Bekheirnia et al., 2010) and C183 (Wilson et al., 2007). The latter report is our own New Zealand family described here. Patients with other mutations of the NC1 domain either lacked a5(IV) in the GBM, or were clinically more severe than the patients with the C177 and C183 mutations, both of which, interestingly involved mutations in the same disulfide linkage.

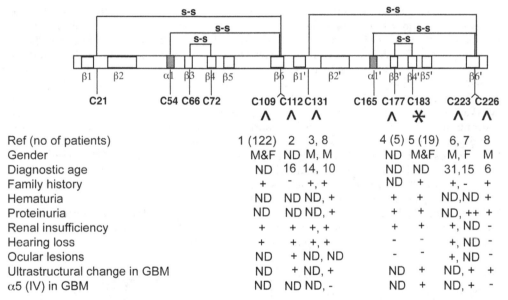

	C109	C112	C131	C165	C177	C183	C223	C226
Ref (no of patients)	1 (122)	2	3, 8		4 (5)	5 (19)	6, 7	8
Gender	M&F	ND	M, M		ND	M&F	M, F	M
Diagnostic age	ND	16	14, 10		ND	ND	31, 15	6
Family history	+	-	+, +		ND	+	+, -	+
Hematuria	ND	ND	ND, +		+	+	ND, ND	+
Proteinuria	ND	ND	ND, +		+	+	ND, ++	+
Renal insufficiency	+	+	+, +		+	+	+, ND	-
Hearing loss	+	+	+, +		-	-	+, ND	-
Ocular lesions	ND	+	ND, ND		-	-	+, ND	-
Ultrastructural change in GBM	ND	+	ND, +		ND	+	ND, +	+
α5 (IV) in GBM	ND	ND	ND, -		ND	+	ND, +	-

Fig. 7. Depiction of NC1 domain showing locations of cysteine sequence alterations, and the clinical details of patients. Shown are the positions of the beta sheet domains (β1-β6, β1'-β6'), and alpha helix (α1, α1') and cysteine residues arranged linearly, and their disulfide linkages. Cysteine residue missense mutations of the NC1 domain that have been previously reported are shown (^), together with the cysteine mutation in the New Zealand family (* under cysteine 183; amino acid numbering in this figure is from the start of the NC1 domain, which is one amino acid longer than in our previous report (Wilson et al, 1997). ND, not determined. +, characteristic is present. -, characteristic is absent. M, male, F, female. Refs; 1 (Zhou et al., 1991); 2 (Knebelmann et al., 1996); 3 (Hertz et al., 2001); 4 (Bekheirnia et al., 2010); 5 (Wilson et al., 1997); 6 (Gross et al., 2002), 7 (Inoue et al., 1999); 8 (Wang et al., 2005).

Kobayashi and colleagues constructed a plasmid containing mutations corresponding to a variety of missense or deletion mutations of the NC1 domain of COL4A5, which were grown in a kidney cell line. The results showed that mutations render the collagen chain defective in terms of heterotrimer formation between the α3, α4 and α5 collagen chains, and/or the secretion of the heterotrimer from cells (Kobayashi et al., 2008). After our publication, these researchers further constructed a plasmid containing the mutation corresponding to Cys1638Tyr into the α5(IV) chain. The results of this experiment showed that heterotrimer formation in the cells and secretion of the α5(IV) chain in the monomeric form from the cells were markedly decreased compared to cells containing the wild-type chain. However, the heterotrimer that was formed from the mutant chain was still secreted from the cells. They concluded that the residual ability of the mutant chain to form and be secreted may have led to the unique mild phenotype formed in the Alport syndrome family with the Cys1638Tyr mutation (Kobayashi & Uchiyama 2010).

7. Renal lesions in carrier women of X-linked Alport Syndrome and Thin Basement Membrane Nephropathy

Thin basement membrane nephropathy (TBMN) is the most common cause of inherited renal disease and its incidence has been reported to be as high as 1% of the world population (Kashtan 2005, Tazon et al., 2003, Wang & Savige 2005). It is defined as diffuse thinning of the GBM characterised by persistent glomerular hematuria, minimal proteinuria, and normal renal function. Genetic studies of TBMN have helped to establish that many patients with benign familial hematuria are actually the carriers of autosomal recessive Alport syndrome, carrying mutations only in the one allele of *COL4A3* or *COL4A4* (Voskarides et al., 2008). A novel missense mutation of *COL4A3* in a Chinese Han consanguineous family was identified and the underlying pathogenic role in the homozygous form was investigated in autosomal recessive Alport syndrome and in the hetrozygous form in TBMN within the identical family (Hou et al., 2007). These studies showed that while TBMN manifest as a dominant disorder in the family with the *COL4A3* mutation, Alport syndrome manifested as a recessive disease in the same family. In our experience, by light microscopy the kidney glomerular features of the carrier females (eg V40) of X-linked Alport syndrome in the New Zealand family were relatively unremarkable. However there was occasional periglomerular fibrosis and focal areas of protein casts in occasional tubules associated with epithelial cell atrophy (Fig 8A and 8B).

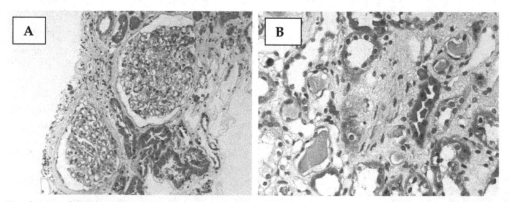

Fig. 8. Histology from a carrier mother (V40) in the New Zealand family with Alport syndrome. (A) Two glomeruli show periglomerular fibrosis. Glomerular tufts are relatively unremarkable. (B) Focal areas show protein casts in occasional tubules that show atrophic epithelial cells.

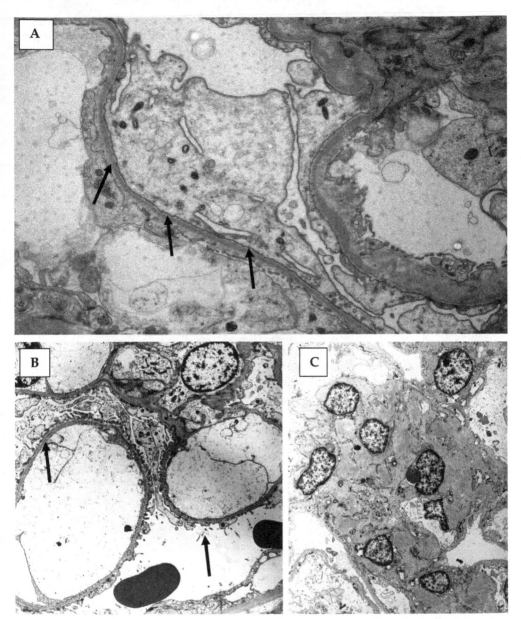

Fig. 9. Electron microscopy of carrier females (V40 and IV28). (A) The same carrier mother (V40) of the Figure 8 and (B) another carrier female (IV28), both showing focal areas of extremely thin GBM (arrows). (C) In addition there are focal areas of irregular GBM thickening. (A x7,400, B x3,000, C x2,100, original magnification respectively).

Electron microscopic findings on one of the carrier women of the New Zealand X-linked Alport syndrome family showed severe thinning of the GBM (Fig 9A) where the thickness was approximately 150 nm, and much thinner than the normal GBM (300-400 nm). Another carrier woman also showed focal areas of severely thin GBM (Fig 9B). In addition there were occasional regional areas of thick segments of GBM (Fig 9C). It is notable that the typical basket weave appearance or splitting was not present in the females. One message to take from these studies is that electron microscopic examination of the kidneys in carrier women with clinical symptoms should be mandatory because the light microscopic observations on their own often provide unremarkable findings or only subtle changes and may not show a full range of pathology.

Although TBMN has been regarded as a benign condition with an excellent prognosis, as high as 38% of *COL4A3/COL4A4* heterozygous mutant carriers, of all ages, develop chronic renal failure and 19.5% progress to ESRF (Voskarides et al., 2008). These authors emphasize a strong association between TBMN and focal segmental glomerulosclerosis (FSGS). Several studies report that TBMN predisposes to premature glomerular obsolescence and that this may then lead to late onset renal insufficiency followed by ESRF (Nieuhof et al., 1997, Nogueira et al., 2000). Other studies suggest that there may be other factors that predispose transition from TBMN to FSGS (Sue et al., 2004). These factors could be due to involvement of modifier genes such as podocyte specific genes or environmental factors.

These findings concur with a previous report (Jais et al., 2003) in that hematuria was observed in 95% of 323 female carriers of X-linked Alport syndrome. Proteinuria, hearing loss, and ocular defects also developed in 75%, 28%, and 15%, respectively. Moreover, the probability of developing ESRF or deafness before the age of 40 yr was 12% and 10%, respectively, in females versus 90% and 80%, respectively in men. In their study ultrastructural change of the GBM were found in 26 of 28 carriers and consisted of typically thick and split or alternatively thick and thin GBM in 19 patients. When taken together, our results and those of Jais et al (2003) suggest that TBMN may frequently develop in carrier women with a heterozygous *COL4A5* mutation.

8. Conclusions

In conclusion, mild forms of Alport syndrome may occur in association with certain mutations in the collagenous domain of the collagen proteins. In addition, we showed a p.Cys1638Tyr mutation occurring within the NC1 domain of *COL4A5* in a New Zealand family was associated with a mild form of Alport syndrome. Mild forms of Alport syndrome also occur in females with *COL4A5* mutations, in whom there is considerable phenotypic variation. In particular, it appears that electron microscopy carried out in female carriers of *COL4A5* mutations reveals much more about the health of their kidneys than does routine light microscopy alone. The abnormalities present in the kidneys of female carriers suggest that with appropriate management of diet and hypertension this could prevent the onset of renal disease in these women. Additional investigations of the pathogenic role of *COL4A5* mutations in female members of Alport families, and of the role of the NC1 domain in the New Zealand family, will further help to better understand the role of collagens in the structure and function of the filtration barrier in the GBM.

9. Acknowledgments

The authors thank Dr Y Sado, for his generous gift of rat monoclonal antibodies H11, H22, H31, H43, H53 and H63 specific for the $\alpha1(IV)$, $\alpha2(IV)$, $\alpha3(IV)$, $\alpha4(IV)$, $\alpha5(IV)$, and $\alpha6(IV)$

collagen, Dr Rob Walker for clinical advice, and Mr Richard Eisenwood and Ms Gillian Maudsley for carrying out electron microscopy and measurement. This work has been supported by the Otago Medical Research Foundation, the Healthcare Otago Charitable Trust, and the NZ Institute for Cancer Research Trust.

10. References

Alport, A. (1927). Hereditary familial congenital haemorrhagic nephritis. *Br Med J*, Vol.1, pp. 504-506, ISSN 0958-8146

Arup Laboratories. ARUP Online Scientific Resource: ALPORT database display gene, 2011. Available at: http://www.arup.utah.edu/database/ALPORT/ALPORT_welcome.php?col=loc. *Accessed April21, 2011*

Barker, D., Denison, J., Atkin, C. & Gregory, M. (1997). Common ancestry of three Ashkenazi-American families with Alport syndrome and COL4A5 R1677Q. *Hum Genet*, Vol.99, No.5, pp. 681–684, ISSN 0304-6717

Barker, D., Pruchno, C., Jiang, X., Atkin, C., Stone, E., Denison, J., Fain, P. & Gregory, M. (1996). A mutation causing Alport Syndrome with tardive hearing loss is common in the Western United States. *Am J Hum Genet*, Vol.58, No.6, pp. 1157–1165, ISSN 0002-9297

Bekheirnia, M., Berenice, R., Gregory, M,, McFann, K, Shamshirsaz, A., Masoumi, A. & Schrier, R. (2010). Genotype–phenotype correlation in X-Linked Alport syndrome. *J Am Soc Nephrol*, Vol.21, No.5, pp. 876-883, ISSN 1046-6673

Borza, D., Bondar, O., Ninomiya, Y., Sado, Y., Naito, I., Todd, P. & Hudson, B. (2001). The NC1 domain of collagen IV encodes a novel network composed of the alpha 1, alpha 2, alpha 5, and alpha 6 chains in smooth muscle basement membranes. *J Biol Chem*, Vol.276, No.30, pp. 28532-28540, ISSN 0021-9258

Boutaud, A., Borza, D., Bondar, O., Gunwar, S., Netzer, K., Singh, N., Ninomiya, Y., Sado, Y., Noelken, M. & Hudson, B. (2000). Type IV collagen of the glomerular basement membrane. Evidence that the chain specificity of network assembly is encoded by the noncollagenous NC1 domains. *J Biol Chem*, Vol.275, No.39, pp. 30716-3024, ISSN 0021-9258

Cosgrove, D., Samuelson, G., Meehan, D., Miller, C., McGee, J., Walsh, E. & Siegel M. (1998). Ultrastructural, physiological, and molecular defects in the inner ear of a gene knockout mouse model for autosomal Alport syndrome. *Hear Res*, Vol.121, No.1-2, pp. 84-98, ISSN 0378-5995

Flinter, F., Cameron, J., Chantler, C., Houston, I. & Bobrow, M. (1988). Genetics of classic Alport's syndrome. *Lancet*, Vol.29, No.2, pp. 1005–1007, ISSN 1089-4969

Gross, O., Netzer, K-O., Lambrecht, R., Seibolt, S. & Weber, M. (2002). Meta-analysis of genotype–phenotype correlation in X-linked Alport syndrome: impact on clinical counselling. *Nephrol Dial Transplant*, Vol.17, No.7, pp. 1218-1227, ISSN 0931-0509

Harvey, S., Zheng, K., Sado, Y., Naito, I., Ninomiya, Y., Jacobs, R., Hudson, B. & Thorner, P. (1998). Role of distinct type IV collagen networks in glomerular development and function. *Kidney Int*, Vol.54, No.6, pp. 1857-1866, ISSN 0391-6510

Hertz, J., Juncker, I., Persson, U., Matthijs, G., Schmidtke, J., Petersen, M., Kjeldsen, M. & Gregersen, N. (2001). Detection of mutations in the COL4A5 gene by SSCP in X-linked Alport syndrome. *Hum Mutat*, Vol.18, No.2, pp. 141–148, ISSN 1098-1004

Hou, P., Chen, Y., Ding, J., Li, G. & Zhang, H. (2007). Novel mutation of COL4A3 presents a different contribution to Alport syndrome and thin basement membrane nephropathy. *Am J Nephrol*, Vol.27, No.5, pp. 538-544, ISSN 0360-7615

Huang, T., Cheng, A., Stupak, H., Liu, W., Kim, A., Staecker, H., Lefebvre, P., Malgrange, B., Kopke, R., Moonen, G. & Van De Water, T. Oxidative stress-induced apoptosis of cochlear sensory cells: otoprotective strategies (2000). *Int J Dev Neurosci*, Vol.18, No.2-3, pp. 259-270, ISSN 0736-5748

Hudson, B., Reeders, S. & Tryggvason, K. (1993). Type IV collagen: structure, gene organization, and role in human disease. Molecular basis of Goodpasture and Alport syndromes and diffuse leiomyomatosis. *J Biol Chem*, Vol.268, No.35, pp. 26033-26036, ISSN 0250-8095

Hudson, B., Tryggvason, K., Sundaramoorthy, M. & Neilson, E. (2003). Alport's syndrome, Goodpasture's syndrome, and type IV collage. *New Engl J Med*, Vol.348, No.25, pp. 2543-2556, ISSN 0250-8095

Hudson, B. (2004). The molecular basis of Goodpasture and Alport syndromes: beacons for the discovery of the collagen IV family. *J Am Soc Nephrol*, Vol. 5, pp. 2514–2527, ISSN 1046-6673

Inoue, Y., Nishio, H., Shirakawa, T., Nakanishi, K., Nakamura, H., Sumino, K., Nishiyama, K., Iijima, K. & Yoshikawa, N. (1999). Detection of mutations in the COL4A5 gene in over 90% of male patients with X-linked Alport's syndrome by RT-PCR and direct sequencing. *Am J Kidney Dis*, Vol.34, No.5, pp. 854–862, ISSN 0272-6386

Jais, J., Knebelmann, B., Giatras, I., De Marchi, M., Rizzoni, G., Renieri, A., Weber, M., Gross, O., Netzer, K-O., Flinter, F., Pirson, Y., Verellen, C., Wieslander, J., Persson, U., Tryggvason, K., Martin, P., Hertz, J., Schröder, C., Sanak, M., Krejcova, S., Carvalho, M., Saus, J., Antignac, C., Smeets, H. & *Gubler, M. (2000)*. X-linked Alport Syndrome: Natural history in 195 families and genotype- phenotype correlations in males. *J Am Soc Nephrol, Vol.11, No.4, pp. 649-657, ISSN 1046-6673*

Jais, J., Knebelmann, B., Giatras, I., De Marchi, M., Rizzoni, G., Renieri, A., Weber, M., Gross, O., Netzer, K-O., Flinter, F., Pirson, Y., Verellen, C., Wieslander, J., Persson, U., Tryggvason, K., Martin, P., Hertz, J., Schröder, C., Sanak, M., Krejcova, S., Carvalho, M., Saus, J., Antignac, C., Smeets, H. & Gubler, M. (2003). X-linked Alport Syndrome: Natural history and genotype-phenotype correlation in girls and women belonging to 195 families: A "European community Alport syndrome concerted action study. *J Am Soc Nephrol*, Vol.14, No.10, pp. 2603-2610, ISSN 1046-6673

Jefferson, J., Lemmink, H., Hughes, A., Hill, C, Smeets, H., Doherty, C. & Maxwell, A. (1997). Autosomal dominant Alport syndrome linked to the type IV collage $\alpha 3$ and $\alpha 4$ genes (COL4A3 and COL4A4). *Nephrol Dial Transplant*, Vol.12, No.8, pp. 1595-1599, ISSN 0931-0509

Kalluri, R., Shield, C., Todd, P., Hudson, B. & Neilson, E. (1997). Isoform switching of type IV collagen is developmentally arrested in X-linked Alport syndrome leading to increased susceptibility of renal basement membranes to endoproteolysis. *J Clin Invest*, Vol.99, No.10, pp. 2470-2478, ISSN 0021-9738

Kalluri, R., Cantley, L., Kerjaschki, D. & Neilson, E. (2000). Reactive oxygen species expose cryptic epitopes associated with autoimmune goodpasture syndrome. *J Biol Chem*, Vol.275, No.26, pp. 20027-20032, ISSN 0021-9258

Kashtan, C. (2005). Familial hematurias: what we know and what we don't. *Pediatr Nephrol*, Vol.20, pp. 1027–1035, ISSN 0391-6510

Knebelmann, B., Breillat, C., Forestier, L., Knebelmann, B., Breillat, C., Forestier, L., Arrondel, C., Jacassier, D., Giatras, I., Drouot, L., Deschênes, G., ., Broyer, M., Gubler, M. & Antignac, C. (1996). Spectrum of mutations in the COL4A5 collagen gene in X-linked Alport syndrome. *Am J Hum Genet*, Vol.59, No.6, pp. 1221–1232, ISSN 0002-9297

Kobayashi, T., Kakihara, T. & Uchiyama, M. (2008): Mutational analysis of type IV collagen alpha5 chain, with respect to heterotrimer formation. *Biochem Biophys Res Commun*, Vol.366, No.1, pp. 60-65, ISSN 0006-291X

Kobayashi, T. & Uchiyama, M. (2010). Mutant-type alpha5(IV) collagen in a mild form of Alport syndrome has residual ability to form a heterotrimer. *Pediatr Nephrol*, Vol.25, No.6, pp. 1169-1172, ISSN 0391-6510

Miner, J. (2003). A molecular look at the glomerular barrier. Nephron. *Exp Nephrol*, Vol.94, pp. 119–122, ISSN 1018-7782

Mochizuki, T., Lemmink, H., Mariyama, M., Antignac, C., Gubler, M., Pirson, Y., Verellen-Dumoulin, C., Chan, B., Schroder, C., Smeets, H. & Reeders, S. (1994). Identification of mutations in the α3(IV) and α4(IV) collagen genes inautosomal recessive Alport syndrome. *Nat Genet*, Vol.8, pp. 77–82, ISSN 1061-0056

Naito, I., Kawai, S., Nomura, S., Sado, Y. & Osawa, G. (1996). Relationship between COL4A5 gene mutation and distribution of type IV collagen in male X-linked Alport syndrome. Japanese Alport Network. *Kidney Int*, Vol.50, No.1, pp. 304–311, ISSN 0391-6510

Naito, I., Ninomiya, Y. & Nomura S. (2003). Immunohistochemical diagnosis of Alport's syndrome in paraffin-embedded renal sections: antigen retrieval with autoclave heating. *Med Electron Microsc*, Vol.36, pp. 1–7, ISSN 0914-4287

Nakanishi, K., Yoshikawa, N., Iijima, K., Kitagawa, K., Nakamura, H., Ito, H., Yoshioka, K., Kagawa, M. & Sado, Y. (1994). Immunohistochemical study of alpha 1-5 chains of type IV collagen in hereditary nephritis. *Kidney Int*, Vol.46, No.5, pp. 1413–1421, ISSN 0391-6510

Netzer, K., Seibold, S., Gross, O., Lambrecht, R. & Weber, M. (1996). Use of psoralen-coupled nucleotide primers for screening of COL4A5 mutations in Alport syndrome. *Kidney Int*, Vol.50, pp. 1363–1367, ISSN 1391-6510

Nieuwhof, C., de Heer, F., de Leeuw, P. & van Breda Vriesman, P. (1997). Thin GBM nephropathy: premature glomerular obsolescence is associated with hypertention and late onset renal failure. *Kidny Int*, Vol.51, No.5, pp. 1596-1601, ISSN 0391-6510

Nogueira, M., Cartwright, J.Jr., Horn, K., Doe, N., Shappell, S., Barrios, R., Coroneos, E. & Truong, L. (2000). Thin basement membrane disease with heavy proteinuria or nephritic syndrome at presentation. *Am J Kidney Dis*, Vol.35, No.4, E15, ISSN 0272-6386

Reddan, J., Steiger, C., Dziedzic, D. & Gordon, S. (1996). Regional differences in the distribution of catalase in the epithelium of the ocular lens. *Cell Mol Biol* (Noisy-le-grand), Vol.42, No.2, pp. 209-219, ISSN 0145-5680

Smeets, H., Melenhorst, J., Lemmink, H., Schröder, C., Nelen, M., Zhou, J., Hostikka, S., Tryggvason, K., Ropers, H., Jansweijer, M., Monnens, L., Brunner, H. & van Oost, B. (1992). Different mutations in the COL4A5 collagen gene in two patients with different features of Alport syndrome. *Kidney Int*, Vol.42, No.1, pp. 83-88, ISSN 0391-6510

Sue, Y., Huang, J., Hsieh, R. & Chen, F. (2004). Clinical features of thin basement membrane disease and associated glomerulonephritis. *Nephrology*, Vol.9, No.1, pp. 14-18, ISSN 1320-5358

Tazon, V., Badenas, C., Ars, E., Lens, X., Mila, M., Darnell, A. & Torra, R. (2003): Autosomal recessive Alport's syndrome and benign familial hematuria are collagen type IV diseases. *Am J Kidney Dis*, Vol.42, pp. 952–959, ISSN 0272-6386

Timpl, R., Wiedemann, H., van Delden, V., Furthmayr, H. & Kühn, K. (1981). A network model for the organization of type IV collagen molecules in basement membranes. *Eur J Biochem*, Vol.120, No.2, pp. 203–211, ISSN 0014-2956

Voskarides, K., Pierides, A. & Deltas, C. (2008). *COL4A3/COL4A4* mutations link familial hematuria and focal segmental glomerulosclerosis. Glomerular epithelium destruction via basement membrane thinning? *Connect Tissue Res*, Vol.49, No.3. pp. 283-288, ISSN 0074-767X

Wang, Y. & Savige, J. (2005). The epidemiology of thin basement membrane nephropathy. *Semin Nephrol*, Vol.25, pp. 136-139, ISSN 0270-9295

Wang, F., Wang, Y., Ding, J., Yang, J. ((2005). Detection of mutations in the COL4A5 gene by analyzing cDNA of skin fibroblasts. *Kidney Int*, Vol 67, pp. 1268-1274, ISSN 0391-6510

Wilson, J., Yoon, H-S., Walker, R. & Eccles, M. (2007). A novel Cys1638Tyr NC1 domain substitution in a5(IV) collagen causes Alport syndrome with late onset renal failure without hearing loss or eye abnormalities. *Nephrol Dial Transplant*, Vol.22, No.5, pp. 1338-1346, ISSN 0931-0509

Yoshioka, K., Hino, S., Takemura, T., Maki, S., Wieslander, J., Takekoshi, Y., Makino, H., Kagawa, M., Sado, Y. & Kashtan, C. (1994). Type IV collagen alpha 5 chain. Normal distribution and abnormalities in X-linked Alport syndrome revealed by monoclonal antibody. *Am J Pathol*, Vol.144, No.5, pp. 986-96, ISSN 0002-9440

Zhou, J., Barker, D., Hostikka, S., Gregory, M., Atkin, C. & Tryggvason, K. (1991). Single base mutation in alpha 5(IV) collagen chain gene converting a conserved cysteine to serine in Alport syndrome. *Genomics*, Vol.9, No.1, pp. 10–18, ISSN 1471-2164

Zhou, J. & Reeders, S. (1996). The α chains of type IV collagen, In: *Molecular Pathology and Genetics of Alport Syndrome*, Tryggvason K, pp. (80-104), Karger, ISBN 0302-5144, Basel, Switzerland

Part 3

Miscellaneous Topics

11

Blood Pressure Control in Patients with Glomerulonephritis

Toshihiko Ishimitsu
Department of Hypertension and Cardiorenal Medicine,
Dokkyo Medical University, Mibu, Tochigi,
Japan

1. Introduction

Although the expanding prevalence of lifestyle-related diseases such as diabetes mellitus and hypertension which ultimately cause renal dysfunction, glomerulonephritis still remains as one of the major causes of end-stage renal failure in most countries all over the world. In addition to the immunological therapy using corticosteroids and immunosuppressants, management of non-immunological risk factors such as hypertension, obesity and disorders of glucose and lipid metabolism greatly affect the prognosis of renal function in the treatment of patients with glomerulonephritis. Especially, hypertension is a pivotal risk factor for the progression of renal injuries and the adequate blood pressure control is a matter of primary importance in order to prevent the development of renal dysfunction.

In this chapter, the importance of blood pressure control is stressed referring the evidence thus far, and current topics and future prospects are discussed as to the matters such as target blood pressure levels and choices of antihypertensive agents.

2. Target blood pressure

Generally, hypertension is diagnosed when the systolic blood pressure is higher than 140mmHg and/or the diastolic blood pressure is higher than 90mmHg. However, this is an arbitrary definition and the linear relation between the blood pressure level and the risk of renal dysfunction can be extended even in the normotensive range in epidemiological studies. Figure 1 shows the relations of blood pressure level categories and the risk of developing end-stage renal failure in 17-year follow-up study of Okinawa prefecture residents in Japan (1). Naturally, hypertension increases the risk of renal failure with elevating grade of blood pressure levels. Moreover, blood pressure levels lower than 140/90mmHg but higher than 130/85mmHg, namely the high-normal blood pressure, offers a significant risk for future development of renal failure.

As for the target blood pressure level in the treatment of glomerulonephritis patients, Figure 2 depicts the outcomes of Modification of Diet in Renal Disease (MDRD) study (2) in which the blood pressure control level less than 125/75mmHg brought about slower GFR reduction than the level less than 140/90mmHg in subjects with nondiabetic renal diseases especially when the proteinuria was prominent. Similarly, Figure 3 plots the annual decrease rates of GFR against achieved blood pressure levels in hypertensive subjects with renal diseases (3). In patients whose hypertension was not treated, GFR decreased by more than 10mL/min per year. When the blood pressure was lowered to 140/90mmHg, the rate of annual GFR decline was reduced by half. However, considering that the physiological annual GFR decline with aging is about 1mL/min, the annual GFR decline in 140/90mmHg subjects is faster than the natural rate. As compared with this, strict blood pressure lowering to 130/85mmHg or 130/80mmHg yielded retardation of GFR decline to a nearly physiological level in subjects with renal diseases.

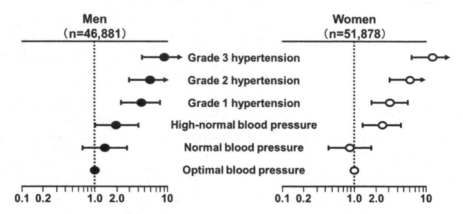

Fig. 1. Relationship between the incidence of end-stage renal failure and the blood pressure level (1). The incidence of end-stage renal failure is increased not only in hypertensive subjects but also in subjects with high-normal blood pressure ranging 130-139/85-89 mmHg as compared with lower normal blood pressure subjects.

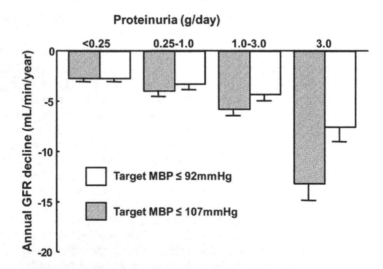

Fig. 2. The annual decrease in glomerular filtration rate (GFR) in nondiabetic renal disease patients of The Modification of Diet in Renal Disease(MDRD) Study. (2)

Thus, it is suggested that the blood pressure should be lowered below the high-normal level in glomerulonephritis patients in order to maximally slow the progression of renal dysfunction. Therefore, the American, European and Japanese guidelines for the management of hypertension recommend the target blood pressure level of less than 130/80mmHg in patients with chronic kidney disease (CKD) (4-6).

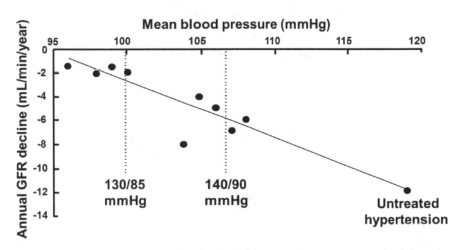

Fig. 3. Relationship between the annual decrease in glomerular filtration rate (GFR) and the achieved mean blood pressure level in studies treated hypertensive patients with renal diseases (3). The GFR decline rate was suppressed to the level near to the physiological decrease with aging in patients whose blood pressure was lowered under 130/85mmHg.

3. Glomerular hypertension and hyperfiltration

According to the hyperfiltration theory proposed by Hostteter and Brenner (7,8), increases in glomerular capillary pressure, referred to as glomerular hypertension, play an important role in the development and the progression of glomerular injuries ultimately resulting in glomerular sclerosis and the loss of its nephron. As indicated in Figure 4, not only high blood pressure but also increased salt intake and decreased urinary sodium excretion resulting in body fluid volume expansion raise intraglomerular capillary pressure and cause glomerular hypertension. In addition, the increases in protein intake and glomerular efferent arteriolar resistance are also the factors that contribute to the elevation of intraglomerular capillary pressure. Long-lasting of sustained glomerular hypertension impairs glomerular capillary endothelium and allows filtration of plasma protein molecules, followed by widening of mesangial area, obstruction of capillary lumen, hyalinosis of glomerular tuft and finally resulting in glomerular sclerosis, abolition of blood flow and filtration function. The loss of glomeruli brings about the atrophy of following renal tubules and nephrons themselves. Once a certain proportion of nephrons fall into atrophy, the intraglomerular capillary pressure and the single nephron filtration glomerular filtration rate of remaining glomeruli increase in order to compensate the reduced renal blood flow and maintain the glomerular filtration rate, which consequently promote further development of glomerular hypertension.

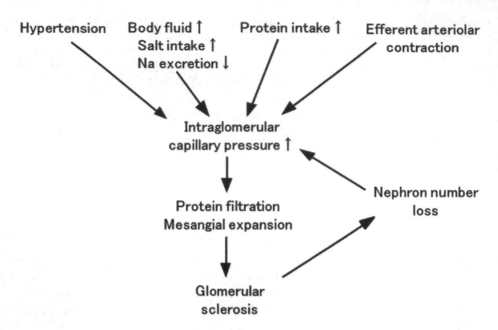

Fig. 4. Relations of factors contributing to the increase in intraglomerular capillary pressure and progression of glomerular sclerosis.

In order to stop the progression of this vicious cycle, comprehensive control of factors influencing the intraglomerular capillary pressure elevation such as arterial hypertension and intakes of salt and protein is needed. As mentioned concerning the target blood pressure, strict blood pressure control is important in patients with glomerulonephritis. In controlling the blood pressure, it should be kept in mind that reduction of intraglomerular capillary pressure as well as systemic arterial pressure is essential in order to achieve maximally effective inhibition of glomerular injuries and renal dysfunction. With regard to the hemodynamic aspect of renal microcirculation, intraglomerular capillary pressure is regulated by the balance between vascular resistances of afferent and efferent glomerular arterioles as depicted in Figure 5. A number of neural and humoral factors are known to affect the contraction and dilation of glomerular arterioles. Among them, the renin-angiotensin-aldosterone (RAA) system indicated in Figure 6 is assumed to play a pivotal role in the regulation of glomerular hemodynamics. Especially, angiotensin II, a peptide exhibiting prominent bioactivities in the RAA system, induce strong contraction of efferent rather than afferent glomerular arterioles. In addition, angiotensin II facilitates mesangial cell proliferation, increases oxidative stress by activating NAD(P)H oxidase, and induce proinflammatory transcription factor NF-κB (9,10). These versatile effects of angiotensin II also contribute to the progression of renal tissue injuries.

On the other hand, angiotensin II stimulates the adrenal cortex to secrete aldosterone, a major mineralocorticoid, which facilitates renal tubular reabsorption of sodium resulting in blood and body fluid volume expansion and blood pressure elevation. Besides this well-known effect, aldosterone has been shown to promote renal tissue fibrosis and production of extracellular matrices such as collagen (9-11). Moreover, aldosterone injures endothelial, epithelial and mesangial cells of glomeruli. In addition, aldosterone, like angiotensin II, constricts the efferent arterioles preferably to the afferent arteriole and increase the intraglomerular capillary pressure and filtration of plasma protein molecules. Thus, aldosterone is also assumed to be a factor exerting detrimental effects to the progression of glomerular diseases.

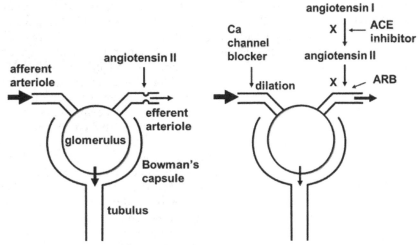

Fig. 5. The structure of glomeruli and factors relating to the hemodynamics and hydrauric pressure of glomeruli and glomerular arterioles.

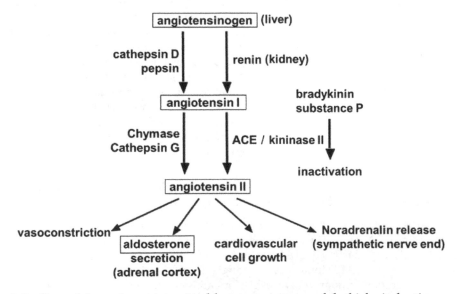

Fig. 6. Outlines of the renin-angiotensin-aldosterone system and the biological actions elicited by its components.

Several other hormones and autacoids are known to elicit dilation or contraction of the glomerular arterioles. Atrial natriuretic peptide (ANP), produced by the heart, dilates the afferent arteriole and preserves renal and glomerular blood flow in the state of heart failure (12). This action is supposed to work also in glomerulonephritis patients with reduced renal function because the plasma ANP level is increased by body fluid volume increase and reduced clearance in the kidney. Vascular endothelium produces vasoactive substances such as nitric oxide (NO) and endothelin (ET). NO preferentially dilates and ET preferentially contract the afferent arterioles (13,14). NO is supposed to participate in the mechanism of increased glomerular filtration in the early stage of diabetic nephropathy, however, the NO synthase inhibition has been shown to increase intraglomerular capillary pressure in experimental glomerulonephritis (15,16). The pathophysiological implication of ET in the glomerular circulation is not well understood. The kidney has abundant ability to produce prostaglandins (PG) from arachidonic acid and PGE_2 which facilitates natriuresis and dilates the afferent arterioles is the major PG produced in the kidney. As compared with this, PGI_2 produced by vascular endothelium dilates both the afferent and the efferent arterioles (17). Nonsteroidal anti-inflammatory drugs such as indomethacin, which inhibit cyclooxygenase and PG production, can cause renal dysfunction as the adverse effect. The inflammatory process in the pathogenesis of glomerulonephritis is supposed to stimulate PG production in the kidney. This possibly increases glomerular and renal blood flow on one hand, however, may rather increase intraglomerular pressure on the other hand by preferentially dilating the afferent arterioles. However, it has been reported that the long-term administration of PGI_2 analogue mitigated the progression of renal dysfunction without increasing intraglomerular capillary pressure in patients with chronic glomerulonephritis (18).

Taken these together into consideration, it is suggested that the enhancement of RAA system is harmful to the glomeruli and the kidney via the nocuous actions of angiotensin II and aldosterone. Reductions in renal function generally cause an increase in body fluid volume which inhibits plasma renin activity and concentrations of angiotensin II and aldosterone. Therefore, the circulating components of RAA system is supposed to be rather suppressed in patients with advanced glomerulonephritis. However, the renal and cardiovascular cells have been shown to produce components of RAA system such as renin, angiotensin converting enzyme (ACE) and aldosterone. In addition, angiotensinogen produced by the liver is abundant in plasma. Therefore, it is thought that angiotensin II and aldosterone are locally produced in the renal and cardiovascular systems and their concentrations in the tissues may be higher than in plasma. And, it is possible that the renal tissue RAA system is rather enhanced and contributes to the progression of renal injuries in patients with advanced glomerulonephritis although the circulating components of RAA system are suppressed.

4. Inhibitors of renin-angiotensin-aldosterone system in antihypertensive drug therapy for patients with glomerulonephritis

The precedent sections stressed the importance of strict blood pressure control and the implications of RAA system in the management of renal diseases in order to prevent the progression of renal dysfunction efficiently and effectively. In this context, inhibitors of RAA system such as ACE inhibitors and angiotensin II receptor antagonists (ARB) are supposed to provide renoprotective effects in addition to their hypotensive effects by inhibiting the detrimental actions of angiotensin II and aldosterone. Especially, these inhibitors of RAA system preferentially dilate the efferent arterioles as compared to the afferent arterioles and thereby lower intraglomerular capillary pressure effectively (Figure 5). Anderson et al. (19) have shown that an ACE inhibitor lowers intraglomerular capillary pressure, reduces proteinuria and inhibits the progression of glomerular sclerosis more prominently than other antihypertensive drugs in rats with reduced renal mass in which the circulating RAA system is thought to be suppressed.

In human, it is a distinctive feature that the intraglomerular capillary pressure is elevated and the GFR is increased at the early stage of diabetic nephropathy. This glomerular hypertension facilitates the progression of diabetic nephropathy stages, namely, microalbuminuria, overt proteinuria, a GFR reduction, a serum creatinine increase and end-stage renal failure. Taguma et al. (20) have first reported that an ACE inhibitor reduces proteinuria in patients with diabetic nephropathy, and it is suggested that the suppression of angiotensin II generation brings about alleviation of glomerular hypertension and reduce hydrauric transcapillary filtration pressure of protein. After that, Lewis et al. (21) performed the multi-center collaborative prospective study evaluating the renoprotective effects of an ACE inhibitor in patients with type 1 diabetes mellitus presenting overt proteinuria and demonstrated that captopril inhibited the serum creatinine increase and the incidence of end-stage renal failure. As well as ACE inhibitors, multiple lines of later clinical studies have indicated that ARB are effective in retarding the progression of nephropathy at each stage in patients with type 2 diabetes (22-24).

With regard to the non-diabetic renal disease such as glomerulonephritis, the ACE Inhibition in Progressive Renal Insufficiency (AIPRI) study (25) and Ramipril Efficacy in Nephropathy (REIN) study (26) showed that ACE inhibitors delay the progression of renal insufficiency in European patients with non-diabetic renal disease. Furthermore, African American Study of Kidney Disease and Hypertension (AASK) (27) suggested that ACE inhibitors slow renal disease progression in African American patients with hypertensive renal disease. Also as for the Asian population, we have reported that an ACE inhibitor and an ARB are effective in reducing proteinuria and slowing the deterioration of renal function in Japanese patients with chronic glomerulonephritis (28,29). Namely, an ACE inhibitor, benazepril, or an ARB, valsartan, inhibited the increase in serum creatinine and reduced proteinuria by 30-40% as compared with placebo (Figure 7,8). In addition, there is another study reported that an ACE inhibitor improved renal outcomes in Chinese patients with advanced stage of non-diabetic renal disease whose serum creatinine ranged 3.1 to 5.0mg/dL (30).

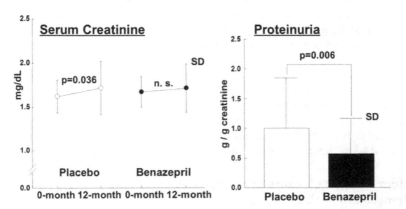

Fig. 7. Changes in serum creatinine concentrations and urinary protein excretions in glomerulonephritis patients given the ACE inhibitor or the placebo (28).

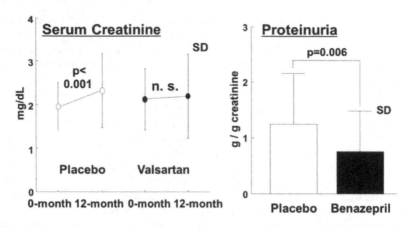

Fig. 8. Changes in serum creatinine concentrations and urinary protein excretions in glomerulonephritis patients given the angiotensin II receptor blocker (ARB) or the placebo (29).

As compared with ACE inhibitors and ARB, clinical evidence of other inhibitors of RAA system, such as renin inhibitors and aldosterone blockers seems less abundant regarding their renoprotecitve effects in patients with glomerulonephritis. In the cascade of RAA system indicated in Figure 6, conversion of angiotensinogen to angiotensin I by the enzymatic action of renin is assumed to be a rate-limiting step. Therefore, renin inhibitors such as aliskiren are thought to be theoretically effective in suppressing the activity of RAA system. Aliskiren, alone or in combination with ARB, has been shown to reduce albuminuria and proteinuria in patients with diabetic nephropathy (31,32), however, its efficacy in patients with glomerulonephritis is to be studied.

ACE inhibitors are widely used in the treatment of hypertension and renal disease. They reduce plasma levels of angiotensin II and aldosterone. However, it has been shown that the plasma aldosterone concentration rather increases in a certain portion of patients after month of long-term administration and this phenomenon is recognized as aldosterone breakthrough. Sato et al. (33) have reported that the long-term ACE inhibitor treatment failed to reduce albuminuria in patients with diabetic nephropathy who had developed aldosterone breakthrough, however, the albuminuria significantly reduced after adding spironolactone, an aldosterone blocker. Although spironolactone can cause adverse effects by its partially estrogenic actions such as gynecomastia and menstrual disorder which sometimes hamper the continuation of administration, eplerenone, a newly developed aldosterone blocker, is much more specific to the mineralocorticoid receptor and almost free from such estrogenic side effects. There is paucity of clinical evidence as to the effects of aldosterone blockers in glomerulonephritis patients, however, the use of an aldosterone blocker in addition to an ACE inhibitor or an ARB would be expected to exhibit protective effects against the progressions of glomerular injuries and renal dysfunction.

5. Calcium channel blockers in antihypertensive drug therapy for patients with glomerulonephritis

Although the guidelines for hypertension management recommend strict blood pressure control in order to prevent organ injuries and cardiovascular diseases, the target blood pressure is generally achieved only in less than a half of hypertensive patients under treatment. In terms of lowering blood pressure, the hypotensive effect of CCB, directly dilating vascular smooth muscle, is consistently reliable in various conditions including glomerulonephritis patients. Therefore, the addition of CCB to RAA system inhibitors is expected to bring about effective blood pressure reduction with few chances to cause impeding adverse effects.

Ca channels residing in the plasma membrane of cells are composed five subunits; $\alpha 1$, $\alpha 2$, β, γ and δ. Among them, the $\alpha 1$ subunit conforming Ca^{2+} ion pathway has isoforms of L, N, P/Q, R and T. There are three isoforms of $\alpha 1$ subunit, L, N and T in the cardiovascular tissues, and Table 1 shows their distributions, functions and pharmacological blockers. Dihydropyridine (DHP) CCB, which are generally used as hypertensive drugs, blocks the L-type Ca channels existing in the arterial smooth muscle. With regard to the glomerular arterioles, because the afferent but not the efferent arterioles have the L-type channels, DHP CCB generally preferentially dilate the afferent arterioles. Therefore, it is supposed that the reduction in intraglomerular capillary pressure may not be so prominent as compared with the reduction in systemic arterial pressure. In this respect, the N-type and the T-type channels exist both in the afferent and the efferent arterioles and the blockers of these Ca channels are assumed to dilate both glomerular arterioles. This property is expected to contribute to the reduction in intraglomerular capillary pressure. Indeed, the N-type CCB, cilnidipine, and the T-type CCB such as efonidipine and azelnidipine have been shown to reduce proteinuria significantly in patients with glomerulonephritis as compared with L-type CCB (Figure 9), suggesting these CCB are effective in alleviating glomerular hypertension (34-36).

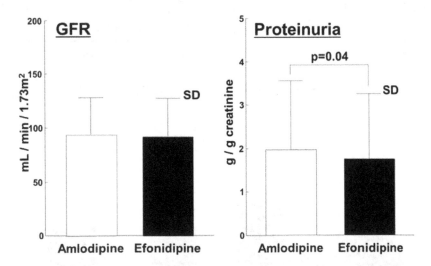

Fig. 9. The glomerular filtration rate (GFR) and the urinary excretions of protein in glomerulonephritis patients given the L-type Ca channel blocker (CCB), amlodipine, or the L- and T-type CCB, efonidipine (35).

As listed in Table 1, T-type Ca channels exist also in the adrenal and the in vitro experiments using cultured adrenal cells have shown that the T-type CCB suppress the expression of aldosterone synthase gene (CYP11B2) and production of aldosterone (37,38). In harmony with this, clinical studies in healthy subjects and hypertensive patients have shown that the acute or the chronic administrations of T-type CCB lower plasma aldosterone levels (39,40). We have compared the effects of L- and T-type CCB efonidipine and L-type CCB amlodipine in patients with glomerulonephritis and observed that efonidipine reduces plasma aldosterone concentration as compared with amlodipine while the plasma angiotensin II concentrations were comparable (Figure 10)(35). It is mentioned in the previous section of this chapter that aldosterone is supposed to promote the progression of glomerular injuries and the aldosterone blocker can reduce albuminuria. Considering that the mechanism of aldosterone suppression by T-type CCB is different from those by ACE inhibitors, ARB and aldosterone blockers, this property of T-type CCB would be expected to provide an additive benefit, when combined with the RAA system inhibitors, against the progression of renal dysfunction in the antihypertensive treatment of glomerulonephritis patients.

Ca channel	Tissue distribution	Function	Blocker
L-type	vascular smooth muscle intestinal smooth muscle	vasocontraction intestinal contraction	nifedipine nicardipine nitrendipine amlodipine etc.
N-type	brain nerve end	facilitation of signal transmission	cilnidipine
T-type	vascular smooth muscle cardiac muscle adrenal	vasocontraction stimulation of excitement conduction aldosterone secretion	manidipine efonidipine benidipine azelnidipine mibefradil

Table 1. Subtypes of Ca channel and their locations, functions and blockers.

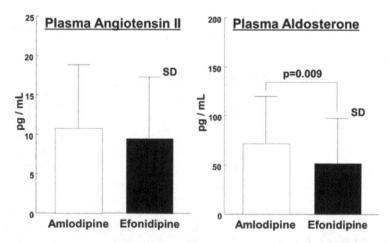

Fig. 10. The plasma concentrations of angiotensin II and aldosterone in glomerulonephritis patients given the L-type Ca channel blocker (CCB), amlodipine, or the L- and T-type CCB, efonidipine (35).

6. Summary and conclusions

Strict blood pressure control over 24 hours is of primary importance in preventing progression of renal injuries and deterioration of renal function in patients with glomerular diseases. In addition, it is important to lower not only systemic blood pressure but also intraglomerular capillary pressure in order to protect glomeruli from sclerosis because the increase in intraglomerular capillary pressure, glomerular hypertension, causes filtration of albuminuria and proteinuria which are dose-dependently related to the progression of renal injuries. Therefore, the antihypertensive therapy in patients with glomerulonephritis should aim not only the normalization of blood pressure but also the reduction of proteinuria and albuminuria. In order to lower intraglomerular capillary pressure, inhibitors of RAA system such as ACE inhibitors and ARB are effective as antihypertensive drugs because angiotensin II greatly contribute to the contraction of the efferent arterioles of glomeruli. In addition, interests are attracted as to the usefulness aldosterone receptor blockers and renin inhibitors as novel agents protecting the kidney. CCB are potent hypotensive agents, however, they rather dilate the afferent arterioles and may not be so effective as RAA system inhibitors in lowering intraglomerular capillary pressure. In this respect, some dihydropyridine CCB which block not only L-type Ca channel but also N- or T-type Ca channel have been shown to dilate efferent arterioles in addition to dilating afferent arterioles and are expected to be beneficial to protect glomeruli as well as lowering blood pressure effectively.

Prognosis of renal function in glomerulonephritis may be largely dependent on the nature of its pathohistological diagnosis and the therapeutic effects of immunosuppressive agents. In addition to these, efforts to lessen and minimize risk factors for renal injuries should be continuously made in order to inhibit the deterioration of renal function. Such efforts would be expected to contribute to inhibit not only the development of renal failure but also the incidence of cardiovascular diseases and to improve the prognosis of glomerulonephritis patients. Among the various risk factors for real injuries hypertension has great influence and the adequate blood pressure control is a pivotally important issue.

7. References

[1] Tozawa M, Iseki K, Iseki C, Kinjo K, Ikemiya Y, Takishita S. Blood pressure predicts risk of developing end-stage renal disease in men and women. Hypertension 2003; 41: 1341-1345.

[2] Peterson JC, Adler S, Burkart JM, Greene T, Hebert LA, Hunsicker LG, King AJ, Klahr S, Massry SG, Seifter JL. Blood pressure control, proteinuria, and the progression of renal disease. The Modification of Diet in Renal Disease Study. Ann Intern Med 1995; 123: 754-762.

[3] Bakris GL, Williams M, Dworkin L, Elliott WJ, Epstein M, Toto R, Tuttle K, Douglas J, Hsueh W, Sowers J. Preserving renal function in adults with hypertension and diabetes: a consensus approach. National Kidney Foundation Hypertension and Diabetes Executive Committees Working Group. Am J Kidney Dis 2000; 36: 646-661.

[4] National Heart, Lung, and Blood Institute Joint National Committee on Prevention, Detection, Evaluation, and Treatment of High Blood Pressure; National High Blood Pressure Education Program Coordinating Committee. The Seventh Report of the

Joint National Committee on Prevention, Detection, Evaluation, and Treatment of High Blood Pressure: the JNC 7 report. JAMA 2003; 289: 2560-2572.

[5] The task Force for the Management of Arterial Hypertension of the European Society of Hypertension and European Society of Cardiology. 2007 Guidelines for the Management of Arterial Hypertension. J Hypertens 2007;25: 1105-1187.

[6] Ogihara T, Kikuchi K, Matsuoka H, Fujita T, Higaki J, Horiuchi M, Imai Y, Imaizumi T, Ito S, Iwao H, Kario K, Kawano Y, Kim-Mitsuyama S, Kimura G, Matsubara H, Matsuura H, Naruse M, Saito I, Shimada K, Shimamoto K, Suzuki H, Takishita S, Tanahashi N, Tsuchihashi T, Uchiyama M, Ueda S, Ueshima H, Umemura S, Ishimitsu T, Rakugi H; Japanese Society of Hypertension Committee. The Japanese Society of Hypertension Guidelines for the Management of Hypertension (JSH 2009). Hypertens Res 2009; 32: 3-107.

[7] Hostetter TH, Olson JL, Rennke HG, Venkatachalam MA, Brenner BM. Hyperfiltration in remnant nephrons: a potentially adverse response to renal ablation. J Am Soc Nephrol 2001; 12: 1315-1325.

[8] Brenner BM, Meyer TW, Hostetter TH. Dietary protein intake and the progressive nature of kidney disease. The role of hemodynamically mediated glomerular injury in the pathogenesis of progressive glomerular sclerosis in aging, renal ablation, and intrinsic renal disease. N Engl J Med 1982; 307: 652-659.

[9] Remuzzi G, Perico N, Macia M, Ruggenenti P. The role of renin-angiotensin-aldosterone system in the progression of chronic kidney disease. Kidney Int Suppl 2005; 99: S57-S65.

[10] Brewster UC, Setaro JF, Perazella MA. The renin-angiotensin-aldosterone system: cardiorenal effects and implications for renal and cardiovascular disease states. Am J Med Sci 2003; 326: 15-24.

[11] Rafiq K, Hitomi H, Nakano D, Nishiyama A. Pathophysiological roles of aldosterone and mineralocorticoid receptor in the kidney. J Pharmacol Sci 2011; 115: 1-7.

[12] Lanese DM, Yuan BH, Falk SA, Conger JD. Effects of atriopeptin III on isolated rat afferent and efferent arterioles. Am J Physiol. 1991; 261: F1102-F1109.

[13] Patzak A, Lai E, Persson PB, Persson AE. Angiotensin II-nitric oxide interaction in glomerular arterioles. Clin Exp Pharmacol Physiol 2005; 32: 410-414.

[14] Naicker S, Bhoola KD. Endothelins: vasoactive modulators of renal function in health and disease.Pharmacol Ther 2001; 90: 61-88.

[15] Sugimoto H, Shikata K, Matsuda M, Kushiro M, Hayashi Y, Hiragushi K, Wada J, Makino H. Increased expression of endothelial cell nitric oxide synthase (ecNOS) in afferent and glomerular endothelial cells is involved in glomerular hyperfiltration of diabetic nephropathy. Diabetologia 1998; 41: 1426-1434.

[16] Ferrario R, Takahashi K, Fogo A, Badr KF, Munger KA. Consequences of acute nitric oxide synthesis inhibition in experimental glomerulonephritis. J Am Soc Nephrol 1994; 4: 1847-1854.

[17] Edwards RM. Effects of prostaglandins on vasoconstrictor action in isolated renal arterioles. Am J Physiol 1985; 248: F779-F784.

[18] Fujita T, Fuke Y, Satomura A, Hidaka M, Ohsawa I, Endo M, Komatsu K, Ohi H. PGI2 analogue mitigates the progression rate of renal dysfunction improving renal blood flow without glomerular hyperfiltration in patients with chronic renal insufficiency. Prostaglandins Leukot Essent Fatty Acids 2001; 65: 223-227.

[19] Anderson S, Rennke HG, Brenner BM. Therapeutic advantage of converting enzyme inhibitors in arresting progressive renal disease associated with systemic hypertension in the rat. J Clin Invest 1986; 77: 1993-2000.

[20] Taguma Y, Kitamoto Y, Futaki G, Ueda H, Monma H, Ishizaki M, Takahashi H, Sekino H, Sasaki Y. Effect of captopril on heavy proteinuria in azotemic diabetics. N Engl J Med 1985; 313: 1617-1620.

[21] Lewis EJ, Hunsicker LG, Bain RP, Rohde RD. The effect of angiotensin-converting-enzyme inhibition on diabetic nephropathy. The Collaborative Study Group. N Engl J Med 1993; 329: 1456-1462.

[22] Lewis EJ, Hunsicker LG, Clarke WR, Berl T, Pohl MA, Lewis JB, Ritz E, Atkins RC, Rohde R, Raz I; Collaborative Study Group. Renoprotective effect of the angiotensin-receptor antagonist irbesartan in patients with nephropathy due to type 2 diabetes. N Engl J Med 2001; 345: 851-860.

[23] Brenner BM, Cooper ME, de Zeeuw D, Keane WF, Mitch WE, Parving HH, Remuzzi G, Snapinn SM, Zhang Z, Shahinfar S; RENAAL Study Investigators. Effects of losartan on renal and cardiovascular outcomes in patients with type 2 diabetes and nephropathy. N Engl J Med. 200; 345: 861-869.

[24] Parving HH, Lehnert H, Bröchner-Mortensen J, Gomis R, Andersen S, Arner P; Irbesartan in Patients with Type 2 Diabetes and Microalbuminuria Study Group. The effect of irbesartan on the development of diabetic nephropathy in patients with type 2 diabetes. N Engl J Med 2001; 345: 870-878.

[25] Maschio G, Alberti D, Janin G, Locatelli F, Mann JF, Motolese M, Ponticelli C, Ritz E, Zucchelli P. Effect of the angiotensin-converting-enzyme inhibitor benazepril on the progression of chronic renal insufficiency. The Angiotensin-Converting-Enzyme Inhibition in Progressive Renal Insufficiency Study Group. N Engl J Med 1996; 334: 939-945.

[26] The GISEN Group. Randomised placebo-controlled trial of effect of ramipril on decline in glomerular filtration rate and risk of terminal renal failure in proteinuric, non-diabetic nephropathy. Lancet 1997; 349: 1857-1863.

[27] Agodoa LY, Appel L, Bakris GL, Beck G, Bourgoignie J, Briggs JP, Charleston J, Cheek D, Cleveland W, Douglas JG, Douglas M, Dowie D, Faulkner M, Gabriel A, Gassman J, Greene T, Hall Y, Hebert L, Hiremath L, Jamerson K, Johnson CJ, Kopple J, Kusek J, Lash J, Lea J, Lewis JB, Lipkowitz M, Massry S, Middleton J, Miller ER 3rd, Norris K, O'Connor D, Ojo A, Phillips RA, Pogue V, Rahman M, Randall OS, Rostand S, Schulman G, Smith W, Thornley-Brown D, Tisher CC, Toto RD, Wright JT Jr, Xu S; African American Study of Kidney Disease and Hypertension (AASK) Study Group. Effect of ramipril vs amlodipine on renal outcomes in hypertensive nephrosclerosis: a randomized controlled trial. JAMA 2001; 285: 2719-2728.

[28] Ishimitsu T, Akashiba A, Kameda T, Takahashi T, Ohta S, Yoshii M, Minami J, Ono H, Numabe A, Matsuoka H. Benazepril slows progression of renal dysfunction in patients with non-diabetic renal disease. Nephrology 2007; 12: 294-298.

[29] Ishimitsu T, Kameda T, Akashiba A, Takahashi T, Ando N, Ohta S, Yoshii M, Inada H, Tsukada K, Minami J, Ono H, Matsuoka H. Effects of valsartan on the progression of chronic renal insufficiency in patients with nondiabetic renal diseases. Hypertens Res 2005; 28: 865-870.

[30] Hou FF, Zhang X, Zhang GH, Xie D, Chen PY, Zhang WR, Jiang JP, Liang M, Wang GB, Liu ZR, Geng RW. Efficacy and safety of benazepril for advanced chronic renal insufficiency. N Engl J Med 2006; 354: 131-40.

[31] Persson F, Rossing P, Reinhard H, Juhl T, Stehouwer CD, Schalkwijk C, Danser AH, Boomsma F, Frandsen E, Parving HH. Renal effects of aliskiren compared with and in combination with irbesartan in patients with type 2 diabetes, hypertension, and albuminuria. Diabetes Care 2009; 32: 1873-1879.

[32] Parving HH, Persson F, Lewis JB, Lewis EJ, Hollenberg NK; AVOID Study Investigators. Aliskiren combined with losartan in type 2 diabetes and nephropathy. N Engl J Med 2008; 358: 2433-2446.

[33] Sato A, Hayashi K, Naruse M, Saruta T. Effectiveness of aldosterone blockade in patients with diabetic nephropathy. Hypertension 2003; 41: 64-68.

[34] Fujita T, Ando K, Nishimura H, Ideura T, Yasuda G, Isshiki M, Takahashi K; Cilnidipine versus Amlodipine Randomised Trial for Evaluation in Renal Desease(CARTER) Study Investigators. Antiproteinuric effect of the calcium channel blocker cilnidipine added to renin-angiotensin inhibition in hypertensive patients with chronic renal disease. Kidney Int 2007; 72: 1543-1549.

[35] Ishimitsu T, Kameda T, Akashiba A, Takahashi T, Ohta S, Yoshii M, Minami J, Ono H, Numabe A, Matsuoka H. Efonidipine reduces proteinuria and plasma aldosterone in patients with chronic glomerulonephritis. Hypertens Res 2007; 30: 621-626.

[36] Nakamura T, Sugaya T, Kawagoe Y, Suzuki T, Ueda Y, Koide H, Inoue T, Node K. Azelnidipine reduces urinary protein excretion and urinary liver-type fatty acid binding protein in patients with hypertensive chronic kidney disease. Am J Med Sci 2007; 333: 321-326.

[37] Tanaka H, Shigenobu K. Pathophysiological significance of T-type Ca2+ channels: T-type Ca2+ channels and drug development. J Pharmacol Sci 2005; 99: 214-220.

[38] Imagawa K, Okayama S, Takaoka M, Kawata H, Naya N, Nakajima T, Horii M, Uemura S, Saito Y. Inhibitory effect of efonidipine on aldosterone synthesis and secretion in human adrenocarcinoma (H295R) cells. J Cardiovasc Pharmacol 2006; 47: 133-138.

[39] Okayama S, Imagawa K, Naya N, Iwama H, Somekawa S, Kawata H, Horii M, Nakajima T, Uemura S, Saito Y. Blocking T-type Ca2+ channels with efonidipine decreased plasma aldosterone concentration in healthy volunteers. Hypertens Res 2006; 29: 493-497.

[40] Tanaka T, Tsutamoto T, Sakai H, Fujii M, Yamamoto T, Horie M. Comparison of the effects of efonidipine and amlodipine on aldosterone in patients with hypertension. Hypertens Res 2007; 30: 691-697.

12

Nephrotic Syndrome in Children – Studies from South Africa

Gertruida van Biljon
University of Pretoria, Department of Paediatrics
South Africa

1. Introduction

Worldwide research has shown that racial differences occur with regard to the histological subtypes, response to treatment and outcome of idiopathic nephrotic syndrome (INS) in children (Bhimma et al. 2006:1847; Bhimma, R. 2009:15; Ingulli &Tejani 2001:393). Several reasons have been suggested to explain these differences such as a higher prevalence of infections, lower socio-economic status and inequalities in access to health care resources, genetics, and environmental factors but none of these have been substantiated by data. Results from the International Study of Kidney Disease in Children (International Study of Kidney Disease in Children ISKDC 1978:159) showed that the majority of children with INS have minimal change nephrotic syndrome (MCNS) which responds to corticosteroid treatment and that a kidney biopsy is not indicated. Based on these findings empiric corticosteroid treatment was recommended, without performing a kidney biopsy. The study population consisted of predominantly white children from North America, Europe and Asia. These recommendations have been implemented worldwide as standard of care for the past 40 years despite the lack of prospective renal biopsy studies to substantiate this recommendation and which may not be applicable to other settings with a predominance of black patients. An increasing incidence of focal segmental glomerulosclerosis (FSGS) in children and adults with INS has been reported recently (Borges et al. 2007:1309; Filler et al. 2003 :1107; Srivastava et al. 1991:13). Studies reporting the outcome of INS associated with FSGS are variable, which is not surprising, as differences in the population mix, aetiology, pathogenesis and duration of disease are often not taken into consideration. This begs the question whether the recommendation of the International Study of Kidney Disease in Children for the management of INS should still be adhered to. Or should it be revised taking into consideration different racial groups? On the other hand, in the light of the rising incidence of FSGS, it may be prudent to withdraw the recommendation.

Paediatric nephrologists from developing countries, and specifically Africa, need to formulate guidelines specific to their patients with INS. To this end, relevant clinical characteristics such as the antenatal and family history, birth weight, feeding and nutrition, growth and onset of disease should be documented and analysed in their reports. Low birth weight (LBW) which has been shown to be associated with decreased glomerular endowment (Manalich et al. 2007:770, Vehaskari , VM. 2007:490) and subsequent increased risk for the development of chronic kidney disease (CKD), is a case in point, since it is more common in impoverished population groups living in Africa. However, most publications describing the influence of LBW on CKD come from developed countries. (Teeninga et al. 2008:1615)

Limited resources are often the stumbling block for clinicians in developing countries. For the standard care of a child with INS the minimum investigations necessary in the work-up include urine biochemistry, urine microscopy and investigations to exclude infectious and immune disorders. A kidney biopsy is recommended for all children and should include light microscopy, immuno-histochemistry or immunofluorescent studies and electron microscopy. These investigations are costly, but essential to make a definitive diagnosis. Without a specific diagnosis of the underlying pathology and the associated complications it will not be possible to make reliable recommendations for targeted treatment in a child with INS in a developing country.

2. Aim

The aim of the study is to describe the clinical characteristics, histological subtypes, response to treatment and outcome of children with INS treated at the paediatric renal unit of the Steve Biko Academic Hospital (SBAH). This is a level 3 South African hospital, affiliated to the University of Pretoria and the referral centre for the surrounding multiracial population of roughly 5 million children under the age of 14 years.

3. Methods

A retrospective audit was performed of consecutive children admitted with a clinical diagnosis of INS. The latter was defined as ≥2+ proteinuria on a urine dipstick test, hypoalbuminaemia of <25 g/L and oedema. Children who had macroscopic haematuria (red or brownish discolouration of urine) substantiated by >2+ blood on a urine dipstick test and hypertension in addition to the criteria for INS, were also included and were categorised as nephritic-nephrotic. Hypertension was diagnosed according to the 4th Report of the National High Blood Pressure Education Program Working Group on High Blood Pressure in Children and Adolescents. (The Fourth Report of the National High Blood Pressure Education Program Working Group on High Blood Pressure in Children and Adolescents. 2004:555).

The racial groups were documented as black, white, Indian, and mixed. The Indian and white racial groups were pooled and categorised as white. The black and mixed racial groups were similarly pooled and categorised as black. This grouping was done because of known similarities in clinical presentation, response to treatment and outcome in the respective groups. (Bhimma et al.1997:429).

The clinical characteristics analysed were age at presentation, gender, anthropometry (height/length for age and weight for age), and blood pressure.

The following investigations were analysed: urine dipstick tests, urine protein:creatinine ratio (mg/mg), s-albumin and s-cholesterol, s-creatinine and estimated glomerular filtration rate (eGFR) in ml/min/1.73m2. eGFR was calculated using a modified Schwartz formula (Schwartz. et al. 1987:571), i.e.: [40 x height (cm)/s-creatinine (μmol/L)]. Kidney function at presentation was categorised according to the National Kidney Foundation Kidney Disease Outcomes (K/DOQI clinical practice guidelines 2002:S1). Investigations to rule out secondary nephrotic syndrome include: the third and fourth components of complement (C3 and C4), immunologic tests for systemic lupus erythematosus (antinuclear antibodies and anti-double-stranded DNA antibodies), antistreptolysin O and anti DNase B titers, hepatitis B and C serology, cytomegalovirus (CMV) antibodies and HIV enzyme-linked immunosorbent assay (ELISA).

The indications for a kidney biopsy were: a family history of kidney disease, congenital and infantile nephrotic syndrome, children with clinical features suggestive of nephrotic syndrome (NS) other than MCNS, children who failed to respond to an 8-week course of corticosteroids, prior to the administration of cyclophosphamide, children with persisting elevated s-creatinine levels and all black children.

4. Treatment

The mainstay of treatment was corticosteroids with the aim to achieve and maintain remission rather than adhering to a standardised protocol. For this reason a higher dose and a longer course were used (daily dose versus alternate day treatment) compared to the ISKDC guidelines (International Study of Kidney Disease in Children 1978:159). The primary contraindications for corticosteroid treatment were children with CNS, secondary NS (e.g. hepatitis B associated nephropathy, Henoch-Schönlein purpura), children with CKD Stage 3 or more associated with stunting and wasting, cardiomegaly, anaemia and bone mineral disease and presumably immune-compromised children.

Second line immunosuppressive therapy was initiated in a selective group of children, influenced by compliance and socio-economic factors, and only after parental consent had been obtained. Indications for second line immunosuppressive therapy included children with steroid dependent or frequently relapsing NS, those who developed secondary steroid resistance and a selective group of children with partial response. Exclusion criteria for cyclophosphamide treatment included children with underlying chronic infections, e.g. untreated *Mycobacterium tuberculosis* or HIV infection and those at increased risk of developing acute or chronic infections due to poor nutritional status.

4.1.1 Corticosteroid treatment

Prednisone was administered as a single daily dose at 2 mg/kg/day and tapered to 1 mg/kg/day after 4 weeks in children who responded and achieved remission. Further tapering was only initiated after another 4 weeks and treatment stopped after a total of 20 weeks. For those who had not responded to corticosteroid treatment at a dose of 2 mg/kg/day by the 4th week – which occurred commonly in the event of black children - this high dose was continued for a maximum of 8 weeks when the dose was tapered according to the response of the child.

Response to treatment was classified as: remission, partial response and steroid resistant. Remission was defined as no or trace proteinuria on dipstick test for three consecutive days or urine protein:creatinine ratio of <0.2 mg/mg. Relapse was defined as proteinuria of ≥ 2+ on dipstick test for three consecutive days or urine protein:creatinine ratio of ≥ 2.0 mg/mg. Partial response was defined as ≤ 2+ proteinuria on urine dipstick or urine protein:creatinine ratio < 2.0 mg/mg after a maximum of 8 weeks of high dose steroid treatment (2 mg/kg/day). Steroid resistance was defined as persistent proteinuria ≥2+ and urine protein:creatinine ratio ≥ 2.0 mg/mg after a maximum of 8 weeks of high dose steroid treatment (2 mg/kg/day). Steroid dependence was defined as relapse when the dose of corticosteroid treatment was decreased or within two weeks after stopping it. Frequent relapse was defined as ≥2 relapses per 12-month period.

4.1.2 Cyclophosphamide treatment

The total course of oral cyclophosphamide for an individual child was calculated as 168 mg/kg over 8 or 12 weeks administered as 3 mg/kg/day for 8 weeks or 2 mg/kg/day for 12 weeks (=168 mg/kg). Cyclophosphamide tablets are sugar coated and contain 50 mg cyclophosphamide/tablet. It cannot be crushed or divided. The dose to be taken per 7-day week was therefore calculated for each patient and was limited to a maximum dose of 3 mg/kg/day. Tablets were administered for fewer than seven days per week for smaller patients weighing less than 25 kg who required <50 mg/day (i.e. no treatment on weekend days).

A kidney biopsy was performed in all children before cyclophosphamide treatment was initiated. No child received a second course of cyclophosphamide.

4.1.3 Intravenous methylprednisolone pulse treatment

A course of intravenous methylprednisolone was administered in three scenarios, i.e. children with anasarca and who were resistant to their first course of oral corticosteroid treatment, children who became steroid dependent or developed frequent relapses after having had a course of cyclophosphamide treatment and children with partial response to oral corticosteroid and cyclophosphamide treatment. Selection of patients for this form of treatment was further influenced by their ability or willingness to frequently return to the hospital and by the absence of recurrent infections.

Intravenous corticosteroid treatment consisted of methylprednisolone 30 mg/kg/dose (maximum dose of 1000 mg) administered according to established guidelines (Mendoza et al 1990:303), but excluding cyclophosphamide treatment (Table 1).

It was discontinued when a patient experienced unacceptable adverse effects, e.g. progressive fluid retention or volume overload, with worsening hypertension or when proteinuria remained unchanged after 6 to 8 weeks.

Week	M-P[a]	N	Prednisone
1-2	30 mg/kg thrice weekly	6	None
3-10	30 mg/kg per week	8	2 mg/kg/day [b]
11-18	30 mg/kg per 2 weeks	4	1.5mg/kg/day tapered slowly
19-52	30 mg/kg per 4 weeks	8	1 mg/kg/day tapered slowly
53-78	30 mg/kg per 8 weeks	4	0.5mg/kg/day tapered slowly

a = Maximum dose 1000 mg
b = Maximum dose 60 mg

Table 1. Intravenous methylprednisolone (M-P) pulse regimen

4.1.4 Adjunctive treatment

Adjunctive treatment included diuretics for symptomatic management of oedema, antihypertensive drugs, multivitamin and folic acid supplementation, alpha-calcidol for children on high-dose corticosteroid treatment and with persisting nephrotic-range proteinuria. Treatment with an angiotensin converting enzyme inhibitor (ACE-inhibitor) was given for its antiproteinuric effect to alleviate persistent proteinuria and as an antihypertensive drug if needed. Other antihypertensive drugs used included a β-blocker (atenolol), calcium antagonist (amlodipine), α-blocker (prazosin) and a vasodilator (hydralazine). Angiotensin receptor blockers were not prescribed because of unavailability.

Diuretics of all classes, namely furosemide, hydrochlorothiazide and spironolactone were used in combinations if needed for children with diuretic-resistant NS. Hydroxy-methylglutharyl coenzyme A reductase inhibitors (statins) were selectively prescribed to children older than 5 years with persistent NS associated with an elevated total cholesterol level of >10 mmol/L. All children received a diet containing reduced salt and saturated fat. Protein intake was not restricted.

5. Ethical approval

The study was approved by the University of Pretoria Research Ethics Committee and permission was obtained from the chief executive officer of the hospital to access hospital files.

6. Statistical analysis

Categorical data was reported as proportions and quantitative data as means (standard deviations) and medians (range).
Frequencies of variables within groups were compared using the two-sided Fisher exact test and a p-value <0.05 was regarded as significant. Renal and patient survival in the two population groups were assessed using Kaplan Meier non parametric life table survival analysis.

7. Results

Over a period of 23 years (1986 – 2009) 358 children with a clinical diagnosis of NS were admitted and comprised the study group. Of these 278/358 (77.7%) were black and 80/358 (22.3%) white. The median age was 58 months (range 0.5 – 144 months) and the male: female ratio 1.3:1.
The age at presentation was categorised in 4 groups as depicted in table 2. Twenty seven children were ≤ 12 months of age at the time of presentation, of whom 15/27 (4%) presented within the first 3 months of life and were diagnosed with CNS. An additional ten children were also diagnosed with CNS but were referred later, when they were older than 3 months. Fifty percent (179/358) of the children were in the age group >12-72 months.

Age category (months)	Number	%
0-3	15	4.2
>3-12	12	3.3
>12 - 72	179	50.0
>72	152	42.5
Total	358	100%

Table 2. Age Categories of Children at Presentation

Stunting (height/length for age z-score > -2SD) was present in 88/358 (24.6%) children. Microscopic haematuria was present in 52/109 (47.7%) and macroscopic haematuria in 34/109(9.5%) children with MCNS.
A constellation of clinical and laboratory features including, age >12 months to 72 months, normal blood pressure, absence of haematuria, normal renal function and normal levels of

serum C_3 have been quoted as suggestive of MCNS with an expected good prognosis (International Study of Kidney Disease in Children 1978:159). In this study 67% of the children with MCNS fulfilled the criteria for the diagnosis, apart from not having a normal blood pressure. This finding has been described by others (Habib et al 1971) which questions the validity of the criteria for diagnosing MCNS.

Hypertension was present in 227/358 (63.4%) children at presentation of whom 171/227 (47.8%) required treatment with antihypertensive drugs for at least 6 weeks. Diuretics were used for symptomatic management of oedema and were often used as a first line antihypertensive drug in children considered to have volume overload. Of those with persistent hypertension 146/171 (85.4%) received an ACE-inhibitor as the preferred antihypertensive drug. Overall 213/358 (59.5%) received an ACE-inhibitor for its anti-proteinuric effect. Renal function and s-potassium were monitored in all children who were treated with an ACE-inhibitor. No child experienced an allergic response or developed significant coughing with this treatment. An acute increase in s-creatinine levels occurred in some patients, usually in association with volume contraction, which was reversible in all cases with fluid resuscitation.

The mean s-albumin level at the time of presentation was 13.2 ± 5.2 g/L. Some patients had below detectable s-albumin levels and for these the lowest value documented was an arbitrary level of 10g/L for the purpose of statistical analysis. This means that the true mean level was in fact lower. The mean s-cholesterol at the time of presentation was 11.4 ± 7.3 mmol/L. As already stated above, statins were only prescribed to a limited number of older children with persistent hypercholesterolaemia. The main reason why younger children with similar high cholesterol levels were not treated with statins is the lack of long-term safety information on the effects of these drugs on the developing brain, immune functions, hormones and energy metabolism.

Kidney function was monitored using change in eGFR over time. Despite its limited accuracy, especially in children with poor muscle bulk, it was the only feasible test which could be done at regular intervals at follow-up visits. The results of eGFR at the time of presentation and at last follow up for the two race groups are depicted in table 3.

CKD Stage	eGFR[1] (ml/min/1.73m²)	eGFR at presentation n = 358		eGFR last follow up n = 358	
		Black children n=278	White children n=80	Black children n=278	White children n=80
1	≥90	189 (68.0%)	55 (68.8%)	178 (64.0%)	66 (82.5%)
2	60-89	42 (15.1%)	20 (25.0%)	29 (10.4%)	10 (12.5)
3	30-59	27 (9.7%)	4 (5.0%)	18(6.5%)	1 (1.3%)
4 + 5	<29	20 (7.1%)	1(1.3%)	53(19.0%)*	3 (3.8%)

eGFR = Estimated glomerular filtration rate
*One black child with CKD stage 5 who had a successful kidney transplant is included in the number of black children with stage 4 and 5 CKD.

Table 3. eGFR at the Time of Presentation and During Follow Up in the Two Race Groups

Significantly more black compared to white children had stage 4 or 5 CKD on presentation, 7.1% vs. 1.3% respectively (p=0.03), or had developed stage 4 or 5 CKD at the time of last follow up, 19.0% vs. 3.8% respectively (p= 0.000).

A secondary cause for NS was identified in 26 (7.2%) children including Henoch-Schönlein purpura, systemic lupus erythematosus, chronic hepatitis B infection, HIV infection and IgA glomerulonephritis. Ten children (2.8%) had chronic hepatitis B associated nephropathy. None of them were given any immunosuppressive treatment, interferon or other specific antiviral treatment. In eleven children a genetic cause of NS was suspected.

CNS was diagnosed in 25/358 (7%) children, none of whom had a syndromic form of CNS. Investigations for mutations of *NPHS1, NPHS2* and *WT1* were not done in any of the children with CNS or suspected familial NS because of unavailability.

Kidney biopsies were performed in 318/358 (89%) children. The main histological diagnoses are depicted in table IV. Eighteen children had inconclusive histology which was reported as "FSGS cannot be excluded." In these cases there was a chronic inflammatory cell infiltrate in the interstitium, interstitial fibrosis and tubulo-interstitial atrophy suggestive of FSGS but the biopsy sample did not have glomeruli with focal sclerosis. If this group of children is added to the group with definite FSGS, the frequency of FSGS increases to 98/318 (31%). Eleven children (10 black, 1 white) were diagnosed with immune complex glomerulonephritis (ICGN), based on the presence of immune deposits in the basement membrane on electron microscopy examination and another 26 (25 black, 1 white) had ICGN with secondary glomerular sclerosis.

Histological diagnosis	White Number (%)	Black Number (%)	Total (%)	p-value
MCNS	42(66)	67(26.4)	109 (34.2)	<0.001*
Focal segmental glomerulosclerosis (FSGS)	9 (14)	71(28)	80 (25)	0.01*
MCNS – FSGS **	7(11)	11 (4.3)	18 (5.7)	0.048*
Immune complex glomerulonephritis (ICGN)	1(1.6)	10 (4)	11(3.4)	0.31
ICGN and secondary FSGS	1 (1.6)	25(9.8)	26 (8.2)	0.02*
Membranous nephropathy (MN)	0 (0)	14 (5.5)	14 (4.4)	0.04*
Mesangiocapillary glomerulonephritis	1 (1.6)	12 (5)	13 (4)	0.22
Congenital nephrotic syndrome (CNS)	0 (0)	25 (9.8)	25 (8)	0.02*
Other	3 (4.7)	19 (7.5)	22 (7)	
Total ***	64(100)	254 (100)	318 (100)	

*Statistically significant
**MCNS-FSGS: Histology was reported as "FSGS cannot be excluded" and was therefore inconclusive but very suggestive of FSGS due to the presence of a chronic inflammatory cell infiltrate in the interstitium, interstitial fibrosis and tubular atrophy on the biopsy.
***Includes all children who had kidney biopsies, including the children with congenital nephrotic syndrome.

Table 4. Main Histological Subtypes of Nephrotic Syndrome (n = 318)

In table 5. the frequencies of all the histological subtypes excluding CNS are depicted, which is in line with the procedure followed by the ISKDC. CNS is considered a distinct form of NS with a unique etio-pathogenesis and a high frequency of underlying genetic mutations and is therefore usually not analysed with other forms of INS. Kidney biopsies were done in 318 children (64 white and 254 black). After exclusion of the 25 children with CNS, all of whom were black, the frequencies of the histopathological subtypes of only the remaining 229 black children changed.

Histological diagnosis	White Number (%)	Black Number (%)	Total (%)	p-value
MCNS	42(65.6)	67(29.3)	109 (37.2)	<0.000*
Focal segmental glomerulosclerosis (FSGS)	9 (14.0)	71(31.0)	80 (27.3)	0.004*
MCNS – FSGS **	7(10.9)	11 (4.8)	18 (6.1)	0.07
Immune complex glomerulonephritis (ICGN)	1(1.6)	10 (4.4)	11(3.7)	0.26
ICGN and secondary FSGS	1 (1.6)	25(11.0)	26 (8.9)	0.01*
Membranous nephropathy	0 (0)	14 (6.1)	14 (4.8)	0.03*
Mesangiocapillary glomerulonephritis	1 (1.6)	12 (5.2)	13 (4.4)	0.18
Other	3 (4.7)	19 (8.3)	22 (7.5)	
***Total	64 (100)	229 (100)	293 (100)	

*Statistically significant
**MCNS-FSGS: Histology was reported as "FSGS cannot be excluded" and was therefore inconclusive but very suggestive of FSGS due to the presence of chronic inflammatory cell infiltrate in the interstitium, interstitial fibrosis and tubular atrophy on the biopsy.
***All children who had kidney biopsies, but excluding the children with congenital nephrotic syndrome.

Table 5. Histological Subtypes of Nephrotic Syndrome Excluding Children with Congenital Nephrotic Syndrome (n=293)

The incidences of the four major histological subtypes (MCNS, FSGS, membranous nephropathy, mesangiocapillary glomerulonephritis were significantly higher in the black children (Table 5).

7.1 Results of treatment

Remission with oral corticosteroid treatment was achieved in 33/41(81%) white vs 33/59(56%) black children (p=0.02) who had MCNS. The response rate of the black children is similar to the 60% response rate in black children reported previously from Kalafong Hospital (Prinsloo JG. 1986:375) but lower than the 78% response rate reported a decade later in children from the Chris-Hani Baragwanath Hospital (Johannesburg), both tertiary hospitals in South Africa (Thomson 1997:402). Oral corticosteroid treatment resulted in remission in 3/9 white children and 8/40 black children with FSGS (p=0.6). In the combined group of children with FSGS and MCNS-FSGS 9/13 (69.2%) white children vs 4/14 (28.5%) (p<0.05) black children went into remission with this treatment. Twenty five children who failed to respond to oral corticosteroid treatment were treated with a course of intravenous methylprednisolone of whom only 4 (one white and 3 black children) went into complete remission. This form of treatment was abandoned because of its poor efficacy, high toxicity and cost and the disruptive effect it had on school attendance. Hundred children were treated with cyclophosphamide, 46 were white and 54 black. The response rate to this treatment was statistically significantly different in the white and black children. Sustained remission was achieved in 37/46 (80%) white and in 23/54 (43%) black children (P=0.002; 95% CI 2.2 – 13.7). The ISKDC reported no benefit of orally administered cyclophosphamide and prednisone compared to prednisone alone for the treatment of steroid resistant NS (Tarshish, P et al. 1996: 590). Their report and the poor response of children with steroid resistant NS in this study prompted discontinuation of cyclophosphamide treatment in children with steroid resistant NS since 2007. No patient experienced side effects of cyclophosphamide treatment, but they were all monitored at least every 10 to 14 days throughout the duration of the treatment. Several children who had been in contact with chicken pox were given human varicella-zoster immune globulin and/or acyclovir prophylactically, but none developed serious chicken pox.

7.2 Morbidity and mortality

Acute reversible renal failure occurred in 35/358 (9.8%) children and thrombotic complications, other than strokes in 9/358 (2.5%). Six children (1.7%) developed strokes, one of whom developed bilateral sequential middle cerebral artery thromboses a few months apart. She was one of a family of 3 children who all had steroid resistant NS. At the time that she developed the first stroke she was not dehydrated, but had a mild lower respiratory tract infection, iron deficiency anaemia and a thrombocytosis, which are known risk factors for thrombo-embolic complications in children with nephrotic syndrome.

Fourty eight percent of all children experienced acute invasive bacterial infections, including pneumonia, peritonitis and septicaemia. In those with steroid sensitive NS acute bacterial infections occurred during relapses. The frequency of infection was inversely related to age and was particularly high in children younger than 3 months. Of these children 87% developed serious infections compared to 39% of children older than 6 years. Streptococcus pneumoniae was the predominant causal organism, followed by Escherichia coli and other gram negative organisms. Twenty six children (7.3%) developed peritonitis of whom three demised due to pneumococcal septicaemic shock. Pneumococcal infections occurred in 7/80 (8.7%) white children vs 19/278 (6.8%) black children (p=0.6). Until recently pneumococcal polysaccharide vaccine was given to all children younger than 5 years at the time of their first presentation, despite its limited efficacy in children younger than 2 years. Since 2009 the pneumococcal conjugate vaccine is available in South Africa which is used for revaccination of this group of children. Long term prophylactic penicillin was not used.

Chronic hepatitis B infection (positive HBsAg and/or HBeAg) occurred in 10/358 (2.8%) children, all of whom were black. Hepatitis B vaccine was included in the routine immunization schedule of children in South Africa since 1991 and since that time no child was diagnosed with hepatitis B related NS. No child had hepatitis C related NS. Investigations to rule out CMV infection were only done in children with CNS and in those with atypical clinical features of NS, including anaemia, hepatosplenomegaly, skin rash or positive central nervous system signs. In most cases only CMV IgM and IgG were done, which were often both positive due to unexplained reasons at the time, because the test for CMV viral load was not available. Should a CMV infection be diagnosed it is not necessarily proof of the causality of the NS.

All children were screened for underlying Mycobacerium tuberculosis infection with a chest X-ray, gastric aspirates or induced sputum cultures and Mantoux test (skin prick test with intradermal injection of purified protein derivative of Mycobacterium tuberculosis). Because children uncommonly have sputum positive tuberculosis, several of our patients received empiric anti-tuberculous treatment for 6 months when the diagnosis could not be unequivocally excluded. A high prevalence of tuberculosis associated with a deleterious effect on renal function was reported in black children with FSGS. (Kala et al.1993:392). It has been postulated that immune responses mediated by infections with Mycobacterium tuberculosis and HI-virus may contribute to glomerulosclerosis. Mycobacterium tuberculosis infection was present in too few patients in this study to draw any conclusion.

Investigations for HIV infection were only done in children who had clinical features suggestive of the disease and whose parents had given consent to testing. It is therefore not possible to report on the true incidence of NS associated with HIV infection. Patients with HIV infection had a variety of histological lesions, including, immune complex glomerulonephritis, immunotactoid and fibrillary glomerulonephritis and FSGS. No patient had HIV collapsing glomerulopathy which has been reported as one of the commonest histological lesions in black adult patients with HIV infection. Recently HIV- associated kidney disease has been reported to have become the most common form of kidney disease in children seen in the renal unit at one of the academic hospitals in South Africa. (Bhimma R, 2009:15)

Only one infant with CNS had congenital syphilis and treatment with penicillin did not result in cure of the disease. Chronic "quartan malarial nephropathy" or other parasitic related forms of NS did not occur.

7.3 Outcome

At presentation 21/358 children had CKD stage 4 or 5. Of the black children 20/278 (7.2%) had CKD stage 4 or 5 compared to 1/80(1.3%) white children (p=0.03). Over the period of follow up more black children (53/278) (19%) developed stage 4 or 5 CKD compared to white children (3/80)(3.8%)(p= 0.000). Kaplan-Meier estimation of renal survival depicting the difference in renal survival in black and white children is demonstrated in Fig1. One black child was successfully transplanted during the follow up period and had normal renal function at last follow up. Persistent nephrotic range proteinuria is associated with a rapid progression to end-stage kidney disease. Several children in this study had long standing suboptimal management of nephrotic range proteinuria when presenting to the SBAH which contributed to a more rapid progression to end stage kidney disease.

Forty three patients died during the follow up period. Three (3.7%) white children died of whom 2 succumbed to complications of renal failure (renal deaths) and one died due to pneumococcal septicaemia (non renal death). Forty black children died during the follow up period, mostly due to end stage renal failure. In the black children infectious related deaths occurred mostly in the children with congenital NS. Black children had a significantly higher mortality compared to white children (40/268 vs. 3/80) (p<0.001). Kaplan-Meier patient survival estimate depicting the difference in patient survival for black and white children is demonstrated in Fig 2.

8. Discussion

This study population differs in several aspects from those reported from developed countries. The majority of patients are black with an inherent risk of CKD due to a genetic predisposition aggravated by poor socio-economic circumstances and chronic infections. Poor prognostic indicators namely stunting, profound hypoalbuminaemia, long standing nephrotic-range proteinuria, hypertension and impaired kidney function are common at presentation against a background of tuberculosis and HIV infection.

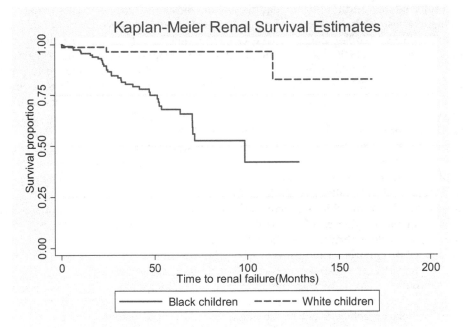

Fig. 1. Kaplan-Meier estimation of renal survival

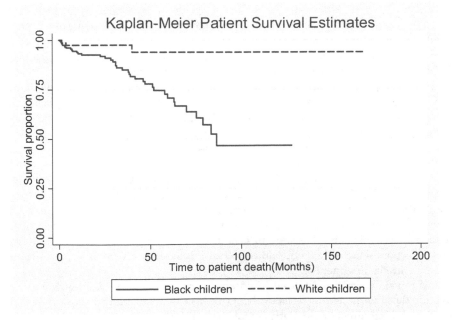

Fig. 2. Kaplan-Meier estimation of patient survival

The results of this audit confirm that significant racial differences exist in the clinical presentation, histological subtypes, response to treatment and outcome in South African children with NS. Similar findings have been reported by other study groups in South Africa (Bhimma et al. 2006: 1847; Bhimma R, 1997: 429), from other countries in Africa (Yao Doe, J. et al. 2006: 672; Olowu et al. 2010:200) and also from elsewhere in the world (Ingulli, E. & Tejani, A. 2001:393). In their study on idiopathic FSGS in children Ingulli et al. (Ingulli, E. & Tejani, A. 2001:393) reported that the rate of FSGS was higher (32.2% vs. 20%), and progress to end stage kidney disease was more common (78% vs. 33%) in black and Hispanic compared to white children. Olowu et al. (Olowu et al. 2010:200) reported an incidence of 18.5 % MCNS and 25.9% FSGS in their study of black Nigerian children with INS. Ethnic differences in the incidences of FSGS have now been well established. Over the past 10 years there have been several reports of an increasing incidence of FSGS in children (Borges et al. 2007:1309; Filler et al. 2003: 1107)

In this study 77% of the children were black and 23% were white. There was a significant difference in the incidences of the main histological subtypes (MCNS, FSGS, immune complex glomerulonephritis, secondary FSGS and membranous nephropathy) between black and white children. The incidence of MCNS was 65.6% and 29.3% (p<0.000) and of FSGS, 14% and 31% (p=0.004) in white and black children respectively.

The first course of corticosteroid treatment was often longer or more intense than that recommended by the ISKDC (International Study of Kidney Disease in Children: 1978:13) because of delayed achievement of remission or only partial response after the first four weeks. Corticosteroid treatment was also often given daily rather than on alternate days because parents failed to understand alternate day dosing schemes. White children with MCNS had a better response to oral corticosteroid treatment compared to black children with MCNS (80% vs 56%; p=0.02). Remission with oral corticosteroid treatment was achieved in more white children with FSGS compared to black children with FSGS, although this difference did not reach statistical significance (33% vs 20 %; p=0.6). Response rates in both race groups in this study were much lower compared to the 93.1% response rate reported by the ISKDC (International Study of Kidney Disease in Children: 1978:13).

After 2000 we stopped using high dose intravenous methylprednisolone for the treatment of steroid resistant NS in our patients for several reasons. It is too costly, it places a heavy burden on the family and child, and only 4 of 25 children (16%) went into remission with this treatment. This very poor response rate compared to that of Mendoza et al (Mendoza, S.A. et al. 1990:303), who reported complete remission in 52% of their patients, can possibly be explained by the fact that we omitted an alkylating agent in our treatment regimen. Adhikari et al (Adhikari et al. 1997:423) reported a dismal outcome in 12 South African children with FSGS who were treated with a combination of intravenous methylprednisolone and an alkylating agent. Although they considered this treatment as "promising," their patients developed serious side effects including alopecia, cataracts, leukopaenia, systemic candidiasis, gram negative septicaemia, and one child demised of a serious infection which was undoubtedly caused by the severe immune suppression associated with the treatment.

Infections remain a serious risk to all children during a relapse of NS, which is practically always for those with steroid resistant NS. This risk is intensified in those living in poor socio-economic circumstances. Forty eight percent of our patients experienced acute invasive bacterial infections and three succumbed to documented pneumococcal septicaemia. Management of the children with CNS was particularly challenging, due to their serious immune compromised state and high frequency of recurring infections. All children with CNS were black and screening for a possible infectious cause was not very fruitful. Genetic studies were not undertaken in any of our patients as we do not have access to genetic laboratory services. Kidney biopsy revealed idiopathic FSGS or secondary glomerular sclerosis in 15/25 children with CNS. A very dense chronic inflammatory cell infiltrate was present in all cases. Children with CNS were not treated with corticosteroids or other immunosuppressive drugs. Most of them remained in hospital for long periods or required frequent admissions for treatment of bacterial infections or gastroenteritis. An ACE inhibitor was not prescribed to any child less than 3 months old and was usually only given to children older than 12 months.

Because of the lower incidence of MCNS in black children in South Africa first reported in 1979, (Bhimma et al. 1997:429; Lewin, et al. 1979: 88) it has been our practice to biopsy all black children at the time of their first presentation. For the same reason paediatric nephrologists elsewhere in Africa have also advocated pre-treatment renal biopsies in their patients. Olowu et al. (Olowu et al. 2010:200] reported that only 18.5% of the black children with INS in their study of Nigerian patients had MCNS.

Most centres in developed countries are still following the ISKDC recommendation regarding biopsies despite worldwide reports of an increasing incidence of FSGS in both children and adults. Filler et al (Filler et al. 2003 :1107) reported a declining incidence of MCNS from 81.1% to 64% and an increasing incidence of FSGS from 10.8 to 24.7% of FSGS in their childhood population in Ontario, over two time periods 1985-1993 and 1993-2002. The incidence of MCNS in the first period did not differ significantly from that reported by the ISKDC (International Study of Kidney Disease in Children 1978: 13) and although not specifically reported, the inference is made that the majority of their patients responded to corticosteroid therapy. The incidence of FSGS in their patients has more than doubled over 17 years while the population under study remained stable. Race is not mentioned in their study. Despite an alarming increase in the incidence of FSGS in their patients, they argue that empirical steroid treatment with a cut-off point at 28 days is still justifiable. During the second period of their study the incidence of MCNS is similar to the incidence of MCNS in white children in our study, 64.7% vs. 65.6 % and the incidence of FSGS slightly less than that of FSGS in black patients in our study 24.7% vs. 31%.

Already in 1997 Thomson et al. (Thomson, P.D. 1997:508), performing pre-treatment biopsies in all their black patients, reported an incidence of FSGS in 31.3% which is identical to the 31% incidence of FSGS in black patients in this study. It appears that there has not been an increase in the incidence of FSGS in black children in Gauteng Province in South Africa over this period.

It can be expected that the HIV epidemic has contributed to the incidence of CKD in South Africa in general, but its possible role in the development of FSGS, or its contribution to an increase in the incidence of FSGS, is uncertain. Local multi-centre prospective research studies in patients with HIV-associated nephropathy will be necessary to explore this question.

Primary FSGS is a spectrum of podocytopathies caused by a variety of contributing etiologies, including genetics, infections, environment, including the intra-uterine environment, drugs and toxins. It is an aggressive disease, more so in black children compared to white children. The rationale of performing a kidney biopsy at presentation is that it confirms the histological subtype and may give clues to the stage and type of initial injury. It has been suggested that the different variants of FSG may respond differently to treatment (Valeri. et al. 1996: 1734). Immuno-histochemistry and electron microscopy may also help in differentiating primary and secondary forms of FSGS. It is well known that patients with extensive involvement of glomeruli, advanced tubulo-interstitial fibrosis and tubular atrophy are less likely to respond to corticosteroid treatment compared to those with no interstitial involvement. It is questionable whether it is justifiable to expose such a patient who may also happen to be malnourished and have poor social circumstances to aggressive immune suppression for a disease which may not have an immunological background. The possible departure of many of our black patients from a hostile intra uterine environment resulting in low birth weight and low glomerular endowment is an aspect which has not been investigated systematically.

9. Conclusions

Compared to the ISKDC report black children have a lower incidence of MCNS and a higher incidence of FSGS. Black children also have a more aggressive form of FSGS which responds poorly to corticosteroid and other immuno-suppressive treatment. More black children develop CKD stage 4 and 5 compared to white children and black children have a higher mortality compared to white children. The results of this study and similar evidence from the rest of Africa suggest that the ISKDC recommendation of empiric corticosteroid treatment in children with INS should not be followed in the management of black children with INS. We suggest that a kidney biopsy should be done at presentation to allow a definitive diagnosis and targeted treatment from the outset.

10. References

Adhikari, M. et al. 1997. Intensive pulse therapies for focal glomerulosclerosis in South African children. *Pediatr Nephrol*, 11:423-428.

Bhimma, R. 2009. HIV-associated renal disease in children. The Pediatric Quarterly, 1(4), 15-18.

Bhimma, R. et al. 2006. Steroid–resistant nephrotic syndrome: the influence of race on cyclophosphamide sensitivity. *Pediatr Nephrol*, 21, 1847-1853.

Bhimma, R. et al. 1997. Nephrotic Syndrome in South African Children: changing perspectives over 20 years. *Pediatr Nephrol*, 11, 429-434.

Borges, FF. et al. 2007. Is focal segmental glomerulosclerosis increasing in patients with nephrotic syndrome ? *Pediatr Nephrol*, 22, 1309-1313.

Filler, G. et al. 2003. Is There Really an Increase in Non Minimal Change Nephrotic Syndrome in Children? *Am J Kidney Dis*, 42(6), 1107-1114.

Habib, R. & Kleinknecht, C. 1971. The primary nephrotic syndrome of childhood: Classification and clinicopathologic study of 406 cases. Pathology Annual, 6, 417-474.

Hodson, E.M. et al. 2006. Intervention for idiopathic steroid-resistant nephrotic syndrome in children. Cochrane Database Sys Rev, 2, CD003594

Ingulli, E. & Tejani, A. 2001. Racial differences in the incidence and renal outcome of idiopathic focal segmental glomerulosclerosis in children. *Pediatr Nephrol,* 5, 393-397.

International Study of Kidney Disease in Children. 1978. Nephrotic syndrome in children: Prediction of histopathology from clinical and laboratory characteristics at the time of diagnosis. A report of the International Study of Kidney Disease in Children. Kidney Int, 13, 159-165.

Kala, U. et al. 1993. Impact of tuberculosis in children with idiopathic nephrotic syndrome. *Pediatr Nephrol,* 7, 392-395.

K/DOQI clinical practice guidelines for chronic kidney disease: evaluation, classification, and stratification. 2002. Kidney Disease Outcome Quality Initiative. Am J Kidney Dis, 39, S1-S246

Lewin, J.R. et al. 1979. The differing histology in black and white children with nephrotic syndrome (abstract). *Kidney Int,* 16, 88.

Manalich, R. et al. 2000. Relationship between weight at birth and the number and size of renal glomeruli in humans: a histomorphometric study. *Kidney Int, 58,* 770-773.

Mendoza, S.A. et al. 1990. Treatment of steroid-resistant focal segmental glomerulosclerosis with pulse methylprednisolone and alkylating agents. Pediatr Nephrol, 4, 303-307.

Olowu, W.A. et al. 2010. Reversed Clinical and Morphologic Characteristics of Idiopathic Childhood Nephrotic Syndrome. Int J Nephrol Urol. 2(1), 200 – 211.

Prinsloo, J.G. 1986. The nephrotic syndrome in black children at Kalafong Hospital. SAMJ, 70:375.

Schwartz, G.J. et al. 1987. The use of plasma creatinine concentration for estimating glomerular filtration rate in infants, children and adolescents. Pediatr Clin North Am, 34, 571-590.

Srivastava, T. et al. 1991. High incidence of focal segmental glomerulosclerosis in nephrotic syndrome of childhood. *Pediatr Nephrol,* 13, 13-18.

Tarshish, P. et al. 1996. Cyclophoshamide does not benefit patients with focal segmental glomerulosclerosis: Report of the International Study of Kidney Diseases in Children. *Pediatr Nephrol,*10:590-593.

Teeninga, N. et al. 2008. Influence of low birth weight on minimal change nephrotic syndrome in children, including meta-analysis. *Nephrol Dial Transplant,* 23, 1615-1620.

The Fourth Report of the National High Blood Pressure Education Program Working Group on High Blood Pressure in Children and Adolescents. 2004. Pediatrics, 114(2), 555-575.

Thomson, P.D. 1997. Renal problems in black South African children. Pediatr Nephrol, 1, 508-512.

Valeri, A. et al. 1996. Idiopathic collapsing focal glomerulosclerosis: A clinicopathologic study. Kidney Int, 50, 1734-1746

Vehaskari, V.M. 2007. Developmental origins of adult hypertension: new insights into the role of the kidney. Pediatr Nephrol, 22, 490-495

White, R.H.R. et al. 1970. Clinicopathologic study of nephrotic syndrome in childhood. Lancet, 1,1353-1359.

Yao Doe, J. et al. 2006. Nephrotic syndrome in African children: lack of evidence of "tropical nephrotic syndrome". Nephrol Dial Transplant, Vol. 21, 672-676.

Permissions

The contributors of this book come from diverse backgrounds, making this book a truly international effort. This book will bring forth new frontiers with its revolutionizing research information and detailed analysis of the nascent developments around the world.

We would like to thank Richard J. Glassock, MD, MACP, for lending his expertise to make the book truly unique. He has played a crucial role in the development of this book. Without his invaluable contribution this book wouldn't have been possible. He has made vital efforts to compile up to date information on the varied aspects of this subject to make this book a valuable addition to the collection of many professionals and students.

This book was conceptualized with the vision of imparting up-to-date information and advanced data in this field. To ensure the same, a matchless editorial board was set up. Every individual on the board went through rigorous rounds of assessment to prove their worth. After which they invested a large part of their time researching and compiling the most relevant data for our readers. Conferences and sessions were held from time to time between the editorial board and the contributing authors to present the data in the most comprehensible form. The editorial team has worked tirelessly to provide valuable and valid information to help people across the globe.

Every chapter published in this book has been scrutinized by our experts. Their significance has been extensively debated. The topics covered herein carry significant findings which will fuel the growth of the discipline. They may even be implemented as practical applications or may be referred to as a beginning point for another development. Chapters in this book were first published by InTech; hereby published with permission under the Creative Commons Attribution License or equivalent.

The editorial board has been involved in producing this book since its inception. They have spent rigorous hours researching and exploring the diverse topics which have resulted in the successful publishing of this book. They have passed on their knowledge of decades through this book. To expedite this challenging task, the publisher supported the team at every step. A small team of assistant editors was also appointed to further simplify the editing procedure and attain best results for the readers.

Our editorial team has been hand-picked from every corner of the world. Their multi-ethnicity adds dynamic inputs to the discussions which result in innovative outcomes. These outcomes are then further discussed with the researchers and contributors who give their valuable feedback and opinion regarding the same. The feedback is then collaborated with the researches and they are edited in a comprehensive manner to aid the understanding of the subject.

Apart from the editorial board, the designing team has also invested a significant amount of their time in understanding the subject and creating the most relevant covers. They scrutinized every image to scout for the most suitable representation of the subject and create an appropriate cover for the book.

The publishing team has been involved in this book since its early stages. They were actively engaged in every process, be it collecting the data, connecting with the contributors or procuring relevant information. The team has been an ardent support to the editorial, designing and production team. Their endless efforts to recruit the best for this project, has resulted in the accomplishment of this book. They are a veteran in the field of academics and their pool of knowledge is as vast as their experience in printing. Their expertise and guidance has proved useful at every step. Their uncompromising quality standards have made this book an exceptional effort. Their encouragement from time to time has been an inspiration for everyone.

The publisher and the editorial board hope that this book will prove to be a valuable piece of knowledge for researchers, students, practitioners and scholars across the globe.

List of Contributors

Chi Chiu Mok
Department of Medicine, Tuen Mun Hospital and Center for Assessment and Treatment of Rheumatic Diseases, Pok Oi Hospital, Hong Kong, SAR China

Kouichi Hirayama and Kunihiro Yamagata
Tokyo Medical University Ibaraki Medical Center, University of Tsukuba, Japan

Marco Zaffanello
University of Verona, Italy

Emiko Takeuchi
Kitasato University School of Medicine, Japan

Martin Kimmel, Niko Braun and Mark Dominik Alscher
Department of Internal Medicine, Division of Nephrology, Robert-Bosch-Hospital, Stuttgart, Germany

Mitra Naseri
Mashhad University of Medical Sciences, Islamic Republic of Iran

Mahmoud Barazi and Sharma Prabhakar
Department of Internal Medicine, Texas Tech University Health Science Center, Lubbock, TX

Harneet Kaur
Department of Internal Medicine, New York Medical College, Valhalla, NY, USA

Daniel Fischman, Arvin Parvathaneni and Pramil Cheriyath
Pinnacle Health System-Harrisburg Hospital, Harrisburg, Pennsylvania, United States of America

Hequn Zou
Institute of Nephrology and Urology, The 3rd Affiliated Hospital of Southern Medical University, Guangzhou, China

Yuxin Wang
Department of Nephrology, The No. 2 Hospital of Xiamen, Fu Jian Medical University, Xiamen, China

Guimian Zou
Nephrology Department of Guilin 181 Hospital & Guangxi Provincial Key Laboratory of Metabolic Disease Research, Guilin, China

Jianxin Wan
Department of Nephrology, The No. 1 Hospital of Fu Jian Medical University,Fuzhou, China

Han-Seung Yoon and Michael R. Eccles
Department of Pathology, Dunedin School of Medicine, University of Otago, Dunedin, New Zealand

Toshihiko Ishimitsu
Department of Hypertension and Cardiorenal Medicine, Dokkyo Medical University, Mibu, Tochigi, Japan

Gertruida van Biljon
University of Pretoria, Department of Paediatrics, South Africa

Printed in the USA
CPSIA information can be obtained
at www.ICGtesting.com
JSHW011447221024
72173JS00004B/981